TRAUMA CARE
PRE-HOSPITAL MANUAL

TRAUMA CARE
PRE-HOSPITAL MANUAL

EDITED BY

IAN GREAVES FRCEM FRCP FRCSEd FIMC FASI DTM&H DMCC DipMedEd L/RAMC
Consultant in Emergency Medicine, UK

KEITH PORTER FRCS FRCSEd FRCEM FFSEM FIMC FASI
Professor of Clinical Traumatology, UK

with

CHRIS WRIGHT DIMC FRCEM L/RAMC
Consultant in Emergency Medicine, UK

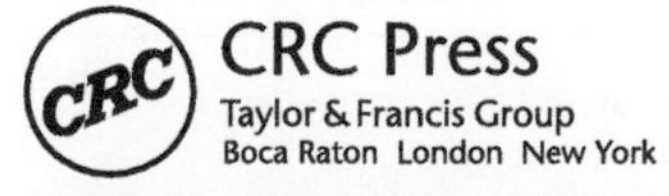

CRC Press is an imprint of the
Taylor & Francis Group, an **informa** business

CRC Press
Taylor & Francis Group
6000 Broken Sound Parkway NW, Suite 300
Boca Raton, FL 33487-2742

Printed on acid-free paper

International Standard Book Number-13: 978-1-138-62684-3 (Paperback)
International Standard Book Number-13: 978-1-138-62457-3 (Hardback)

Library of Congress Cataloging-in-Publication Data

Names: Greaves, Ian, editor. | Porter, Keith M., editor.
Title: The trauma care pre-hospital manual / edited by Ian Greaves, Keith Porter.
Description: Boca Raton : CRC Press, 2018. | Includes bibliographical references and index.
Identifiers: LCCN 2018012347| ISBN 9781138626843 (pbk. : alk. paper) | ISBN 9781138624573 (hardback : alk. paper) | ISBN 9781315212821 (ebook)
Subjects: | MESH: Advanced Trauma Life Support Care | Wounds and Injuries--therapy | United Kingdom
Classification: LCC RD93.95 | NLM WB 105 | DDC 617.1--dc23
LC record available at https://lccn.loc.gov/2018012347

Visit the Taylor & Francis Web site at
http://www.taylorandfrancis.com

and the CRC Press Web site at
http://www.crcpress.com

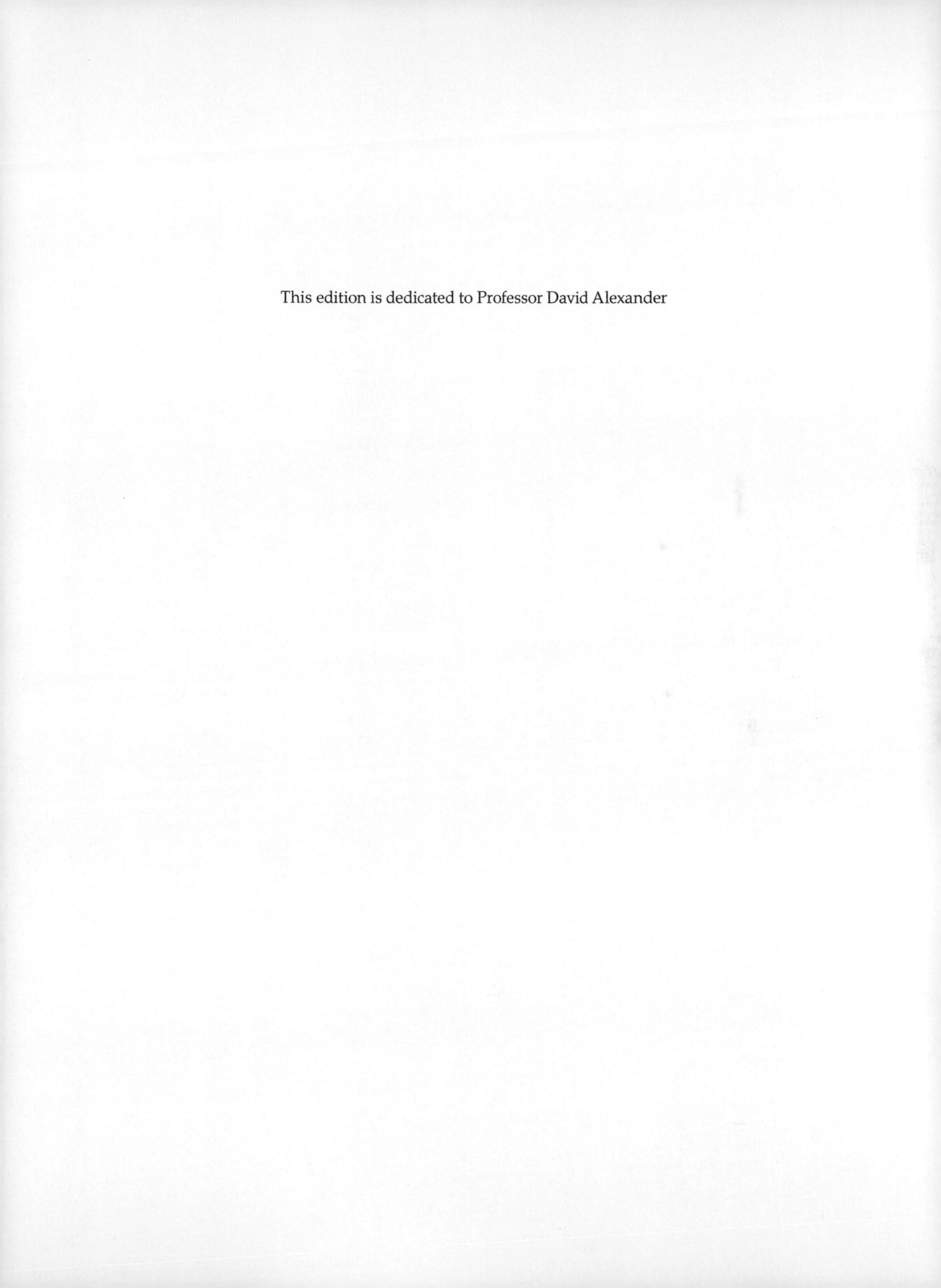

This edition is dedicated to Professor David Alexander

This edition is dedicated to Professor David A [illegible]

Contents

Introduction

When the first edition of the *Trauma Care Manual* was published in 2001, we wrote that it had been prepared to '*begin the process of establishing United Kingdom guidelines for best practice in the management of major trauma*' and expressed a wish that it and future editions would be recognised as 'definitive statements of best practice'. So it has turned out. A second edition of the *Trauma Care Manual* appeared in 2009, and a third edition, focused on care of the victim of trauma in hospital is currently being prepared.

This volume, the *Trauma Care Pre-Hospital Manual,* builds on the earlier books and, like them, offers evidence-based guidelines for the management of major trauma, written by clinicians with many years of trauma experience, and endorsed as authoritative by Trauma Care (UK). As its title suggests, it deals with the management of trauma in the pre-hospital environment and thus complements the upcoming third edition of the *Trauma Care Manual.*

In 2001, few if any of those most involved in the care of victims of trauma could have anticipated the changes and developments that have occurred in the years that followed. The UK now has functioning (and on the evidence to date) effective trauma systems and networks, and clinical developments include the introduction of damage control resuscitation, tranexamic acid, blood product resuscitation, hybrid resuscitation and an emphasis on the control of major external haemorrhage as part of a new <C>ABCDE approach. As a consequence, more patients with major trauma are surviving than ever before. Much of this change has been led by experience from recent conflicts in Iraq and Afghanistan. If this experience has taught one thing more emphatically than any other, it is that optimal pre-hospital care is essential if survival rates are to be improved and morbidity reduced.

We are more aware than ever that trauma victims do not, in a sense, die from the trauma, but from *the effects of trauma*. These include hypoxia, acidosis, embolism, haemorrhage, abnormal clotting, hypothermia, metabolic and immunological derangement. The sooner these harmful processes are arrested (or better still prevented), the better outcomes will be. It is the recognition of this concept as the key to trauma management that underpins these guidelines.

The *Trauma Care Pre-Hospital Manual* offers clear, didactic, evidence-based guidelines for the management of major trauma before arrival at hospital. Where it is available, the evidence base is given, and where it is not, we have indicated a course of action supported by recognised authorities in the field. Needless to say, we have ensured that all the recent advances in care of the trauma victim are included, but we have tempered our recommendations with practical experience of what can realistically be achieved outside hospital. We hope this text will be useful to all practitioners of pre-hospital care whatever their profession or seniority, and we look forward to future editions incorporating the changes that will undoubtedly occur in the next few years.

Abbreviations and acronyms

AAA	abdominal aortic aneurysm
ac	alternating current
ACCOLC	access overload control
ACE	angiotensin converting enzyme
ACS	American College of Surgeons
ACSCT	American College of Surgeons Committee on Trauma
ADI	acute decompression illness
A&E	accident and emergency
AED	automated external defibrillator
AEP	Attenuating Energy Projectile
AF	atrial fibrillation
AIC	ambulance incident commander
AIS	abbreviated injury scale
ALS	advance life support
ALSO	advanced life support obstetrics
AMPLE	Allergies, Medications, Past Medical History, Last ate or drank, Events
AOC	air operations centre
AP	anteroposterior
APACHE	Acute Physiology and Chronic Health Evaluation
APLS	advanced paediatric life support
ARDS	acute respiratory distress syndrome
ASHICE	Age, Sex, History, Injuries sustained, Condition of patient, Estimated time of arrival
ATLS	Advanced Trauma Life Support®
ATMIST	Age, Time of injury, Mechanism of injury, Injuries suspected or known, Signs as recorded, Treatment provided, and its effect
ATOMFC	Airway obstruction, Tension pneumothorax, Open pneumothorax, Massive haemothorax, Flail chest, Cardiac tamponade
AV	atrioventricular
AVLS	automatic vehicle location system
AVNRT	AV nodal re-entrant tachycardia
AVPU	Alert, Voice, Pain, Unresponsive
BA	biological agent
BASICS	British Association for Immediate Care
BAT	burns assessment team
BATLS	Battlefield Advanced Trauma Life Support
BLS	basic life support
BP	blood pressure
BSA	body surface area
BTLS	basic trauma life support

BURP	backward-upward-rightward pressure
BVM	bag, valve, mask
CAA	Civil Aviation Authority
<C>ABCDE	catastrophic external haemorrhage, airway, breathing, circulation, disability, exposure
CAD	computer-aided dispatch
CAT	Combat Application Tourniquet®
CBRN	chemical, biological, radiological, and nuclear
CCA	Civil Contingencies Act
CCC	Civil Contingencies Committee
CCS	casualty clearing station
CH47	Chinook helicopter
CLI	caller line Identification
cm	centimetre
CMACE	Centre for Maternal and Child Enquiries
CNS	central nervous system
CO	carbon monoxide
COBR	Cabinet Office Briefing Room
COPD	chronic obstructive pulmonary disease
CPP	cerebral perfusion pressure
CPR	cardiopulmonary resuscitation
CRM	crew resource management
CSCATT	Command and control, Safety, Communication, Assessment, Triage, Treatment, Transport
CSF	cerebrospinal fluid
CT	computerised tomography
CVA	cerebrovascular accident
DAI	diffuse axonal injury
dc	direct current
DCS	damage control surgery
DCR	damage control resuscitation
DipIMC	Diploma in Immediate Medical Care
DKA	diabetic ketoacidosis
DNR	do not resuscitate
DORA	dynamic operation risk assessment
DSTC	Definitive Surgical Trauma Care®
DVT	deep vein thrombosis
ECG	electrocardiogram
ECT	enhanced care team
EDH	extradural/epidural haematoma
EMD	electromechanical association
EMJ	Emergency Medicine Journal
EPO	emergency planning officer
ePRF	electronic patient report form
ERL	emergency reference level
ET	endotracheal
ETC	European Trauma Course
$ETCO_2$	End-tidal CO_2
FEMA	Federal Emergency Management Agency (US)
FIMC	Fellowship in Immediate Medical Care

FMJ	Full metal jacket
FPOS	first person on scene
GCS	Glasgow Coma Scale
GMC	General Medical Council
GMP	Good Medical Practice
GSW	gunshot wound
GTN	glyceryl trinitrate
HART	hazardous area response team
HAZCHEM	hazardous chemical
HAZMAT	hazardous material
HCPC	Health and Care Professions Council
HEMS	helicopter emergency medical service
HGV	heavy goods vehicle
HITMAN	Hydration, Hygiene, Infection, Tubes, Temperature control, Medication, Analgesia, Nutrition and notes
HIV	human immunodeficiency virus
hr	hour
IBTPHEM	Intercollegiate Board for Training in Pre-Hospital Emergency Medicine
ICH	intracerebral haemorrhage/haematoma
ICP	intracranial pressure
ICRC	International Committee of the Red Cross
IED	improvised explosive device
IHCD	Institute for Health Care Development
IHD	ischaemic heart disease
ILMA	intubating laryngeal mask airway
Im	intramuscular
In	intranasal
ISS	Injury Severity Score
ICU	intensive care unit
ITU	intensive therapy unit
Iv	Intravenous
JESIP	Joint Emergency Services Interoperability Programme
JRCALC	Joint Royal Colleges Ambulance Liaison Committee
JVP	jugular venous pressure
KE	kinetic energy
kg	kilogram
L	litre
LA	local anaesthetic
LEDC	less economically developed country
LEH	local emergency hospital
LMA	laryngeal mask airway
LSD	lysergic acid diethylamide
m	metre
MAC	military aid to the civil powers
MAOI	monoamine oxidase inhibitor
MAP	mean arterial pressure
MCA	Maritime and Coastguard Agency
mcg	microgram

MDI	metered dose inhaler
MERIT	Medical Emergency Response Incident Team
METHANE	Major incident declared or stand by; Exact location; Type of incident; Hazards present and potential; Access, the direction of approach; Numbers of casualties, with nature and type; Emergency services present and required
mg	milligram
MI	myocardial infarction
MIA	medical incident advisor
MICC	major incident coordination centre
MICP	mean intracranial pressure
MIMMS	Major Incident Medical Management and Support
min	minute
mL	millilitre
mm	millimetre
MMMF	man-made material fibre
MRC	Medical Research Council
MRCC	Maritime Rescue Co-ordination Centres
MRSC	Maritime Rescue Sub-Centres
MSK	musculo-skeletal
mTBI	mild traumatic brain injury
MTC	major trauma centre
MTPAS	Mobile Telecommunications Privileged Access System
NAI	non-accidental injury
NAIR	National Arrangements for Incidents involving Radioactivity
NASA	National Aeronautics and Space Administration (US)
NATO	North Atlantic Treaty Organisation
NCEPOD	National Confidential Enquiry into Patient Outcome and Death
NEXUS	National Emergency X-Radiography Utilization Study
NIBP	non-invasive blood pressure
NICE	National Institute for Health and Care Excellence
NIJ	National Institute of Justice (US)
NMC	Nursing and Midwifery Council
NPA	nasopharyngeal airway
NPIS	National Poisons Information Service
NRPB	National Radiological Protection Board
NRS	(verbal) numerical rating scale
NSAID	non-steroidal anti-inflammatory drug
OPA	oropharyngeal airway
ORCON	operational research consultancy
PACS	picture archiving and communication system
PASG	pneumatic anti-shock garment
PCI	percutaneous coronary intervention
PE	pulmonary embolism
PEA	pulseless electrical activity
PEFR	peak expiratory flow rate
PEPP	paediatrics for pre-hospital professionals
PHEA	pre-hospital emergency anaesthesia
PHEC	pre-hospital emergency care

PHEM	pre-hospital emergency medicine
PHPLS	pre-hospital paediatric life support
PHTC	pre-hospital trauma course
PHTLS	pre-hospital trauma life support
PICO	Population (participants), Intervention (or exposure for observational studies), Comparator and Outcomes
PICU	paediatric intensive care unit
PPE	personal protective equipment
PR	per rectum
PRF	patient report form
PTS	paediatric trauma score
RCSEd	Royal College of Surgeons of Edinburgh
REBOA	retrograde endoscopic balloon occlusion of the aorta
RED	Russell extrication device
RICE	rest, ice, compression, and elevation
RNLI	Royal National Lifeboat Institution
RSI	rapid sequence induction (of anaesthesia)
RTC	road traffic collision
RTS	revised trauma score
RVS	Royal Voluntary Service (formerly Women's Royal Voluntary Service)
SAD	supraglottic airway device
SAH	subarachnoid haemorrhage/haematoma
SAMU	Service d'Aide Médicale Urgente
sc	subcutaneous
SCG	Strategic Coordinating Group
SCIWORA	spinal cord injury without radiological abnormality
SDH	subdural haematoma
sec	second
SIDS	sudden infant death syndrome
SIRS	systemic inflammatory response syndrome
SOAP-ME	Suction, Oxygenation, Airway, Pharmacy, Monitoring, Equipment
SOP	standard operating procedure
SSRI	selective serotonin reuptake inhibitors
START	Simple Triage and Rapid Treatment
Stat	Immediately
SUFE	slipped upper femoral epiphysis
SVT	supraventricular tachycardia
TARN	Trauma Audit and Research Network
TBI	traumatic brain injury
TBSA	total burn surface area
TCA	tricyclic antidepressant
tds	three times daily
TED	Telford extrication device
TETRA	Terrestrial Trunked Radio
TIA	transient ischaemic attack
TRA	trauma resuscitation anaesthetist
TREM	transport emergency
TRISS	trauma score – injury severity score

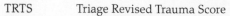

TRTS	Triage Revised Trauma Score
TTL	trauma team leader
TU	trauma unit
TWELVE	Tracheal deviation, Wounds, surgical Emphysema, Larynx, Veins, Exposure
UKIETR	UK International Emergency Trauma Register
USS	ultrasound scanning
V	volts
VAS	visual analogue scale
VF	ventricular fibrillation
VRS	verbal categorical rating scale
VT	ventricular tachycardia
WHA	World Health Assembly
WHO	World Health Organization

Contributors

Neil Abeysinghe MRCP UK FRCA FFICM DIPIMC BSC (HONS) PGCERTMEDED
Consultant Critical Care
Queen Elizabeth Hospital Birmingham,
Birmingham, UK

Colette Augre
Specialist Registrar in Anaesthetics
West Midlands Rotation, UK

David Balthazor DIPIMC MRCS FRCA FFICM
Consultant Anaesthetist and Intensivist
Queen Elizabeth Hospital Birmingham,
Birmingham, UK

Jon Barratt MCEM DMCC DIPIMC RAMC
Specialist Registrar in Emergency Medicine
St Mary's Hospital; London and Defence Medical Services, UK

Emir Battaloglu MBCHB MSC MRCS
Specialist Registrar in Trauma and Orthopaedic Surgery
University Hospitals Birmingham NHS Foundation Trust

Philippa M Bennett MRCS RN
Specialist Registrar in Surgery
Institute of Naval Medicine, Portsmouth, UK

Matt Boylan FRCEM DIPIMC RAMC
Consultant in Emergency Medicine and Pre-Hospital Care
Royal Centre for Defence Medicine, Birmingham, UK

Alasdair Corfield MRCP FCEM DIPIMC
Consultant in Emergency Medicine
Royal Alexandra Hospital; Paisley and Retrieval Doctor with the Emergency Medical Retrieval Service of Scotland

Nick Crombie FRCA FIMC
Consultant Trauma Anaesthetist Resuscitation Service
Clinical Lead, Honorary Researcher, NIHR SRMRC
Queen Elizabeth Hospital Birmingham; Midlands Air Ambulance Service, Birmingham, UK

Paul Dias MRCP FRCA
Consultant Neuroanaesthetist
Queen Elizabeth Hospital Birmingham,
Birmingham, UK

Paul Gates
Consultant Paramedic
North West Ambulance Service, UK

Ian Greaves FRCEM FRCP FRCSED FIMC FASI DTM&H DMCC DIPMEDED L/RAMC
Consultant in Emergency Medicine
James Cook University Hospital, Middlesbrough;
Defence Medical Services, UK

Stephen Hearns FRCS FRCEM FRCP DIPIMC DIPRTM
Consultant in Emergency Medicine
Royal Alexandra Hospital; Paisley and Retrieval Doctor with the Emergency Medical Retrieval Service of Scotland

Kieran M Heil BENG RN
Institute of Naval Medicin, Portsmouth, UK

Simon Horne FRCEM DIPIMC RAMC
Consultant in Emergency Medicine and Pre-Hospital Care
Derriford Hospital Plymouth; Defence Medical Services UK

Amy Hughes MBE DTM&H (LIV) EMDM MRCEM
Lecturer in Emergency Humanitarian Response and Programme Director (Global Health)
Humanitarian and Conflict Response Institute, University of Manchester

Jon Hulme MBCHB MRCP DIPIMC FRCA FFICM
Consultant in Anaesthesia and Intensive Care Medicine
Sandwell and West Birmingham Hospitals NHS Trust

Tim Kilner PHD DIPIMC RCSED PGCERT BN RN
Senior Lecturer
Institute of Health and Society, University of Worcester

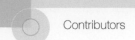

Dhushy Surendra Kumar FCA RCSI FRCA FICM
Consultant in Critical Care, Anaesthesia and Pre-Hospital Emergency Medicine
University Hospital, Conventry, UK

Graham Lawton BSC DMCC MD FRCS (PLAST.) RAMC
Consultant Plastic and Reconstructive Surgeon
Imperial College Healthcare NHS Trust, London; Medical Officer, British Army

Caroline Leech FRCEM FIMC RCSED
Consultant in Emergency Medicine
University Hospitals Coventry and Warwickshire NHS Trust

Simon Leigh-Smith MRCGP FRCSED (A&E) DIPIMC FRCEM RN
Consultant in Emergency Medicine and Pre-Hospital Care
Edinburgh Royal Infirmary; Defence Medical Services, UK

Ari K Leppäniemi MD PHD DMCC
Chief of Emergency Surgery
Department of Surgery, Meilahti Hospital
University of Helsinki, Helsinki, Finland

Rod Mackenzie TD PHD FRCP FRCS FRCEM
Consultant in Emergency Medicine and Pre-Hospital Emergency Care
Addenbrooke's Hospital, Cambridge, UK

David McConnell MRCEM RN
Specialist Registrar in Emergency Medicine
Defence Medical Services, UK

Carl McQueen MB CHB (HONS) MCEM MMED SCI (DIST) DIPIMC RCSED NIHR
Doctoral Research Fellow
Warwick Clinical Trials Unit Warwick Medical School, UK

Robb Moss FRCA DIPIMC
Consultant Anaesthetist
Queen Elizabeth Hospital Birmingham; Mercia Accident Rescue Service, Birmingham, UK

Ross Moy FRSEM DIPIMC RAMC
Consultant in Emergency Medicine and Pre-Hospital Care
John Radcliffe Hospital Oxford; Defence Medical Services, UK

Peter Oakley FRCA
Former Consultant Anaesthetist
University Hospitals of the North Midlands, Stoke-on-Trent, UK

Jowan G Penn-Barwell FRCS (TR & ORTH) RN
Specialist Registrar in Trauma and Orthopaedic Surgery
Institute of Naval Medicine, Portsmouth, UK

Professor Sir Keith Porter FRCS FRCSED FRCEM FFSEM FIMC FASI
Honorary Professor of Clinical Traumatology
University of Birmingham
Consultant Trauma Surgeon
Queen Elizabeth Hospital Birmingham, Birmingham, UK

Paul Reavely FRCEM
Consultant in Emergency Medicine
Bristol Royal Infirmary and Bristol Royal Hospital for Children

Julian Redhead FRCP FRCEM MFSEM
Consultant in Emergency Medicine and Paediatric Emergency Medicine, Medical Director
Imperial College Healthcare NHS Trust

Andy Thurgood MSC FIMC RCSED DIPHS RGN SR PARA
Consultant Nurse in Pre-Hospital Medicine
Advanced Clinical Practitioner (Emergency Department)
Chairman and Clinical Director
Mercia Accident Rescue Service

Darren Walter MPH FRCS(ED) FRCEM FIMC
Consultant in Emergency Medicine
University Hospital of South, Manchester, UK

Matt Wordsworth MA DIPIMC MRCC RAMC
Specialist Registrar in Surgery
Imperial Healthcare NHS Trust; Defence Medical Services, UK

Chris Wright DIPIMC FRCEM RAMC
Consultant in Emergency Medicine, Defence Consultant Advisor in Pre-Hospital Emergency Care
Imperial College Healthcare NHS Trust; Defence Medical Services, UK

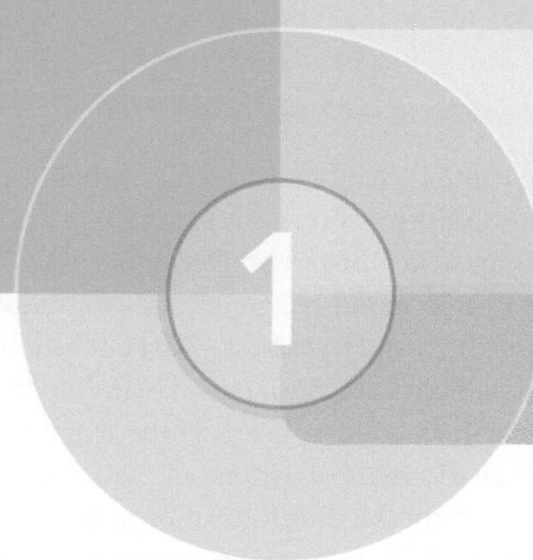

1 Trauma: A global perspective

OBJECTIVES

After completing this chapter the reader will

- Comprehend the scale of the challenge presented by trauma across the world
- Understand the different effects of trauma in developed and less developed societies
- Understand the importance of prevention in reducing the impact of trauma internationally

INTRODUCTION

All we can do in the face of that ineluctable defeat called life is to try to understand it.

Milan Kundera, The Curtain (1)

The aetiology, pathophysiology and management of trauma are complex and challenging. In contrast to a disease process, trauma as an aetiological factor involves more or less immediate external energy transfer into the human body, whether caused by mechanical, thermal or some other form of energy. In order to better understand the multitude of factors involved in the process of traumatic injury, a wider perspective encompassing the context in which the trauma occurs is warranted. When analysing the evolving trends in trauma, a perspective is needed that goes beyond narrow local and clinically orientated views. This chapter considers trauma in its widest context, including other causes of mortality and morbidity, with an emphasis on the causes and manifestations of trauma on a global scale.

THE BIG PICTURE

Many seemingly unrelated events in different parts of the world produce the same end result: one or more people are severely injured or killed as a result of trauma, whether associated with a natural or man-made disaster, a single violent act by an individual, organised crime, an industrial accident, terrorism or warfare. Although easily interpreted as individual and unrelated events, there are many trends in the globalised world that offer at least a partial explanation of the root causes of these occurrences.

Various combinations of fundamentalism, individual and institutional greed, inequality and lack of basic human rights and democracy, just to mention the most obvious factors, can lead to unforeseen consequences. For example, the Arab Spring, which began on December 18, 2010, in Tunisia as a protest against police corruption and ill treatment, triggered demonstrations, protests, riots, civil wars and revolutions all over North Africa and the Middle East culminating in the Syrian civil war that started in 2011. As a consequence of the Syrian civil war, hundreds of thousands of Syrians have sought to escape their war-torn country creating the worst refugee problem in Europe since the Second World War. After 4½ years of war, more than a quarter of a million people have died, many whilst trying to cross the Mediterranean or in the hands of human traffickers. Eleven million have fled their homes (2). In addition to these refugees from war, many others seek better living conditions by trying to enter the United States or the European Union illegally, adding to the already explosive refugee problem.

The financial crisis of September 2008 originating in the United States but having economic consequences throughout the world can be seen just as a temporary setback in continuous globalisation and the success story of the current consumer- and market-orientated way of life. However, it could also be a signal that the current culture based on speculation and immediate reward is no longer sustainable. Immanuel Wallerstein (3) has predicted that after half a millennium of success, the recognisable capitalist world order is coming to an end and is likely to bring chaos for the next 50 years. The main reason he gives is a decrease in profits due to a shortage of cheap labour and natural resources. According to some economists, there are also fundamental flaws in the global monetary and banking system, where independent countries have to increasingly rely on financing their budgets with borrowed money (4). It is also clear that the reactions of individual organisations and states are closely entwined. The current and ongoing political and economic crisis in Greece, for example, was triggered by the fear of losses to major German and French banks. The Greek financial crisis demonstrated that the real global financial (and by extension political) power rests not only in major economies such as the United States, China or Germany, but in the multinational institutions and corporations that also have substantial political influence. Inevitably, unrest and a sense of injustice will lead to changes in the global pattern of trauma.

As stated in a TV interview by Kishore Mahbubai, a leader of the Lee Kuan Yew School of Public Policy in Singapore, 900 million Westerners, 15% of the world population, can no longer dictate world opinion. With the increasing economic power of Asia, especially China and India, it can be expected that their role in the global economy as well as in international organisations will grow at the expense of a Europe that is suffering from shrinkage of its population. According to an estimate by the Berlin Institute, the population of Europe will decrease by 8.3% from 2007 until 2050 and that of Russia by 21.1%. In contrast, the population in Africa, Asia, Latin America (including the Caribbean), the United States and Canada will increase by 105.2%, 30.1%, 37.6% and 30.7%, respectively (5). According to the United Nations Economy and Social Division (DESA), by the end of the year 2008, half of the 6.7 billion people in the world were living in cities and the projection for 2050 is 70%. By 2025 there will be 27 megacities, mostly in Asia and Africa (6). The dark side of rapid economic growth was revealed in one of the fastest growing economies when a huge corruption scandal involving the Brazilian oil company Petrobras emerged in 2013. Top politicians and businesspeople received bribes including luxury yachts, cars, art, fine wines and the services of prostitutes (7). It has been estimated that in 2013 alone the total amount of corruption money was between US$32 billion and US$53 billion.

Another threat to welfare in rich countries is presented by the so-called *frail states*. Almost 50 countries, including Afghanistan, Ethiopia, Georgia, Kenya, Nigeria, Somalia, Sudan and

South Sudan are listed as frail states: they have a total population of 870 million. Such states are characterised by the inability or lack of political will of the state to provide basic services critical to welfare, such as essential social services, security, human rights and the uninterrupted function of basic economic and social institutions. In a typical frail state, poverty increases bringing violence, anarchy and crime, producing uncontrollable refugee flows, epidemics and environmental destruction (8). However, a contrasting view has been presented by the researchers of the World Bank who estimate that the absolute number of the poorest segment of the population in developing countries has decreased by 500 million in the last 50 years (9). In some countries such as Ethiopia, substantial progress has been made in the last decade where the annual economic growth has been around 10%, millions more people have access to clean water, and in spite of the population growing from 40 million in 1984 to 95 million in 2014, the mortality rate among children less than 5 years old has at the same time decreased from 227 to 63 per thousand births (10). Consequently, the life expectancy has increased from 65.3 years in 1990 to 71.5 in 2013.

CLIMATE CHANGE AND ENERGY USE

Climate change is real and becoming critical. Only a few would now deny the contribution of human behaviour to its causation. The sea level rises about 1 mm for every 360 gigatons of water, and during a study period of 1994 to 2013 based on photographs by NASA, the sea level has risen about 4 mm from the melting of Alaskan glaciers alone. The Alaskan coast no longer freezes as it has in the past and storms erode the coastline causing houses to fall into the sea and populations to move inland.

According to the worst-case scenario of the Intergovernmental Panel on Climate Change, the mean temperature of the Earth will increase from 15 to 20 centigrade by the year 2100. Even if this is an overestimate, most scientists agree that the current trend in climate change will bring huge effects including natural disasters and epidemics (11). In the last three decades, over 1000 extreme weather events hit the World Health Organization (WHO) European region alone. Climate change increases the frequency and severity of these events, and according to the latest projections, if global warming is unconstrained (12), the future effects of heatwaves, floods and droughts, worsening air pollution and changes in vector and plant distribution are likely to harm the health of millions of people. As stated by the economist Jeffrey Sachs, climate change is already driving warfare in some Sub-Saharan countries where hungry people clash over scarce food and water (13). Interestingly, it has been shown that long-term fluctuations in war frequency and population changes follow the cycles of temperature change and that relative food scarcity is a fundamental cause of outbreaks of conflict (14).

Besides the long-term effects on climate change through the production of greenhouse gases, the global dependency on oil, especially in the Western world and growing Asian economies, will have major effects in the short term. It has been estimated that the world has utilised about one third of its oil reserves and that the demand for crude oil has permanently surpassed the supply, which means that the price of oil will not consistently decrease in the future (15). The search for alternative fuels has in the last few years focused on bio-fuels made of corn, wheat, soybean or palm oil, for example. This has led to acute food shortages with the risk of food-related unrest in at least 33 countries, as estimated by the former World Bank President Robert Zoellick (16). In the United States, one-third of the corn produced is already used for the production of ethanol, and 75% of the increase in food prices is caused by favouring bio-fuel production (17). Michael Delgado, an agricultural economist from the World Bank, has estimated that the global food reserves per capita are lower than at any time during the last 35 years (18). In addition to food shortages caused by diverting arable land from food production to fuel production, droughts in Australia for example, and speculation in the global food markets have increased the price of food and led to violent uprisings in numerous countries, including Egypt, the Philippines, Yemen, Haiti, Cameroon, Mozambique, Morocco and Indonesia (19).

GLOBAL BURDEN OF TRAUMA

According to the Global Burden of Disease project (20), there will be a projected 40% increase in global deaths due to injury between 2002 and 2030, predominantly due to the increasing number of road traffic collision deaths that, together with increases in population numbers, more than offset small declines in age-specific death rates for other causes of injury. Road traffic collision deaths are projected to increase from 1.2 million in 2002 to 2.1 million in 2030, primarily due to increased motor vehicle fatalities associated with economic growth in low- and middle-income countries (21). The overall increase in injury-related deaths is projected to be from about 5 million to about 7 million by 2030. The changes in rankings for causes of deaths from 2002 to 2030 show an increase in road traffic collisions from 10th to 8th and self-inflicted injuries from 14th to 12th. In disability adjusted life years (DALYs), the ranking change for road traffic accidents is from 8th to 4th, violence from 15th to 13th and self-inflicted injuries from 17th to 14th.

NATURAL DISASTERS

During the last few years, dramatic natural disasters have claimed the lives of hundreds of thousands of people. The 2004 underground earthquake and the following tsunami in South East Asia killed over 230,000 people in 10 countries and the earthquake in October 2005 in northern Pakistan killed 78,000. On May 3, 2008, the floods caused by hurricane Nargis killed 85,000 people and 53,000 went missing in southern Myanmar. The Caribbean and the United States have been hit repeatedly by hurricanes several times a year, with Katrina in 2005 killing 1836 people in New Orleans (22,23).

On March 11, 2011, following a major earthquake, a 15-meter tsunami hit the Japanese coast and disabled the cooling system of three nuclear reactors leading to melting of all three cores and radioactive releases into the air and sea. Although there were no immediate deaths from radiation sickness, over 100,000 people had to be evacuated. The long-term effects on the population and environment remain to be seen.

In large-scale natural disasters with damage or overwhelming of the local and national healthcare facilities, rapid and well-coordinated international relief efforts are of the utmost importance. In some cases, individual countries have opted for evacuating their own citizens from the disaster area (24). In an analysis of the fatalities caused by Hurricane Katrina in Louisiana, the major causes of death were drowning in 40%, injury and trauma in 25% and heat-related illness in 11%. People of 75 years old and older formed the most affected population cohort. The authors recommended that future disaster preparedness efforts should focus on evaluating and caring for vulnerable populations, including those in hospitals, long-term care facilities and their own homes (25).

A new and worrying development in the management of disasters is the increasingly common privatised disaster response, to the extent that disasters themselves have become major new markets, a phenomenon Naomi Klein has called the 'disaster-capitalism complex' (26). Within weeks of hurricane Katrina, several major private companies signed contracts worth millions of dollars for services that included protection of Federal Emergency Management Agency (FEMA) operations and providing mobile homes to evacuees. These companies increasingly regard both the state and non-profit organisations as competitors, while the state has lost the ability to perform its core functions without the help of external agencies. Also on the list of privatised services are the global communication networks, emergency health and electricity services, and the providers of transportation for a global workforce in the midst of a major disaster.

MAN-MADE DISASTERS

Many mass casualty incidents are man-made (or a combination of a natural disaster with man-made elements). In many cases the reason is the lack of appropriate supervision of construction and storage sites by local authorities.

On August 12, 2015, two explosions at a warehouse storing dangerous chemicals devastated an industrial park in the northeastern port city of Tianjin in China killing at least 121 people, including 67 firefighters. More than 700 people were injured and thousands were evacuated because of the risk posed by chemicals stored at the site. On September 11, 2015, at least 87 people died and almost 200 were injured in Mecca in Saudi Arabia when a construction crane fell over the Masjid al-Haram mosque (27). The increasing use of immigrant workforces, especially in some wealthy oil-producing states in the Middle East, has led to a near epidemic of construction site accidents due to deficient safety practices. Added to the reckless driving culture in many of those countries, their trauma centres see many blunt trauma patients every year.

WAR

There were more wars in 2014 than in any other year since 2000. There were 14 conflicts that killed more than 1000 people. Syria, Iraq and Afghanistan were the three deadliest wars with Nigeria being the fourth where the number of deaths almost tripled from the previous year due to the intensification of the conflict with the militant group Boko Haram. While the number of state-based conflicts has remained stable for the last 10 years, the number of non-state conflicts increased from 29 in 2004 to 48 in 2013. Using the Global Peace Index ranking of 162 countries by their relative states of peace, the bottom five countries were Syria, Afghanistan, South Sudan, Iraq and Somalia. In Europe despite the dense web of legal conventions, political agreements, institutions of different kinds and other security instruments in place, political crisis escalated into major conflict in Ukraine in the space of only few months. It has been estimated that by the end of 2014 more than 4300 people had been killed in this conflict and that 500,000 people have been internally displaced. At the time of writing, there appear to be no prospects of a lasting settlement.

In addition to the geopolitical considerations of destabilising neighbouring countries to prevent them joining the opposite political bloc, the persistence of conventional warfare doctrine related to ethnic and resource competition is evident, for example in the war in August 2008 between Georgia and Russia where the control of the oil pipelines from the Caspian Sea area was undoubtedly a major factor. It has been speculated that the vast untapped energy reserves in the Persian Gulf and the Caspian Sea area could provoke great-power warfare even today (28).

An interesting new theory about the causes of conflicts has been presented by the German population scientist Gunnar Heinsohn. The expansion of men aged 15 to 29 years to comprise more than 30% of the adult male population, a so-called *youth bulge,* seems to correlate with the risk of conflict (29). The size of the youth bulge in some of the recent conflict areas is significant: 53% in the Gaza strip, 52% in Kenya and 49% in Afghanistan.

According to a global report on child soldiers, the use of children in wars has decreased during the past few years, but they are still present among the fighters in Myanmar, Chad, the Democratic Republic of Congo, Sudan, Uganda (Lord's Resistance Army), Yemen and Israel where the military has used Palestinian children as human shields and the training of those under the age of 18 is common (30). Another disturbing development is the increasing use of rape as a method of war, as has been witnessed recently in eastern Congo (31). In modern conflicts the great majority of victims are civilians, as seen in the conflict in Syria with millions of civilians fleeing the country and overwhelming neighbouring countries and the whole of Europe with an unprecedented influx of refugees, not forgetting that of the more than 200,000 deaths and more than 800,000 wounded, a large majority were civilians.

One of the uncertain factors potentially destabilising the Middle East is the nuclear program in Iran. In spite of the nuclear agreement with Iran and the reactions of its neighbours, particularly Israel, the strategic balance in the region may shift and lead to a regional and potentially global conflict. The recent decision by the USA to withdraw unilaterally from this agreement has the potential to destabilise an already difficult situation, not least by rendering the situation of Iranian modernisers more difficult. A pre-emptive air strike or other form of attack on the Iranian nuclear facilities would lead to economic and political turmoil which could have worldwide implications. The closure of the Strait of Hormuz, for example, would severely impair global oil availability (32,33).

In 2014, world military expenditure was estimated at US$1776 billion, representing 2.3% of global gross domestic product or US$245 per person. Military spending has continued to increase rapidly in Africa, Eastern Europe and the Middle East, and the conflicts in Ukraine, Syria and Iraq are likely to continue to drive military expenditure in many countries in these regions. Divided by region, military spending in 2014 was largest in North America (US$627 billion) followed by East Asia (US$309 billion) and Western and Central Europe (US$292 billion).

Civil wars continue in many parts of the world and their relationship with the drug trade has become increasingly recognised, at least in Colombia and Afghanistan. According to the United Nations Office on Drugs and Crime (UNODC), the Taliban rebels in Afghanistan received 64 million euros in 2007 from opium growers. The total yield from opium fields was 8000 tons when the average global consumption is 4000 tons. The rest is in storage in unknown locations. Conversely, in Colombia real progress in the FARC conflict may be possible with the release of long term hostages, the death of their leader Manuel Marulanda and the signing of a political accord with the government (31) A political resolution between FARC and the civil government was signed in 2016 but may not ensure permanent peace as large numbers of former FARC members are now leaderless and have lost political and social influence. Illustrative of the difficulties in nation building after a civil war is the double assassination attempt in 2008 on the president and prime minister of East Timor. President Jose Ramos-Horta suffered two abdominal gunshot wounds and was operated on in Australia (34).

The most important major new strand in international terorrism of recent years has been Islamic extremism. The Islamic State of Iraq and Syria (ISIS), or the Islamic State of Iraq and the Levant (ISIL), now known as Islamic State (IS), expanded very rapidly and by the most brutal means to control large areas of the Middle East. Although this geographical dominance is now largely lost, as a result of military intervention by Iraq, Syria and the Western powers, there is no doubt that the spreading of an extremist Islamic ideology will remain prominent in motivating terrorist activity and it seems likely that a consequence of the loss of territory will be the export of violence to states perceived to represent most clearly a decadent western lifestyle and willing to engage militarily with IS. As well as extreme brutality including mass killings, executions and kidnappings, IS was also responsible for destroying ancient temples in Palmyra, possibly for manufacturing or capturing chemical weapons, and using videos advertising a luxury lifestyle to recruit young people to join the five star jihad (35). Another destabilising factor in the area is the complex relationship between Turkey and the Kurdish areas both inside and outside Turkey and in northern Iraq and Syria, mostly driven by domestic political struggle in Turkey between the model of a secular state and an Islamic republic.

TREATMENT OF WAR WOUNDS

In an analysis of 82 US Special Operations Forces fatalities from 2001 to 2004, 19 were non-combat deaths, while of the combat deaths 43% were caused by explosions, 28% by gunshot wounds, 23% by aircraft accidents and 6% by blunt trauma (36). Seventy of the deaths were classified as non-survivable and 12 (15%) as potentially survivable. Of those with potentially survivable injuries, cause of death was identified in 16 cases: 8 (50%) truncal haemorrhage, 3 (19%) compressible haemorrhage, 2 (13%) haemorrhage amenable to tourniquet, and 1 (6%) each from tension pneumothorax, airway obstruction, and sepsis. Structured analysis identified improved methods of truncal haemorrhage control as a principal research requirement. This data and analysis reflects the findings of the very considerable literature arising from medical interventions in Iraq and particularly Afghanistan where there have been significant developments in trauma and particularly shock management which are increasingly being incorporated into civilian practice.

TERRORISM

Since 2000, there has been a more than fivefold increase in the number of deaths from terrorism, rising from 3361 in 2000 to 17,958 in 2013. Over 80% of the lives lost to terrorist activity in 2013 occurred in only five countries – Iraq, Afghanistan, Pakistan, Nigeria and Syria. However, another 55 countries recorded one or more deaths from terrorist activity (37). On July 22, 2011, a deranged Norwegian man exploded a truck bomb adjacent to the government building in Oslo and continued by gunning down young people in a summer camp on a nearby island. Overall, 78 people died and more than 150 were injured. In another incident in Finland in 2002, a young man detonated a self-made explosive in a shopping centre killing and injuring 164 people. In 2013, 60% of all attacks involved the use of explosives, 30% used firearms and 10% used other tactics including incendiary devices, melee attacks and sabotage of equipment (37).

To increase the fatality rate from terrorist attacks some innovative methods have recently been used including *spherical metal pellets* propelled by the explosion increasing the severity of injuries and adding a penetrating component to the blast injury and blunt trauma. Potential transmission of infection by body fragments in suicide bombings is also a concern. Medical teams assessing and treating terrorist bomb victims should be trained to recognise these injuries (38).

A *dirty bomb* is a mix of a conventional explosive with radioactive material resulting in dispersion of radioactive material. Although the major medical risk associated with a dirty bomb is blast injury caused by the conventional charge, the casualty profile of such a bomb will include a small group of casualties who may also be contaminated with radioactive material and who may require implementation of decontamination procedures either in the field or at the receiving hospital (39).

The use of a *second hit* (a second bomb designed to explode in the vicinity of the first bomb after a short time period to injure helpers and bystanders) has been recorded in several recent terrorist attacks. It is imperative that in any current terrorist explosion the risks must be minimised by strict security procedures and scene access control. In two cases recorded from Israel, the second bombs exploded 10 to 30 minutes after the first detonation (40). In addition, the discovery in Israel in 2003 of arms and gunmen in some ambulances lead to the practice that all ambulances, even those conveying critically injured victims had to pause for brief inspection at the perimeter of the hospital's grounds (41). Another potential security risk for EMS personnel entering a 'hostile' area is the possibility of a sniper (42).

In addition to the conventional injury pattern associated with explosions (primary, secondary, tertiary and associated blast injuries) the possibility of *biological foreign body implantation* from the suicide bombers or other victims has been recently reported (43,44).

Despite the death of Osama bin Laden in 2011, al-Qaeda and its associated organisations are still thought to have cells in 40 to 50 countries and a membership of 200–500 men. The decentralised structure makes it hard to control and major attacks can be perpetrated with only a handful of members. The biggest threat, however, is thought to be related to the ability of the terrorists to obtain weapons of mass destruction (45). Access through the Internet to the SCADA guidance systems that control many industrial processes and infrastructures could also be serious by inducing malfunctions in nuclear power plants, mass transport systems, oil and gas pipes, and electricity networks (46).

In the long run, the key issue in coping with militant Islamic radicalism is to understand the deep resentment of Western values by the Wahhabist form of Islam that since the 1700s has been the dominating ideology in Saudi Arabia. Wahhabism was founded by Ibn Abdul Wahhab in the 18th century and has militantly asserted the monotheistic roots of Islam. According to Dore Gold, the former Israeli ambassador to the United Nations, the uneasy alliance of the ruling Saudi family and the Wahhabist ulama (religious leadership), and the Saudi state support for its ideology of hatred has provided the framework for promoting Wahhabi ideology and financial support for radical groups in many conflict areas of the world reaching from Bosnia and the Caucasus through the former Soviet republics in Central Asia and the Taliban in Afghanistan to the Philippines and Indonesia (47). The only permanent solution seems to be in trying to engage the rulers of Saudi Arabia in a meaningful dialogue about the peaceful coexistence of different cultures and ideologies, and minimal standards of acceptable international behaviour.

ORGANISED CRIME AND CIVILIAN VIOLENCE

While the organised crime societies in southern Italy seem to be suffering from severe weakening thanks to diligent work by the police, the rampant violence and turf wars of the drug cartels in Mexico seem to be becoming uncontrollable. Since 2006 at least 85,000 people have been killed, and in 2014 alone there were 19,699 murders in Mexico (48). There are many similarities between the actions of the Mexican drug cartels and IS; extremely brutal killings, mass graves, rapes and hangings, with videos distributed through the Internet. Both obtain arms from the United States: IS by stealing equipment from the Iraqi army and cartels by smuggling illegal arms across the border, about 250,000 weapons annually.

School and other mass shootings have occurred with regularity during the last few years. The highest number of victims in such a shooting (33 dead) was recorded in the Virginia Tech massacre on April 16, 2007, but even in Finland an 18 year-old high school student killed 9 people including himself and injured 12 on November 7, 2007. The killer admired school shooters in other countries and left hints of his plans on the Internet 2 days before the shooting (49). A similar incident occurred on September 23, 2008, in the western part of Finland when a 22-year-old student shot 10 people in a training centre for adults and then killed himself (50). The number of gunshot wounds in the victims varied from 1 to 20 reflecting the degree of determination and hatred of the perpetrator. Besides the dangers of marginalisation, alienation and the specific sub-culture of violence glorification among young men in Western countries, the availability of, and lax laws governing the purchase of, handguns need to be urgently revised. Most of the innocent victims of school and other public-place shootings were shot with guns that had been purchased recently and legally (51).

According to a report from the United States, the number of murders has increased rapidly in some of major cities, by 76% in Milwaukee, 60% in St. Louis and 56% in Baltimore (52). The most popular explanation seems to be that the increased criticism of police actions (starting from August 2014 when an unarmed black teenager was shot by a white policeman in Ferguson, Missouri) has resulted in a less aggressive approach by police forces allowing criminals to have the upper hand. In June 2016, 50 people were shot dead in a bar in Orlando frequented by the LGBT community, an event which, with more recent mass shootings, has led to increasing public demands for gun control legislation. To date there seems little political appetite at a central level for such intervention and the 'gun lobby' remains an exceptionally powerful force in US politics.

GLOBALISATION, TRAUMA SYSTEMS AND EDUCATION

Trauma care practices are becoming increasingly uniform all over the world, not in small part due to trauma training programmes, such as *Advanced Trauma Life Support (ATLS®)*, the *European Trauma Course (ETC®)* and *Definitive Surgical Trauma Care (DSTC™)*. Although some countries are ahead of others, the principles vary little from continent to continent (53–58).

A landmark event in global trauma care occurred on May 23, 2007, when the World Health Assembly (WHA) adopted Resolution 60.22, 'Health Systems: Emergency Care Systems', which called on the World Health Organization (WHO) and governments to adopt a variety of measures to strengthen trauma and emergency care services worldwide (59). This resolution constitutes the highest level of attention ever devoted to trauma care on a global scale.

There are signs, however, that medical systems have increasing difficulty in providing adequate emergency care to their populations. In the United States some hospitals have had to close their emergency departments (60). In 2007, the National Academy of Science and Institute of Medicine published its report 'Future of Emergency Care for the US Health System' which identified the following problems: poorly coordinated and chaotic pre-hospital care ambulances being regularly turned away from hospital doors; overcrowded emergency departments, long waiting times, lack of senior decision makers in emergency departments, poor facilities for paediatric patients and lack of space for continuation of patient care. One of the solutions offered is reorganisation and regionalisation of emergency care along the trauma system model, with improvement in resourcing, training, leadership and research (61).

In Europe, the WHO has observed that emergency departments are overcrowded with cases that cannot be considered urgent and has urged the development of daytime emergency services, better coordination and selection of emergency patients, and more training of the doctors and nurses treating emergency patients (62). In the UK the alleged pressure on the National Health Service resulting from European Union migration was a major area of controversy in the referendum regarding the EU membership debate and there is an opposite political lobby demanding, in effect, ever-increasing health spending with no recognised limit.

One key issue is the level of expertise in the emergency department. Experiences from the United Kingdom and New Zealand show that increasing availability of specialist-level physicians in emergency departments shortens emergency department and hospital lengths of stay, increases daytime and decreases night-time emergency operations, and decreases costs (63,64).

In the United States the combination of trauma surgery, emergency general surgery and surgical critical care into one *acute care surgery* model and curriculum has progressed rapidly (65). Initial experiences show that the acute care surgery model does not compromise the care of the injured patients, and improves the care of some emergency surgery patient groups, such as acute appendicitis or ruptured abdominal aortic aneurysms (66–68). This new paradigm is also having an influence on clinical practice, for example by extending the concept of damage control surgery to emergency general surgery (69,70). Based on a report from various hospitals with similar complication rates but highly variable mortality rates, the concept of failure to rescue has been introduced, and surgical rescue has been included as the fifth pillar of acute care surgery (in the United States) or emergency surgery (in Europe) alongside trauma, critical care, emergency surgery and elective general surgery (71,72).

Finally, the paradigm change will also affect patient care on a system level. A message from the president, Timothy Fabian, in the *American Association for the Surgery of Trauma* newsletter stated: *'For delivery of Emergency Surgical Services, it is time to 'circle the wagons' and regionalize care in the same fashion as healthcare is being regionalized for many disease processes. The future will hold Regional Emergency Surgery Hospitals'* (73).

SUMMARY

In spite of significant advances in clinical practice, economical, educational and organisational limitations prevent us from providing the best available care for many of our patients, at least on a global scale. Fresh solutions and new paradigms are needed in order to approach the key issues successfully. Trauma and emergency clinicians can and should play a key role in identifying the problems and challenges in providing adequate trauma care to the population. To do it, however, requires a view encompassing the wider trends and challenges of the world we live and work in.

REFERENCES

1. Kundera M. *The Curtain*. New York: Harper Collins Publishers, 2005.
2. Huusko J. Pakolaiskriisin jäljet johtavat Syyriaan. *Helsingin Sanomat*, August 22, 2015.
3. Nieminen T. 2008a. Tohtori Wallersteinin hirviö. *Helsingin Sanomat*, March 9, 2008.
4. Immonen P. 2015. Tsunami avasi silmät. Raha-aktivisti Ville Iivarinen kertoo ihmisille rahajärjestelmän ongelmista. *Helsingin Sanomat*, September 2, 2015.
5. Ahtiainen I. 2008. Euroopan väestökehitys maahanmuuton varassa. *Helsingin Sanomat*, August 22, 2008.
6. Sillanpää S. Kaupungistumisesta tulee kiivainta Aasiassa ja Afrikassa. *Helsingin Sanomat*, June 29, 2008.

7. Manner M. Suurpetos järisytti Brasiliaa. *Helsingin Sanomat,* September 14, 2015.
8. Ruohomäki O. Valtioiden haurastuminen uhkaa hyvinvointia rikkaissakin maissa. *Helsingin Sanomat,* December 3, 2007.
9. Baer K. Maailman köyhien määrä kasvoi 400 miljoonalla. *Helsingin Sanomat,* September 4, 2008.
10. Sillanpää S. Rahat menivät kaivoon. *Helsingin Sanomat,* September 5, 2015.
11. Isomäki R. Millainen paikka maapallo on vuonna 2100 ilmaston lämmettyä viidellä asteella? *Duodecim* 2007;123:2795–2801.
12. World Health Organization. Protecting health from climate change: WHO experts call for health systems to play a greater role. Press release, April 4, 2008.
13. Sachs J. 2005. Climate change and war. Global Policy Forum. Project syndicate, March 1, 2005.
14. Zhang DD, Brecke P, Lee HF, He Y-Q, Zhang J. Global climate change, war, and population decline in recent human history. *PNAS* 2007;104:19214–19219.
15. Rossi J. Öljyn kysynnän tyydyttäminen vaikeutuu tulevaisuudessa. *Helsingin Sanomat,* May 14, 2008.
16. Saksa M. 2008. Uusi öljykriisi. *Helsingin Sanomat,* April 27, 2008.
17. Välimaa M. 2008. Maailmanpankki: Biopolttoaineet suurin syy ruuan hinnannousuun. *Helsingin Sanomat,* July 5, 2008.
18. Baer K. Ruuan kysyntä on jo vuosia kasvanut tuotantoa nopeammin. *Helsingin Sanomat,* April 17, 2008.
19. Virtanen J. Ruokamellakat leviävät ympäri maailmaa. *Helsingin Sanomat,* April 8, 2008.
20. Murray CJL, Lopez AD. Mortality by cause for eight regions of the world: Global Burden of Disease Study. *Lancet* 1997;349:1269–1276.
    Murray CJL, Lopez AD. Global mortality, disability, and the contribution of risk factors: Global Burden of Disease Study. *Lancet* 1997;349:1436–1442.
    Murray CJL, Lopez AD. Alternative projections of mortality and disability by cause 1990–2020: Global Burden of Disease Study. *Lancet* 1997;349:1498–1504.
21. Mathers CD, Loncar D. Projections of global mortality and burden of disease from 2002 to 2030. *PLoS Medicine* 2006;3:2011–2030.
22. Sillanpää S. Kiinan maanjäristyksessä kuoli ainakin 10000. *Helsingin,* 2008.
23. Nieminen T. Tulvatuhon silminnäkijä. *Helsingin Sanomat,* August 31, 2008.
24. Leppäniemi A, Vuola J, Vornanen M. Surgery in the air – Evacuating Finnish tsunami victims from Thailand. *Scandanavian Journal of Surgery* 2005;94:5–8.
25. Brunkard J, Namulanda G, Ratard R. Hurricane Katrina deaths, Louisiana, 2006. *Disaster Medicine and Public Health Preparedness.* August 27, 2008. [Epub ahead of print].
26. Klein N. 2007. Disaster capitalism. The new economy of catastrophe. *Harper's Magazine,* October 2007, 47–58.
27. Hiiro J. 2015. Lähes sata ihmistä kuoli nosturin kaaduttua moskeijan päälle Mekassa. *Helsingin Sanomat,* September 12, 2015.
28. Klare MT. 2004. *Blood and oil: How America's thirst for petrol is killing us.* New York: Henry Holt and Company.
29. Huusko J. Nuorten miesten runsaus ruokkii konflikteja. *Helsingin Sanomat,* March 21, 2008.
30. Huusko J. Raportti: Lapsisotilaiden käyttö sodissa vähentynyt. *Helsingin Sanomat,* May 30, 2008.
31. Lehtniemi N. 2008. Itä-Kongossa raiskauksesta on tullut sodankäynnin väline. *Helsingin Sanomat,* January 7, 2008.

32. Duffy M. What would war look like? *Time*, September 25, 2006.
33. Aro J. Israelin isku Iraniin aiheuttaisi kaaoksen Lähi-Idässä. *Helsingin Sanomat*, July 10, 2008.
34. Kovanen I. 2008. Itä-Timor tuotti pettymyksen kansainväliselle yhteisölle. *Helsingin Sanomat*, February 12, 2008.
35. Pettersson M. 2015. Viiden tähden jihad houkuttelee nuoria. *Helsingin Sanomat*, August 31, 2015.
36. Holcomb JB, McMullin NR, Pearse L, Caruso J, Wade CE, Oetjen-Gerdes L, Champion HR et al. Causes of death in U.S. Special Operations Forces in the global war on terrorism 2001–2004. *Annals of Surgery* 2007;245:986–991.
37. Global Terrorism Index. Measuring and understanding the impact of terrorism. Institute for Economics & Peace, 2014.
38. Kluger Y, Mayo A, Hiss J, Ashkenazi E, Bendahan J, Blumenfeld A, Michaelson M et al. 2005. Medical consequences of terrorist bombs containing spherical metal pellets: Analysis of a suicide terrorism event. *European Journal of Emergency Medicine* 2005;12:19–23.
39. Schecter WP. Nuclear, biological and chemical weapons: What the surgeon needs to know. *Scandanavaian Journal of Surgery* 2005;94:293–299.
40. Stein M, Hirshberg A. Medical consequences of terrorism: The conventional weapon threat. *Surgical Clinics of North America* 1999;79:1537–1552.
41. Shapira SC, Cole LA. 2006. Terror medicine: Birth of a discipline. *JHSEM* 2006;3:1–6.
42. Sullivan JP. Medical responses to terrorist incidents. *Prehospital and Disaster Medicine* 1990;5:151–153.
43. Eshkol Z, Katz K. Injuries from biologic material of suicide bombers. *Injury* 2005;36:271–274.
44. Wong JM-L, Marsh D, Abu-Sitta G, Lau S, Mann HA, Nawabi DH, Patel H. Biological foreign body implantation in victims of the London July 7th suicide bombings. *Journal of Trauma* 2006;60:402–404.
45. Kähkönen V. Al-Qaida murenee sisältä päin. *Helsingin Sanomat*, July 6, 2008.
46. Huusko J. Maailma valmistautuu kybersotien aikakauteen. *Helsingin Sanomat*, June 11, 2008.
47. Gold D. *Hatred's Kingdom: How Saudi Arabia Supports the New Global Terrorism*. Washington, DC: Regnery Publishing, 2003.
48. Koskinen M. Huumekartellit muistuttavat Isisiä. *Helsingin Sanomat*, August 24, 2015.
49. Saarinen J. 2007. Auvinen kertoi hyökkäyksestä etukäteen verkossa. *Helsingin Sanomat*, November 8, 2007.
50. Jokelan tragedia toistui Kauhajoella. Yksitoista kuoli verilöylyssä. *Helsingin Sanomat*, September 24, 2008.
51. Wintemute GJ. Guns, fear, the Constitution, and the public's health. *NEJM* 2008;358: 1421–1424.
52. Similä V. Murhat lisääntyneet rajusti USA:ssa. *Helsingin Sanomat*, September 2, 2015.
53. Uranues S, Lamont E. 2008. Acute care surgery: The European model. *World Journal Surgery* 32: 1605–1612.
54. Joshipura MK. Trauma care in India: Current scenario. *World Journal of Surgery* 2008;32: 1613–1617.
55. Christey GR. Trauma care in New Zealand: It's time to move ahead. *World Journal of Surgery* 2008;32:1618–1621.
56. Goosen J, Veller M. Trauma and emergency surgery: South African model. *World Journal of Surgery* 2008;32:1622–1625.

57. Poggetti RS. Acute care surgeon South American model. *World Journal of Surgery* 2008;32: 1626–1629.
58. Hoyt DB, Kim HD, Barrios C. Acute care surgery: A new training and practice model in the United States. *World Journal of Surgery* 2008;32:1630–1635.
59. Mock C, Arafat R, Chadbunchachai W, Joshipura M, Goosen J. 2008. What World Health Assembly Resolution 60.22 means to those who care for the injured. *World Journal of Surgery* 2008;32:1636–1642.
60. Mitchell A, Krmpotic D. What happens when a hospital closes it's emergency department: Our experience. *Journal of Emergency Nursing* 2008;34:126–129.
61. Committee on the Future of Emergency Care in the United States Health System. Emergency medical services: At the crossroads. 2007. htpp://www.nap.edu/catalog/11629.html.Committee on the Future of Emergency Care in the United States Health System. Hospital based emergency care. At the breaking point. 2007. htpp://www.nap.edu/catalog/11629.html.
62. WHO Europe. What are emergency medical services? 2008. 1htpp:/www.euro.who.int /emergservices/About/20020226_3.
63. Sorelli PG, El-Masry NS, Dawson PM, Theodorou NA. The dedicated emergency surgeon: Towards consultant-based acute surgical admission. *Annals of the Royal College of Surgeons of England* 2008;90:104–108.
64. Harvey M, Al Shaar M, Cave G, Wallace M, Brydon P. Correlation of physician seniority with increased emergency department efficiency during a resident doctor's strike. *New Zealand Medical Journal* 2008;121:59–68.
65. The Committee on Acute Care Surgery American Association for the Surgery of Trauma. The acute care surgery curriculum. *Journal of Trauma* 2007;62:553–556.
66. Pryor JP, Reilly PM, Schwab CW, Kauder DR, Dabrowski GP, Gracia VH, Braslow B, Gupta T. Integrating emergency general surgery with a trauma service: Impact on the care of injured patients. *Journal of Trauma* 2004;57:467–473.
67. Earley AS, Pryor JP, Kim PK, Hedrick JH, Kurichi JE, Minogue AC, Sonnad SS, Reilly PM, Schwab CW. An acute care surgery model improves outcomes in patients with acute appendicitis. *Annals of Surgery* 2006;244:498–504.
68. Utter GH, Maier RV, Rivara FP, Nathans AB. Outcomes after ruptured abdominal aortic aneurysms: The "halo effect" of trauma center designation. *Journal of the American College of Surgeons* 2006;203:498–505.
69. Stawicki SP, Brooks A, Bilski T, Scaff D, Gupta R, Schwab CW, Gracias VH. The concept of damage control: Extending the paradigm to emergency general surgery. *Injury* 2008;39:93–101.
70. Leppäniemi A, Kimball EJ, De Laet I, Malbrain ML, Balogh ZJ, De Waele JJ. Management of abdominal sepsis – A paradigm shift? *Anaesthesiology Intensive Therapy.* May 14, 2015. doi: 10.5603/AIT.a2015.0026. [Epub ahead of print]
71. Ghaferi AA, Birkmeyer JD, Dimick JB. Complications, failure to rescue, and mortality with major inpatient surgery in medicare patients. *Annals of Surgery* 2009;250:1029–1034.
72. Peitzman AB, Leppäniemi A, Kutcher ME, Forsythe RM, Rosengart MR, Sperry JL, Zuckerbraun BS. Surgical rescue: An essential component of acute care surgery (editorial). *Scandinavian Journal of Surgery* 2015;104:135–136.
73. Fabian TC. Message from the President. *Newsletter of the American Association for the Surgery of Trauma* 2008:1–2.

2 Safety

OBJECTIVES

After completing this chapter the reader will

- Be aware of the full range of hazards associated with responding to an incident
- Understand the simple steps which will reduce the hazards associated with an incident scene
- Be aware of the importance of honest and open review of adverse events and the need to continuously update practices in the light of lessons learnt

INTRODUCTION

The aim of pre-hospital emergency care is to deliver prompt clinical care to patients within a robust and safe framework. A robust clinical governance framework ultimately keeps everyone safe. Much is made of the need for clinical safety in today's modern healthcare system and this is entirely correct. However, some aspects of safety can be overlooked by the pre-hospital practitioner, particularly when they are faced with the multiple challenges of a critically ill patient. Nevertheless, the pre-hospital environment is challenging and some degree of risk must be considered acceptable: an obsessively safe culture has to be avoided and clinical effectiveness maintained.

It is all too easy to be drawn on arrival into dealing with the clinical aspects of the situation with the result that the pre-hospital practitioner becomes too patient centred too soon: complete focus on dealing with the patient can make the practitioner unsafe as scene safety issues develop around them unnoticed. It is therefore essential that the practitioner has a structure for dealing with these aspects of safety whilst working.

GETTING TO THE SCENE SAFELY

No emergency call is so urgent as to justify an accident. Emergency care providers must comply with the appropriate road traffic acts and avoid putting themselves, other road users and pedestrians at risk. Wherever possible the location of the incident and route to it should be established before responding. Every responder should drive within their capabilities and must take account of road, weather and ground conditions. Response driver training is mandatory. However tempting the alternative might be, it is essential to focus on the journey not the scene, making steady progress without delay, and using headlights and warning lights where permitted.

PRACTICE POINT

Get to the scene safely – do not take risks, do not become a casualty!

When close to the scene, it should be approached slowly, with awareness of possible debris or patients on the roadway. Police instructions should be followed and access or egress must not be obstructed by either vehicle or equipment. Arrival should be notified to control, noting the time. If first on scene, warning lights should be left on; if the other emergency services are present, the warning lights can be switched off and the vehicle parked beyond the incident. Wherever the vehicle is parked, it must be secured. Theft from emergency services vehicle is far from unknown. Having arrived, it is essential to identify the resource leaders and to make oneself known to them. Appropriate personal protective equipment must be worn and it is vital to look out for hazards including moving traffic.

THE SAFETY 123

There are three facets of safety (see Box 2.1).

BOX 2.1: Facets of Safety

- Safety of the practitioner
- Safety of the scene
- Safety of the patient

This is known commonly as *safety 123.* This 123 approach implies a linear progression, starting from the point of arrival at the scene (Figure 2.1). However, attention to safety actually starts well before the practitioner even begins work and continues throughout the care offered, beyond pre-hospital care and into the hospital handover phase.

PRACTICE POINT

Hazards can change over time.

Safety has an important time aspect to it: dangers and threats can evolve on scene as time passes and the situation develops, and if not reassessed may put the practitioner at risk. It is vital therefore to think in three dimensions (or four including time).

This chapter considers the elements of safety that need to be considered before, during and after working in the pre-hospital environment. A SAFE approach is summarised in Box 2.2.

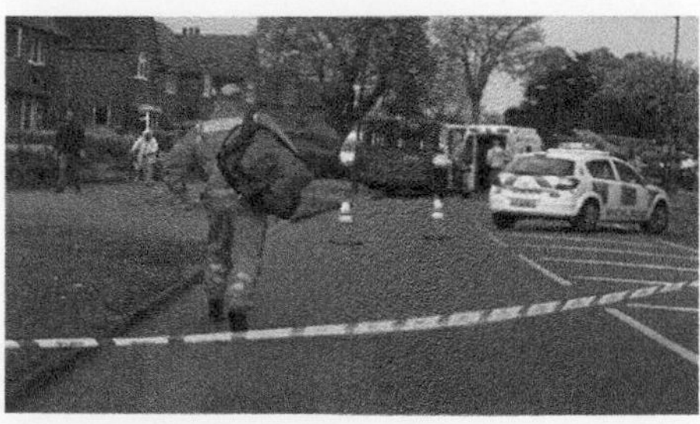

Figure 2.1 The approach to the scene – Safety 123.

BOX 2.2: SAFE

Remember SAFE

- S – Standards
- A – Awareness
- F – Follow SAFETY 123
- E – Evaluation and re-evaluation

S – STANDARDS

The professions involved in the provision of pre-hospital care produce and distribute their own standards for safe practice. With the establishment of pre-hospital emergency medicine (PHEM) as a medical sub-speciality, such standards are now also available for medical practitioners (1). Whatever an individual's background, they must be aware of the aspects of safety standards mandated for their professional group.

A – AWARENESS

Any practitioner working within pre-hospital emergency care must be aware of the dangers and risks inherent in the pre-hospital arena. This awareness can be developed by working with the emergency services on joint exercises using the Joint Emergency Services Interoperability Programme (JESIP; www.jesip.org.uk). Training together allows safe exposure to risks in a controlled manner, together with structured education and rehearsal of those risks. Those starting out in pre-hospital emergency care can develop awareness by doing observer shifts with senior experienced pre-hospital emergency care practitioners. Much of the necessary awareness is gained by exposure to the environment and learning through experience, which is why it is important that new practitioners in pre-hospital emergency care are closely supported. Working with those who have this experience is key to developing the foundation of awareness of dangers and risks.

F – FOLLOW THE 123

1 – SELF

Being healthy and fit for the pre-hospital role is important, and good occupational support and screening will help keep the practitioner safe. Every practitioner must be fit enough to work in the physically challenging environments they will face. Fitness levels vary across different agencies and it is important to establish what the expectations are for each role before starting. All new healthcare workers must now undergo health clearance, including screening for blood-borne viruses for those performing 'exposure prone procedures' (2). Other key issues which must be considered under *self* are transmission of infection, and personal protective equipment (see later).

2 – SCENE

The scene is by definition unsafe. Until an assessment has been made, it should never be assumed that the scene is safe. On arrival, simple steps will reduce the risks (as well as creating a professional impression) (Box 2.3).

Looking at the road on the approach will allow the practitioner to identify any hazards which may be in the road (most commonly debris); spotting these early will prevent injury

BOX 2.3: First Steps on Arrival at the Scene

- Park at the scene as directed by emergency services.
- Do not ignore instructions from the police!
- If the responder is the first to arrive at the incident, consider protecting the scene by the use of the 'fend off position'.
- To do this, site the vehicle at a safe distance from the incident at an angle of 40 degrees into the direction it would be safe for the vehicle to go if it were hit from behind; this is most likely to be the verge with the wheels angled towards the verge. Should another vehicle subsequently strike the stationary vehicle it should deflect the impact from the scene and protect the responders forward of the impact point.
- Do not partially obstruct a traffic lane. If in doubt, fully close that lane as well.

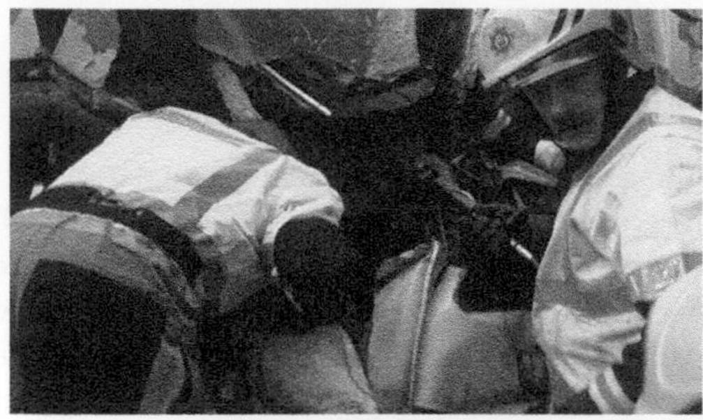

Figure 2.2 Scene hazards: sharps from a road traffic collision and confined space working.

or damage to those arriving (Figures 2.2 and 2.3). Importantly, the trail of debris laid in the road from a road traffic collision is precious forensic evidence that must be protected for the subsequent police accident investigation team; it should not be kicked aside. There may also be sounds and smells which will provide warning of hazards such as unstable vehicles or spilt fuel.

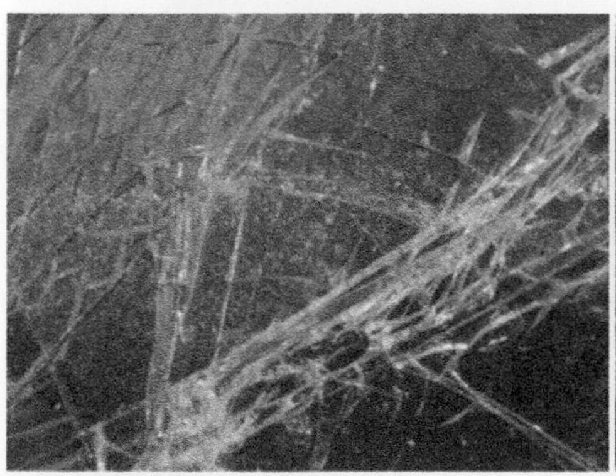

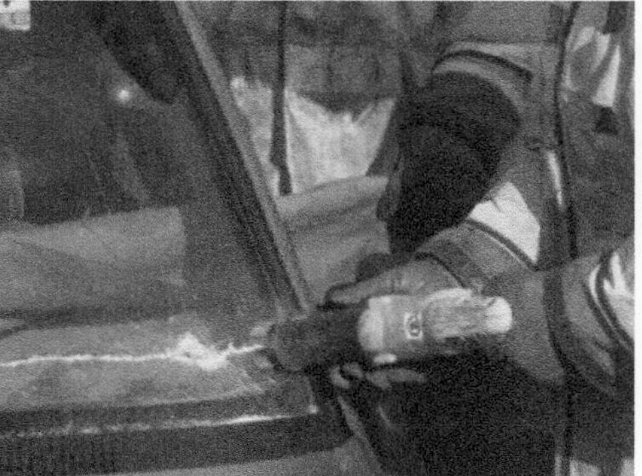

Figure 2.3 Glass dust from a road traffic collision.

3 – PATIENT

A logical structured approach to the patient is essential (Figure 2.4). Rapid access to the patient may require assistance from the fire and rescue service with stabilisation of the vehicle and glass management. A rapid assessment using the <C>ABCDE process will identify life-threatening conditions and allow a judgement regarding the necessary speed of evacuation of the patient: will there be a need for a 'snatch rescue' or a planned and staged removal? Initial communication with the patient will generally very rapidly provide useful information. Once the patient has had analgesia and is ready to move, they must be protected from noise and sharps, and care must be taken that vascular access is not dislodged. Appropriate levels of monitoring are essential. Trip hazards must be avoided.

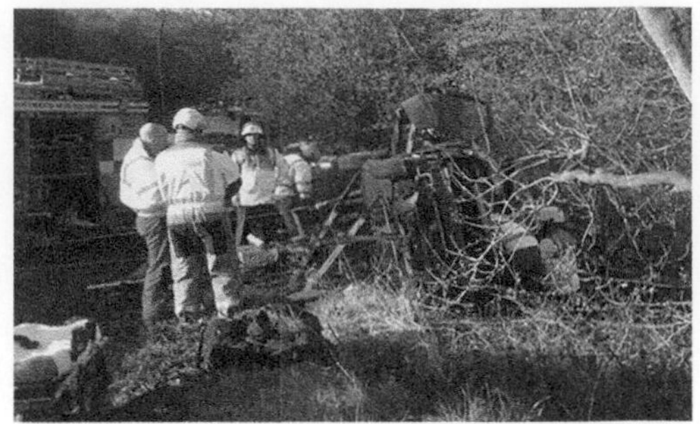

Figure 2.4 Assessing the scene before approaching the patient.

E- EVALUATION AND RE-EVALUATION

Regular reassessment of the scene for developing (or resolving) hazards is essential throughout the assessment treatment and evacuation process. In addition, reassessment of the <C>ABCDE sequence is essential, as the patient's condition may change at any time. In the light of this new information, decisions may change regarding the ultimate destination of the patient. Whatever the destination, all lines must be secured, the patient must be safe and secure in whatever carrying or immobilisation device is used, and a clear plan for their safe removal from the scene to the vehicle must be established and clear to all involved. Hypothermia must be prevented or treated, and splints must be in situ and correctly applied where necessary. Monitoring will allow the rapid recognition of any suggestion of deterioration.

PRACTICE POINT

Blowing three long blasts on a whistle should clear the scene of all personnel if any danger is seen or expected.

An overall evaluation or re-evaluation of the scene will include the wind direction to assess the impact of fumes, as not all fumes are visible. As long as the approach is upwind the risk is reduced, bearing mind that wind direction can change at any time (Figure 2.5).

If possible, odours that may give a clue to potential dangers should be identified, the obvious one being petrol fumes following a road traffic collision (RTC). Strong-smelling chemicals found in a factory may mean that the environment is oxygen-depleted and any entry into this scene could result in rescuer hypoxia and collapse. It should

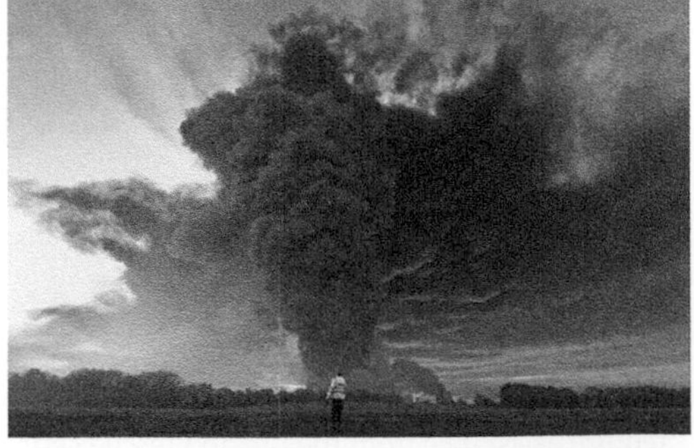

Figure 2.5 The Buncefield fire at the Hertfordshire Oil Storage Terminal, December 11, 2005. A knowledge of wind direction was vital for safe working at this scene.

also be remembered that some fumes such as carbon monoxide do not have a scent and the only clue may come from the situational context of the injured patient, for example in an old house with a poorly maintained gas appliance.

Looking at the posture of those standing around the scene (or running away) may give a clue to the presence of danger, for example a crowd suddenly rushing away from the scene may indicate that someone has just produced a weapon or become aggressive.

PRACTICE POINT

Always have an escape route in case things deteriorate.

TRANSMISSION OF INFECTION

OCCUPATIONAL EXPOSURE TO BLOOD-BORNE PATHOGENS

There is a small but significant risk of transmission of infection in pre-hospital care. When evaluating occupational exposures to fluids that might contain *hepatitis B virus (HBV), hepatitis C virus (HCV), or human immunodeficiency virus (HIV),* PHEM practitioners should consider that all blood, body fluids, secretions, and excretions except sweat may contain transmissible infectious agents and adopt appropriate precautions. Blood contains the greatest load of infectious particles of all body fluids and is the most critical transmission vehicle in the health-care setting (Box 2.4).

BOX 2.4: Blood-Borne Pathogens

What is the risk of infection after an occupational exposure?

Hepatitis B virus (HBV)

PHEM practitioners who have received hepatitis B vaccine and have developed immunity to the virus are at very slight risk of infection. For an unvaccinated person, the risk from a single needle-stick or a cut exposure to HBV-infected blood ranges from 6% to 30% and depends on the hepatitis B e antigen (HBeAg) status of the source individual. Individuals who are both hepatitis B surface antigen (HBsAg) positive and HBeAg positive have more virus in their blood and are more likely to transmit HBV.

Hepatitis C virus (HCV)

Based on limited studies, the estimated risk for infection after a needle-stick or cut exposure to HCV-infected blood is approximately 1.8%. The risk following a blood splash is unknown but is believed to be very small; however, HCV infection from such an exposure has been reported.

Human immunodeficiency virus (HIV)

The average risk for HIV infection after a needle-stick or cut exposure to HIV-infected blood is 0.3% (about 1 in 300). The risk after exposure of the eye, nose, or mouth to HIV-infected blood is estimated to be, on average, 0.1% (1 in 1000).

The risk after exposure of the skin to HIV-infected blood is estimated to be less than 0.1%. A small amount of blood on intact skin probably poses no risk at all. There have been no documented cases of HIV transmission due to an exposure involving such exposure for a short period of time). The risk may be higher if the skin is damaged (for example by a recent cut), if the contact involves a large area of skin or if the contact is prolonged.

PERSONAL PROTECTIVE EQUIPMENT

Personal protective equipment (PPE) consists of specialised clothing or equipment worn to protect against hazards. Examples include gloves, masks, protective eyewear with side shields, and gowns to prevent skin and mucous membrane exposures. In PHEM, PPE is also needed to protect the practitioner from the environment. Employers have legal duties concerning the provision and use of PPE at work through the *Personal Protective Equipment at Work Regulations 1992.* The risks against which PPE should be worn are given in Box 2.5. Based on a dynamic risk assessment of the situation, the level of PPE depends on the requirements of the situation but may include (Figure 2.6):

- High visibility jacket with clear identification labels
- Waterproof overalls with knee protection and fire retardant as a minimum standard
- Safety helmet and visor
- Safety glasses
- Ear defenders
- Debris/chemical gloves
- Safety boots which are acid resistant with steel-toe caps and reinforced sole
- Head torch
- Whistle
- Clinical gloves

Whilst it is essential to be adequately protected, PPE must be tailored to the situation since wearing PPE can dramatically downgrade performance.

BOX 2.5: Potential Hazards in Pre-hospital Practice

Eyes: Chemical or metal splash, dust, projectiles, gas and vapour, radiation
Head: Impact from falling or flying objects, risk of head bumping, hair entanglement
Breathing: Dust, vapour, gas, oxygen-deficient atmospheres
Body: Temperature extremes, adverse weather, chemical or metal splash, spray from pressure leaks or spray guns, impact or penetration, contaminated dust, excessive wear or entanglement of own clothing
Hands and arms: Abrasion, temperature extremes, cuts and punctures, impact, chemicals, electric shock, skin infection, disease or contamination
Feet and legs: Wet, electrostatic build-up, slipping, cuts and punctures, falling objects, metal and chemical splash, abrasion

PRACTICE POINT

It is essential to prepare equipment prior to deployment: rehearsal is key to being safe.

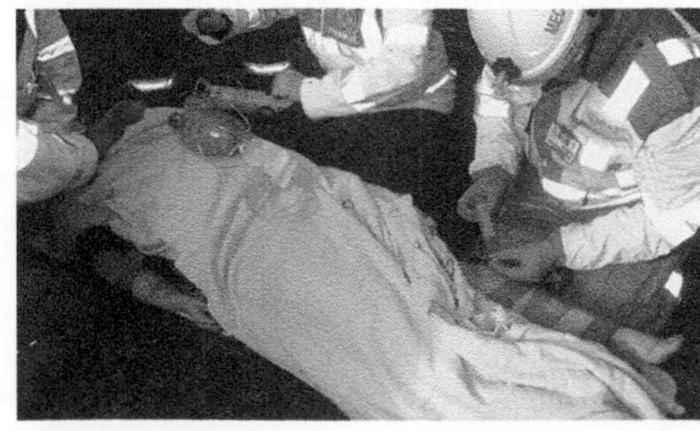

Figure 2.6 Individual personal protective equipment (PPE).

Goggles should provide adequate protection when the risk of splashing is present, and must wrap around the eye area to ensure side areas are protected. Face shields or visors should be considered in place of a surgical mask or goggles when there is a higher risk of splattering or aerosolisation of blood or other body fluids. Gloves must be worn for invasive procedures, contact with sterile sites and non-intact skin or mucous membranes and all activities that have been assessed as carrying a risk of exposure to blood, body fluids, secretions and excretions; and when handling sharp or contaminated instruments (also see Box 2.6).

BOX 2.6: Double Gloving

Double gloving

- Double gloving has been shown to be an effective method for reducing the potential for contact with bodily fluids. In a 1992 study it was reported that surgeons who only single gloved had a 51% hand contamination rate versus a 7% contamination rate for surgeons who double gloved.
- Double gloving (wearing two pairs of gloves) significantly reduces the perforation rate of the inner glove by at least 70% compared to single gloving (3).

SHARPS MANAGEMENT

Sharps injuries do occur on scene and good standards for handling sharps must be observed (Box 2.7). If sharps are used, approved containers for the disposal of sharps (conforming to UN3291 and BS 7320 standards) must be available *before* a procedure is started. Approved sharps containers should be assembled correctly and never over-filled (above the manufacturers' fill line on the box or more than ¾ full).

BOX 2.7: Dealing with a Needle-Stick Injury

Actions in the event of an occupational exposure including needle-stick or similar injury
Perform first aid to the exposed area immediately as follows:

Skin/tissues

- Skin/tissues should be gently encouraged to bleed. Do not scrub or suck the area.
- Wash/irrigate with soap and warm running water. Do not use disinfectants or alcohol.
- Cover the area using a waterproof dressing.

Eyes and mouth

- Eyes and mouth should be rinsed/irrigated with copious amounts of water. Eye and mouth washout kits are usually available in clinical areas.
- If contact lenses are worn, irrigation should be performed before and after removing these. The contact lenses must not be replaced in the eyes.
- Water which has been used for mouth rinsing following mucocutaneous exposure must not be swallowed.

Definitive Management

This will depend on the situation and information regarding the potential infection source but will include blood tests for specific titres, immunisation and less commonly immunoglobulin therapy. Local protocols should be followed and all incidents must be reported.

Sharps should not be passed directly hand to hand, and handling should be kept to a minimum and carried out with care. Needles must not be re-sheathed, re-capped, bent, broken or disassembled after use. Needles or other sharps must never be removed from holding implements using fingers. *Safer sharps* needles (Sharpsafe® or similar) are mandatory.

Sharps boxes should be secured to avoid spillage and appropriately sealed in accordance with the manufacturers' instructions once full. Local waste disposal policy must be followed. Needless to say, items should never be removed from sharps containers. The label on the sharps container must be completed when starting to use the container and again once sealed, to facilitate tracing if required.

EQUIPMENT AND DRUG SAFETY

Arrival at the patient without the necessary equipment can seriously compromise the chances of survival and a good outcome. For every minute that passes following collapse from cardiac arrest before a defibrillation shock is delivered, the chance of survival reduces by 7% to 10%. It is important that kit and drugs are carried safely to maintain clinical effectiveness and can be easily retrieved when needed.

Carriage of materials such as drugs and medical gases must be in accordance with the appropriate regulatory framework as well as being easily accessible and stored in a manner which makes them immediately recognisable and safe from breakage (Figures 2.7 and 2.8). Drugs such as those used for anaesthesia should be pre-drawn at the beginning of each shift, and use of pre-prepared commercial syringes is encouraged. Correct labelling is essential in order to avoid drug errors (Figure 2.9) (4). The use of laminated, easily accessible drug dosage aid memoires is also encouraged (Figure 2.10).

Equipment used in pre-hospital care must be packed and prepared in a way that keeps the equipment safe and accessible. Many equipment-packing systems exist around the world that generally reflect different ways of working.

Many packaging systems are modular, based on the interventions likely to be used by an advanced pre-hospital emergency medical team. These modular systems reduce turnaround times as pre-packed modules that are held in storage can be 'hot swapped' quickly thus keeping the team operational. In addition, location of the required equipment in adverse situations

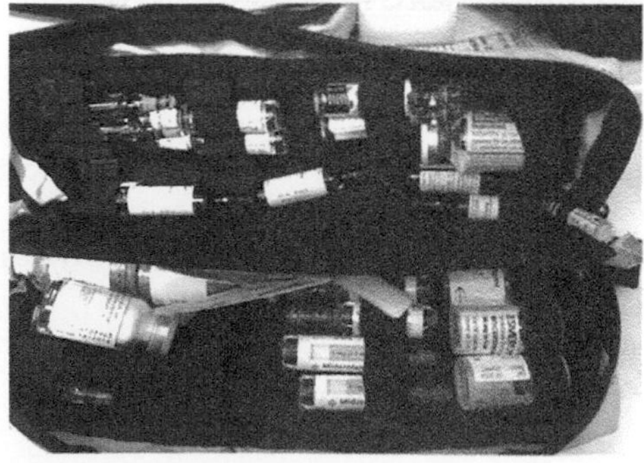

Figure 2.7 Drugs stored in a soft canvass case that leaves drugs prone to breakage (glass on glass).

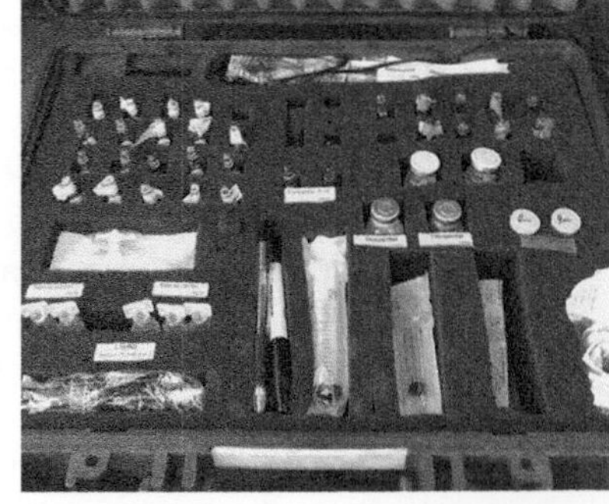

Figure 2.8 Safe carriage of controlled drugs with protection of glass ampoules.

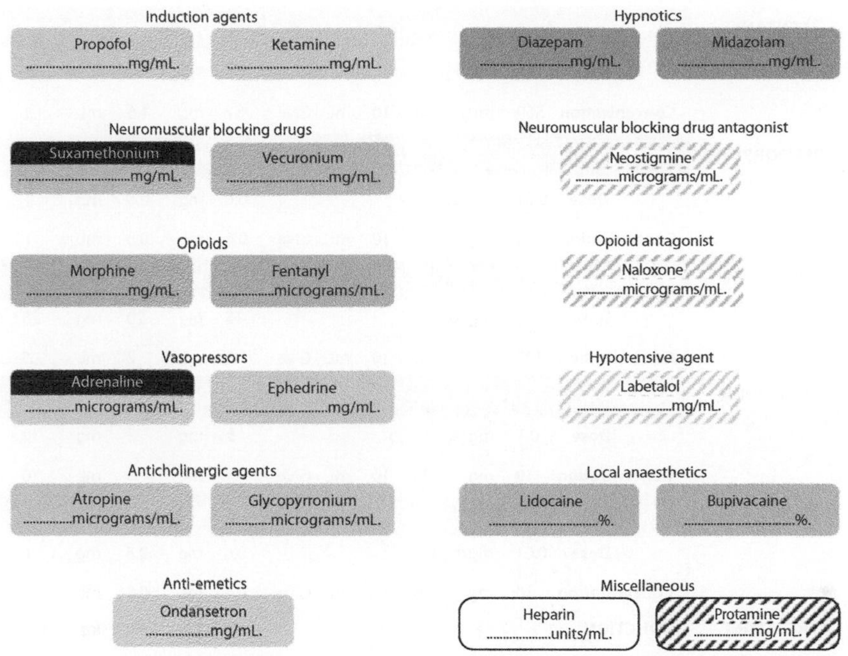

Figure 2.9 Standard drug labelling. (From http://www.rcoa.ac.uk/system/files/SYRINGE-LABELLING-2014_0.pdf.)

is greatly facilitated (Figure 2.11). Using this approach standards of equipment delivery are maintained, as packing and checking are done in a controlled manner.

PRE-DEPLOYMENT CHECKLISTS

Every deploying scheme or individual should have *standard operating procedures* (SOPs) for reference use before deploying to the scene of an incident. These SOPs should aim to ensure that nothing is forgotten and that all necessary safety measures have been put in place. An example of the subjects which should be covered in such an SOP is given in Box 2.8.

HELICOPTER SAFETY

The ability to work safely around helicopters is an essential part of pre-hospital practice and potentially one of its most hazardous components. Each helicopter will be slightly different and the first priority is to be familiar with the airframe used in one's area of practice. Faced with an unfamiliar helicopter, there are certain general principles which are summarised in Figure 2.12 (5). In general however, two points should be remembered: do not approach a helicopter until signalled to do so by the pilot and make sure that unsecured items are unable to cause damage to the airframe. In general, a helicopter should not be approached when the rotors are turning.

FENTANYL	**ANALGESIA**							**60**	**kg**	**80**	**kg**	**100**	**kg**
	Dose	1	mic/kg					60	mcg	80	mcg	100	mcg
	Concentration	500	mcg	in	10	mL	Give	1.2	mL	1.6	mL	2	mL
DIAMORPHINE	**ANALGESIA**							**60**	**kg**	**80**	**kg**	**100**	**kg**
	Dose	0.01	mg/kg					0.6	mg	0.8	mg	1	mg
	Concentration	10	mg	in	10	mL	Give	0.6	mL	0.8	mL	1	mL
KETAMINE	**ANALGESIA**							**60**	**kg**	**80**	**kg**	**100**	**kg**
	Dose	0.25	mg/kg					15	mg	20	mg	25	mg
	Concentration	100	mg	in	10	mL	Give	1.5	mL	2	mL	2.5	mL
MORPHINE	**ANALGESIA**							**60**	**kg**	**80**	**kg**	**100**	**kg**
	Dose	0.1	mg/kg					6	mg	8	mg	10	mg
	Concentration	10	mg	in	10	mL	Give	6	mL	8	mL	10	mL
MIDAZOLAM	**SEDATION**							**60**	**kg**	**80**	**kg**	**100**	**kg**
	Dose	0.01	mg/kg					0.6	mg	0.8	mg	1	mg
	Concentration	10	mg	in	10	mL	Give	0.6	mL	0.8	mL	1	mL
KETAMINE	**INDUCTION**							**60**	**kg**	**80**	**kg**	**100**	**kg**
	Dose	2	mg/kg					120	mg	160	mg	200	mg
	Concentration	100	mg	in	20	mL	Give	12	mL	16	mL	20	mL
SUX	**PARALYSIS**							**60**	**kg**	**80**	**kg**	**100**	**kg**
	Dose	1.5	mg/kg					90	mg	120	mg	150	mg
	Concentration	200	mg	in	2	mL	Give	0.9	mL	1.2	mL	1.5	mL
ROCURONIUM	**PARALYSIS**							**60**	**kg**	**80**	**kg**	**100**	**kg**
	Dose	1	mg/kg					60	mg	80	mg	100	mg
	Concentration	50	mg	in	5	mL	Give	6	mL	8	mL	10	mL
TIDAL VOLUME	**VENTILATION**							**60**	**kg**	**80**	**kg**	**100**	**kg**
	Normal	8	mL/kg					480	mL	640	mL	800	mL
	Pulmonary Protection	6	mL/Kg					360	mL	480	mL	600	mL

Figure 2.10 Drug dosage checking aid memoire for PHEM.

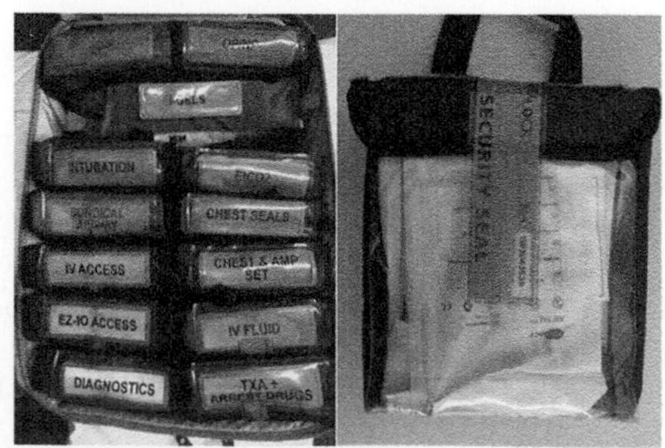

Figure 2.11 A system for equipment layout and packing used in pre-hospital emergency care.

BOX 2.8: SOP for Pre-Hospital Response Team

Personnel

- ID cards
- PPE check
- Ensure head torches are working

Vehicle

- Carry out vehicle check, oil, water, tyres tread and pressures, lights/sirens
- Vehicle work-ticket signed
- Fuel card present
- Check access code and battery level of team tablet and secured to vehicle

Controlled drugs and equipment

- Ensure controlled drugs keys are drawn from keypress
- Check stock and sign controlled drug (CD) register
- Secure small CD pouch on person signing for controlled drugs
- Secure larger CD pouch in car safe
- Check clinical equipment and pouch seals
- Load car using agreed configuration

Communication

- Inform ambulance control of availability and ensure call sign allocated
- Identify consultant clinical support for the team
- Allocate responsibility for radio communications and navigation

Command and control

- Allocate provisional clinical roles before arrival

Record-keeping

- Complete patient report forms (PRFs) for all patients seen and place one copy to patient's hospital records (emergency department), second copy to station for scanning; if applicable, ensure trainee paperwork is present
- Complete case log for all team activity including cancels/stand downs
- Debrief jobs post-incident where necessary

End of shift

- Unload all clinical equipment from car if using vehicle; repack/stock and keep clinical equipment on vehicle
- Return controlled drugs to safe and sign them all back in to controlled drug register.
- Replenish/clean any equipment or leave a message for missing/broken items

SPECIFIC HAZARDS

WEATHER

The most significant weather hazard in pre-hospital care is cold, although even in the UK heat illness is not unknown. Wind chill is the perceived decrease in air temperature felt on exposed skin due to the flow of air. Wind chill will inevitably affect a patient (and practitioner) if they are not protected from it. Appropriate clothing and preparation (including watching the weather reports) before deploying will reduce the risk.

Adding hypothermia to a patient's other problems (through poor control of heat loss) will make the clinical situation worse for the patient, as hypothermia affects the body's ability to regulate

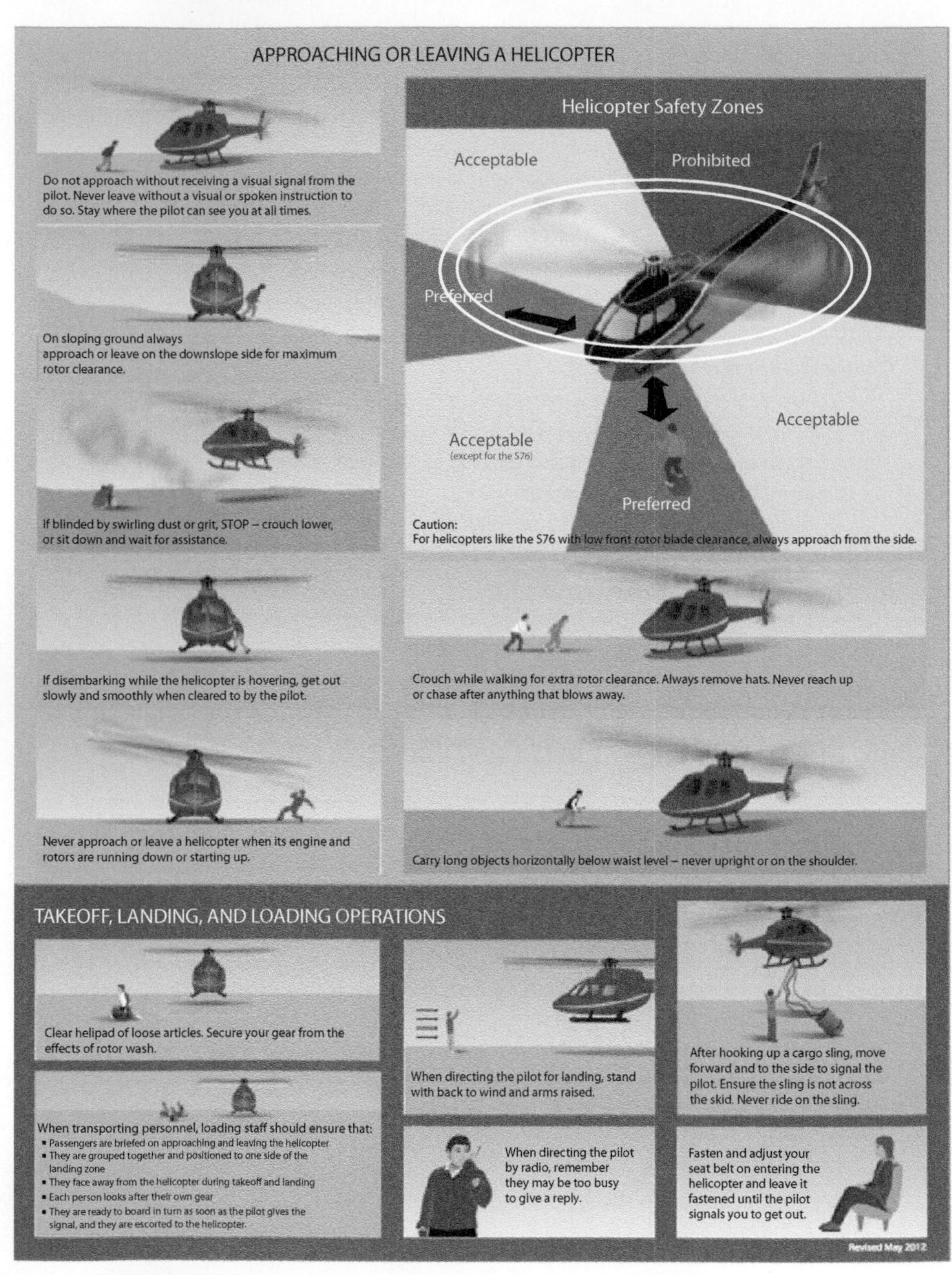

Figure 2.12 Safe working around helicopters. (From https://www.caa.govt.nz/assets/legacy/safety_info/Posters/safety_around_helicopters-industry.pdf.)

Risk of getting hypothermia and frostbite outdoors
Air temperature C

Wind speed m/s	... -10 C							-11 ... -28 C						-29 ... -39 C		
0	10	7	4	1	-2	-5	-8	-11	-14	-17	-20	-23	-26	-29	-32	-35
2	9.2	5.7	2.2	-1.3	-4.8	-8.3	-12	-15	-19	-22	-26	-29	-33	-36	-40	-43
3	8.5	4.9	1.3	-2.3	-5.9	-9.5	-13	-17	-20	-24	-28	-31	-35	-38	-42	-46
4	8	4.3	0.6	-3.1	-6.8	-10	-14	-18	-22	-25	-29	-33	-36	-40	-44	-47
5	7.6	3.8	0.1	-3.7	-7.4	-11	-15	-19	-23	-26	-30	-34	-38	-41	-45	-49
6	7.2	3.4	-0.4	-4.2	-8	-12	-16	-19	-23	-27	-31	-35	-39	-42	-46	-50
7	6.9	3.1	-0.8	-4.6	-8.5	-12	-16	-20	-24	-28	-32	-36	-39	-43	-47	-51
8	6.7	2.8	-1.1	-5	-8.9	-13	-17	-21	-25	-29	-32	-36	-40	-44	-48	-52
9	6.4	2.5	-1.5	-5.4	-9.3	-13	-17	-21	-25	-30	-33	-37	-41	-45	-49	-53
10	6.2	2.2	-1.8	-5.7	-9.7	-14	-18	-22	-26	-30	-34	-38	-42	-46	-50	-53
11	6	2	-2	-6	-10	-14	-18	-22	-26	-30	-34	-38	-42	-46	-50	-54
12	5.8	1.8	-2.3	-6.3	-10	-14	-18	-23	-27	-31	-35	-39	-43	-47	-51	-55
13	5.6	1.6	-2.5	-6.6	-11	-15	-19	-23	-27	-31	-35	-39	-43	-47	-51	-55
14	5.5	1.4	-2.7	-6.8	-11	-15	-19	-23	-27	-31	-35	-40	-44	-48	-52	-56
15	5.3	1.2	-2.9	-7	-11	-15	-19	-24	-28	-32	-36	-40	-44	-48	-52	-56
16	5.2	1	-3.1	-7.2	-11	-16	-20	-24	-28	-32	-36	-40	-45	-49	-53	-57
17	5	0.9	-3.3	-7.5	-12	-16	-20	-24	-28	-32	-37	-41	-45	-49	-53	-57
18	4.9	0.7	-3.5	-7.6	-12	-16	-20	-24	-29	-33	-37	-41	-45	-50	-54	-58
19	4.8	0.6	-3.6	-7.8	-12	-16	-20	-25	-29	-33	-37	-42	-46	-50	-54	-58
20	4.7	0.4	-3.8	-8	-12	-17	-21	-25	-29	-33	-38	-42	-46	-50	-55	-59
21	4.5	0.3	-3.9	-8.2	-12	-17	-21	-25	-29	-34	-38	-42	-46	-51	-55	-59
22	4.4	0.2	-4.1	-8.3	-13	-17	-21	-25	-30	-34	-38	-42	-47	-51	-55	-60

Low risk of hypothermia.
Risk of hypothermia, if being outdoors too long without relevant protection.
Increased risk of hypothermia. Exposed skin gets frostbitten in 10–30 min.
High risk of hypothermia. Exposed skin gets frostbitten in 5–10 min.
Exposed skin gets frostbitten in 2–5 min.
Exposed skin gets frostbitten in less than 2 min.

Figure 2.13 Hypothermia risk.

bleeding and contributes to the trauma *lethal triad* (Figure 2.13). The patient can be wrapped in bubble wrap or cellular blankets; the important thing is to keep the patient out of the wind. Wrapping a patient wearing cold wet clothes in a tinfoil blanket will only exacerbate the problem: cold wet clothes should be removed and replaced where possible, if transfer times are likely to be prolonged.

MOTORWAYS

Motorways are extremely dangerous places to work and deaths of rescuers are sadly not rare. The 20 highest scoring hazards account for around 90% of the total risk and include driver fatigue, speeding, rapid changes of general vehicle speed, tailgating, vehicles stopping in a running lane, pedestrians in running lanes and vehicles recovered from a refuge area.

Some of the hazards can be mitigated, and the design and use of technology to create a controlled environment where drivers comply with signs and speeds have allowed the Highways Agency to manage these risks down to an acceptable level. So, for instance, the hazards of a vehicle being driven too fast or the occurrence of tailgating are mitigated through the use of variable mandatory speed limits and enforcement. As a general principle, one should always adopt a position on the bankside of the safety barrier and watch the approaching traffic (or get someone to spot this aspect of the scene for you) (6).

RAIL INCIDENTS

Unless advised by the fire or ambulance safety officer, or senior representative of Network Rail that the scene is safe, one must not go onto a railway line without prior appropriate training through Network Rail or unless in the company of Network Rail or British Transport Police personnel.

Many rail lines are electrified and access to these sites requires specialist knowledge to manage the risks. For example, the London Underground rail system has a third rail which is charged to around 600 volts. This needs to be isolated before making an approach to a patient on the line. British Transport Police are the agency to refer to for this advice and support.

FIRES

The senior fire officer on scene is in charge of scene safety. The safety of all personnel working on scene is his responsibility. Generally speaking, having arrived on scene the responder should report to the fire officer (white helmet) for a safety briefing (Figure 2.14).

CHEMICAL INCIDENTS

If at a scene one patient appears to have collapsed for unknown reasons, it is usually safe to approach normally. However, if two patients have collapsed for unknown reasons, the approach must be with caution. If three or more patients have collapsed without any obvious reason, then the correct action is to withdraw and report this immediately to control. Having done this, every effort should be made to control scene access and egress until specialist help is available. This latter event maybe a serious chemical incident and requires a specialist response. The recent incidents involving a chemical weapons agent in Salisbury and Amesbury very clearly highlighted the dangers in managing such a situation.

WATER

To prevent drowning and other injuries when working around water, it is crucial to assess the risks and call upon specialist teams who are trained and equipped to deal with this hazard. Some pre-hospital medical schemes that are frequently called to incidents in or around water will allocate personal flotation devices to their staff (7).

ACTS OF AGGRESSION

Managing violence and aggression is a large and important subject and cannot be covered in detail here. If there is a risk of violence, control will advise standing off from the scene until the police have secured it. It is important to ensure familiarity with local

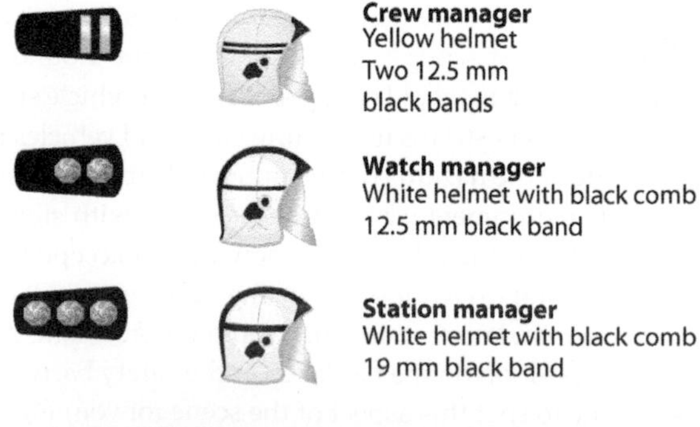

Figure 2.14 Senior fire officers' rank markings.

policies for handling unexpected situations. Sometimes it is not what a person says, but what their body is 'doing' (Box 2.9). There may be situations where contact with the patient is made and it is not obvious at the beginning that there is a threat of violence. Caution is important when someone shows one or more of the 'non-verbal' signs of aggression. Avoidance of specific risk means paying attention to the patient's hands and feet range as well as being aware of the risk of being headbutted! When the risk is identified, the first consideration is 'do I need to leave now?' In many cases this is the first and only option and is entirely correct.

BOX 2.9: Signs of Aggression

- Flushed or pale face
- Sweating
- Pacing, restless or repetitive movements
- Banging/kicking things
- Stamping feet
- Trembling or shaking
- Clenched jaws or fists
- Exaggerated or violent gestures
- Standing too close
- Change in voice
- Loud talking or chanting
- Shallow, rapid breathing
- Scowling, sneering or use of abusive language
- Glaring or avoiding eye contact
- Violating your personal space (they get too close)

Conversely, it is important to be aware of your own body language and present a non-threatening, open stance, keeping good eye contact whilst ensuring this does not appear confrontational.

Make sure you are able to 'escape' at all times when dealing with potentially violent situations. In such situations movements should be slow and steady and actions calm. Personal space should be respected. It is vital to keep calm (8).

POST-INCIDENT DEBRIEFING

Although it might seem unusual to include debriefing and case review in a section on safety, in reality safe and effective practice depends on having an established system for reviewing and changing practise based on experience. Facets of such a structure may include discussion of issues arising from an individual case between a trainee and a supervisor (case-based discussions) and team discussion of critical interventions with review of standard operating procedures in the light of any issues identified. Standard operating procedures which are regularly revised and updated in the light of experience and newly available evidence not only improve performance, but protect the clinician in the event of a serious untoward event. Whenever such an event happens, a full investigation of how and why it happened is mandatory in order to reduce the possibility of it happening again. Honest and constructive analysis of such incidents is essential to non-judgemental learning and a supportive culture.

Equipment governance is also important in maintaining safety standards. All equipment must be ready to use and all personnel must be fully familiar with the checking, maintenance and proper use of equipment and drugs. In addition, systems must be in place to ensure that equipment is safe to use and, where necessary, appropriately calibrated. Equipment failures not infrequently contribute to adverse incidents during PHEM. SOPs must aim to prevent equipment failure through routine checking and maintenance, rapid identification of equipment failures (by checking equipment prior to immediate use and maintaining a high level of vigilance) and by effectively managing an equipment failure (through resolution or replacement).

Failure of equipment should be reported to the appropriate statutory authority. Common causes of equipment failure include lack of training or poor instructions, inappropriate modifications, use in inappropriate circumstances, use outside the manufacturer's specifications, poor maintenance and unsuitable storage conditions (9).

SUMMARY

Safety is a vital aspect of pre-hospital practice. Most risks can be avoided by following very simple rules and by inculcating a safety culture. To do this, it is vital that standard operating procedures reflect accumulated experience and up-to-date knowledge and that a non-judgemental supporting environment allows all those individuals involved to be honest about mistakes and to learn from them.

REFERENCES

1. http://www.ibtphem.org.uk/IBTPHEM/Curriculum.html. Similar standards for the fire and rescue services are at http://www.ukfrs.com/.
2. http://www.gmc-uk.org/education/undergraduate/15_5_health_clearance_and_disclosure.asp.
3. http://www.nhsprofessionals.nhs.uk/download/comms/cg1_nhsp_standard_infection_control_precautions_v3.pdf.
4. Syringe labelling in critical care areas: 2014 review. http://www.rcoa.ac.uk/system/files/SYRINGE-LABELLING-2014_0.pdf.
5. https://www.caa.govt.nz/assets/legacy/safety_info/Posters/safety_around_helicopters-industry.pdf.
6. https://www.gov.uk/government/uploads/system/uploads/attachment_data/file/363993/Smart_motorways_-_Fact_Sheets.pdf.
7. Recognising aggression in others. SkillsYouNeed. http://www.skillsyouneed.com/ps/dealing-with-aggression2.html#ixzz3PGSaSA8l.
8. http://www.mhra.gov.uk/Aboutus/index.htm.

3 The incident scene

OBJECTIVES

After completing this chapter the reader will

- Understand how the scene of an incident is safely managed
- Understand how to function effectively at the scene of an incident
- Be aware of the important information which can be obtained from a careful assessment of the scene of an incident

INTRODUCTION

Pre-hospital practitioners have the opportunity to gain important information from the scene of an incident which may be vital for the effective management of a patient. Equally, the scene of an incident can be a dangerous and inhospitable place. Practitioners *must,* therefore, be able to function effectively at the scene of an incident, including interacting appropriately and professionally with the emergency services and other responders. Practitioners must also be vigilant for those details of the scene which may prove to be important in ensuring optimal management of the patient.

PREPARATION AND RESPONSE

Vehicle and medical equipment checks should take place every day. The most effective way to ensure readiness for service is to use a checklist; a challenge and response checklist with a colleague may prove the most effective system. If an observer or trainee is attending, their role on scene and any expectations of them during the drive or at the scene should be made clear before departing.

TAKING THE CALL AND SETTING OUT

A single responder must inevitably know what the task is, but in a team response some services 'blind' the driver to the type of call in an effort to ensure consistency of driving and avoid a change in speed for the urgent calls.

If a colleague is available to navigate, knowing the exact location of the incident before setting off may not be a priority. A skilled navigator will be able to determine the location of the incident and the most appropriate (not necessarily the fastest) route. As a single responder it is important to have clarity on the location from the outset and use of a satellite navigation system (satnav) is useful (see later), although maps must also be carried.

En route a driver should have the majority of his or her attention or *bandwidth* focused on driving. This means looking out at the road ahead and being aware of the vehicle and how it is responding. To facilitate this, all other distractions should be minimised. If a satellite navigation system is used, its auditory mode should be enabled to avoid the driver being distracted by the map display. Conversation en route should be focused on the task and nothing else. Control should avoid giving unnecessary updates, such as 'the patient has progressed to cardiac arrest'. This will only distract the driver and potentially change their driving style. Important updates such as change of location or safety issues on scene should always be communicated.

THE APPROACH

Accuracy of navigation is vital. A 3 to 4 minute detour because of a wrong turn may have a material effect on outcome in a patient in cardiac arrest. It is better to slow down and stop rather than make hasty navigation decisions. When driving to an incident, any hazards that may require modification of the direction of the approach should be considered. Fires and potential chemical incidents may necessitate a less direct approach depending on the prevailing wind. Consideration should also be given to the time of day, likely flows of traffic, the possibility of traffic build up and gridlock due to the incident. The most direct route may not necessarily be the quickest.

On arrival the vehicle should be parked in a way that will not slow the exit of the ambulance carrying the casualty to hospital or impede other emergency vehicles that may need to be closer to the scene than your own. If the road is not closed and moving traffic threatens those at the scene, the vehicle should be parked in a way that brings traffic to halt and protects the scene. The police will formalise this process on their arrival. It may be appropriate to leave flashing lights active to increase protection. The ignition keys may be left in the vehicle so that the police can move it if necessary, but consideration must be given to the possibility of theft of the vehicle or its contents.

PRACTICE POINT

It is vital to confirm arrival on scene with the operations room.

Arriving by helicopter provides an opportunity to survey the scene. In large-scale incidents, a sketch picture taken from the air may be useful. Such pictures can add significant clarity to people's understanding of the magnitude of an incident and where resources might best be placed.

It is essential to exit the vehicle carefully and safely, especially if traffic is still moving. Risks must not be taken by parking in an unsafe position in an attempt to arrive a few seconds sooner. Ideally, the driver should remind everyone else in the vehicle about the importance of safety before doors are opened. Appropriate personal protective equipment is mandatory.

The walk to the scene is an opportunity to take stock and to survey the scene for immediate hazards. A fall from height through a window or skylight may leave the patient in continued danger from unsecure glass or debris above (Figure 3.1).

If the patient and other rescuers appear in a vulnerable position, any such concerns must be raised as soon as possible and appropriate action taken. A detailed history and examination can

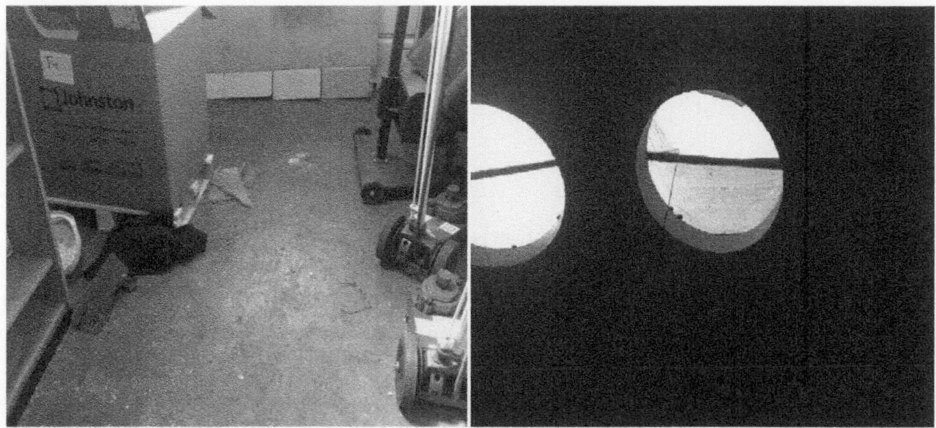

Figure 3.1 (Left) Glass from the skylight is visible on floor. (Right) The patient fell through a skylight.

wait until all are safe. A road traffic collision (RTC) can present many hazards including spilt fuel, an unstable vehicle, sharp metal edges, shattered glass and danger risk from other road users if the road is not closed (Figure 3.2).

If the patient has been injured at height or close to water this may present potential risks, and the use of specialist protective or rescue equipment may be desired or essential. Dynamic risk assessment is vital (Figure 3.3). An unresponsive patient trapped under a car and thought to be in respiratory or cardiac arrest should be removed if resources and manpower will facilitate this. Waiting for dedicated rescue resources may result in a poor patient outcome and public criticism in post-incident analysis.

The final approach on foot is also an opportunity to consider the egress for the patient once the decision to transport has been made. Bystanders can help clear pathways and corridors, or source keys for gates or doors that may be locked. They may also be able to identify an area where the patient can be assessed and treated with 360 degrees of access if the patient was originally injured in a confined space.

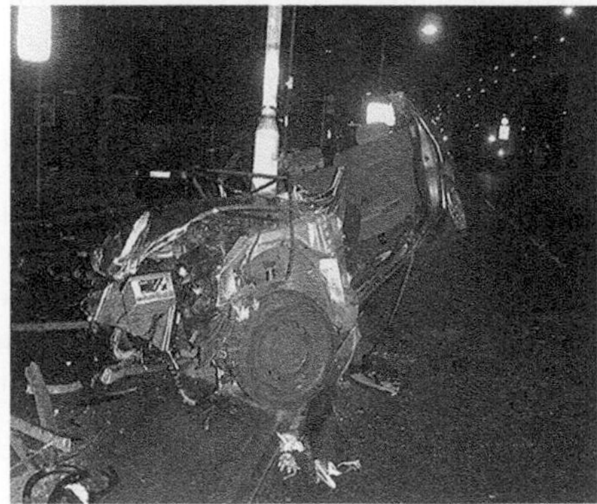

Figure 3.2 Hazards for responding clinicians in this RTC include unstable vehicle, glass, sharp metal fragments, exposed electrics and fuel on the ground, un-deployed airbags.

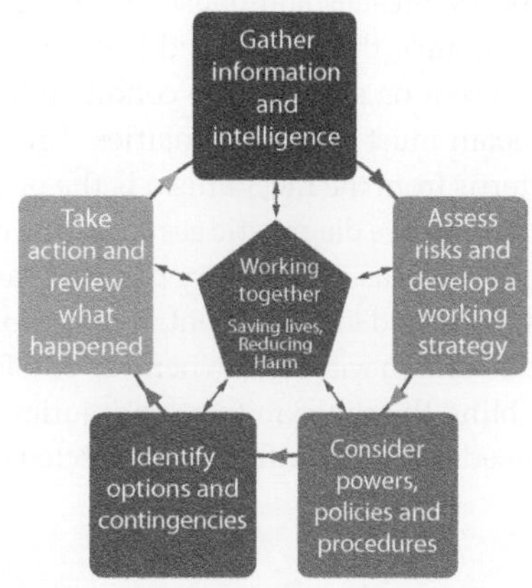

Figure 3.3 The Joint Emergency Services Interoperability Programme (JESIP) Joint Decision Model.

PRACTICE POINT

360 degree access should be obtained at the earliest opportunity.

THE PATIENT

Having made contact with the patient, it is important to establish who else is present. Are those present relatives, friends, work colleagues or simply witnesses? It may be obvious why an ambulance was called but who made the call and exactly why? This may add clarity to the mechanism of the presenting complaint. A witness who saw the crash may intimate there was loss of control before the accident indicating a prodromal medical event.

Questioning the witnesses will also allow the responder to understand the patient's physiology immediately after the injury and whether the patient's condition is improving or deteriorating. Specific questions should be used to clarify the details of any incident which is initially described as being one in which the patient was alleged to have been 'unconscious'. The lay use of the term can be different from the exact clinical definition. It is not unusual for a patient who has not moved their limbs to be deemed unconscious, but closer questioning reveals they had full eye movements and were vocalising seconds after the incident.

WHY MAKING DIAGNOSES IS DIFFICULT IN PRE-HOSPITAL CARE

A clinical consultation in the pre-hospital phase is no different to a consultation in hospital. It is expected that the history will be complete and that examination will elucidate all the clinical findings both positive and negative. However, establishing diagnoses may be harder in the pre-hospital phase. Traditional medical education teaches us that the majority of diagnoses are made from the history and in many cases the primary symptom is pain. Obtaining an accurate history from a trauma patient may be compromised; they may be unconscious, be incapable of feeling pain as a result of spinal cord or brachial plexus injury, or have major distracting injuries. Opiates and adrenaline may mask pain and other symptoms or the patient may be under the effects of alcohol or drugs.

In the pre-hospital phase of trauma management, the injury response will be in evolution. For example the established features of a large pneumothorax or internal bleeding may not be present on scene as the condition may still be developing. For this reason the pre-hospital clinician must anticipate injuries. Understanding the mechanisms of injury and likely injury patterns from the mechanism is the primary way of doing this.

To improve diagnostic accuracy, the examination must be focussed and nuanced using likely injury patterns. Such injury patterns can only be defined when the clinician understands what has happened to the patient, and the exact mechanism of injury is clear. It is necessary, therefore to talk to witnesses wherever possible. Concentration on the predicted injury pattern must not blind the clinician to other injuries which may be present, neither should the examination be used solely to confirm the expected injury pattern.

PRINCIPLES OF SCENE MANAGEMENT

If resources allow, a senior clinician should lead the incident and refrain from touching the patient or undertaking interventions where possible. However, resources are often limited and the clinical lead will be required to undertake patient assessment and specific interventions, recognising that during such times situational awareness is lost. The clinician must make best use of all the resources on scene and tailor the contributions of individuals to their particular skill level; this is part of effective crew resource management. A paramedic should not be left to undertake manual in-line mobilisation of the spine when this could be carried out by a fireman or policeman. The paramedic should be free to use their extended clinical skills appropriately.

Anticipation of the steps in patient care is important and all personnel tending the patient should be aware of what is likely to happen next. When intravenous access is being attempted, another team member should be preparing to secure it and have a primed infusion line ready. The clinical lead should facilitate clinicians working simultaneously around the patient.

UNDERTAKING THE CONSULTATION

If other emergency personnel are tending to the patient, it is entirely inappropriate for a doctor or other senior clinician to behave as if they have primacy and 'own' the patient. Brief introductions to colleagues are important, and knowing who is present and their skill levels will aid communication and teamwork as well as avoiding embarrassment. Careful attention should be paid to any handover, and the plans which have already been put in place must be clearly established and understood. It is good manners and assists with relationships within the team to seek 'permission' to consult the patient.

Introductions to the patient should be appropriate; first names may not be the best approach with an older patient. Whatever the situation, creating the impression that everything is under control will calm the patient, improve their physiology and generally promote effective working. Research shows that conscious patients may have their anxiety raised when they become aware that a helicopter has been sent to the incident with a doctor and specially trained paramedic on board.

Appropriate physical contact is likely to be very reassuring to the patient (Figure 3.4). This is often one of the few things patients remember from the scene. Many patients feel or worry that they may be dying: if they are not, they should be explicitly told so. Appropriate reassurance should always be offered.

The position in which a patient is first found may not be ideal for examination and intervention, In such circumstances, consideration must be given to moving the patient safely in order to facilitate management (Figure 3.5).

Establishing the existence (or otherwise) of significant issues with catastrophic external haemorrhage, airway, breathing or circulation (the *primary survey*) should take place over a few seconds and any necessary interventions carried out as required. A thorough head-to-toe examination should then proceed, again taking only a minute or so, and looking for life- or limb-threatening injuries only. When the clinician has completed this examination the extent of the majority of the injuries should be understood. A plan should be established with regard to further clinical interventions and extrication. At an opportune moment the clinician should meet witnesses to understand the mechanism of injury and may need to return to nuance the examination accordingly.

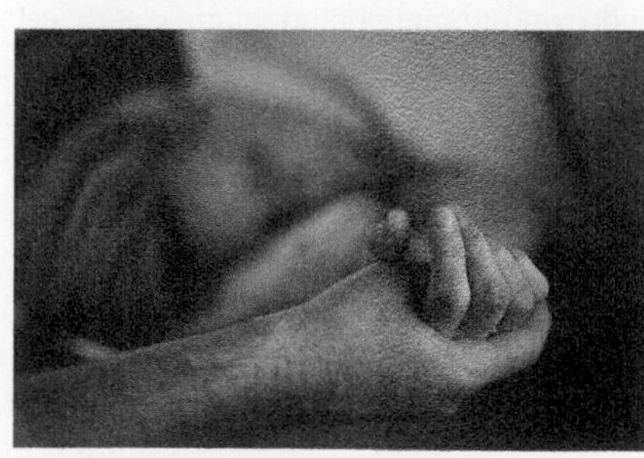

Figure 3.4 Appropriate reassurance is vital.

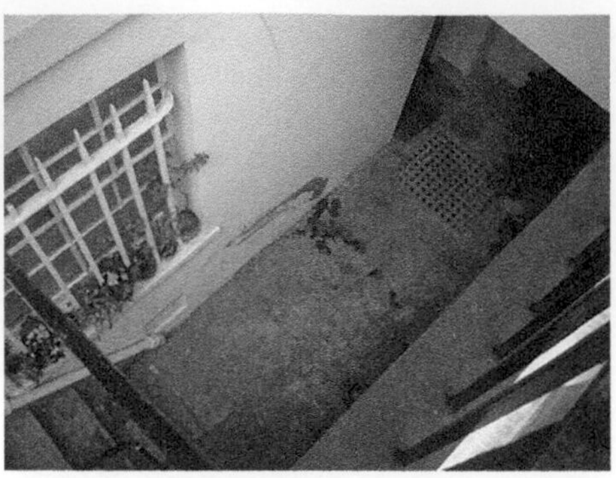

Figure 3.5 Attempts to intubate the patient who had fallen into this basement were unsuccessful until the patient was moved to a more suitable location where 360 degree access was possible.

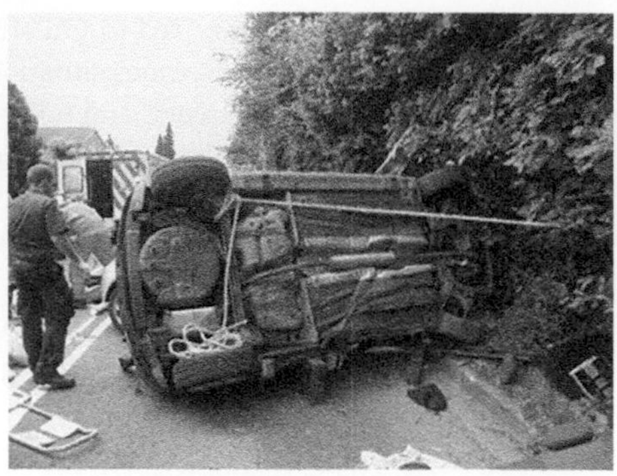

Figure 3.6 Axial skeletal injury from rollover incidents may be asymptomatic and the individual not considered a patient by other emergency services.

It is important to establish how many people have been involved in the incident. Some individuals may not consider themselves to be patients or may not have been 'labelled' as patients by other emergency services on scene (Figure 3.6). Details of who has been involved should be clarified when trying to understand the mechanism of injury and what happened. On initial assessment, patients may appear less badly injured than the circumstances of the accident might suggest. Once the number of patients and their injuries has been established, control must be updated and informed of the resources required.

MANIPULATING THE ENVIRONMENT

The pre-hospital environment can present issues that compromise assessment and interventions. The weather may be windy, cold or wet. It may be very sunny, hampering laryngoscopy or interpretation of ultrasound images on a screen. It is incumbent on the clinician to manage the scene in a way that the effects of the environment are minimised. The fire brigade may have tarpaulin to provide shelter so that the patient can be intubated in an area that is out of bright sunlight, or it might be less windy in the lee of an ambulance vehicle.

VEHICLE ACCIDENTS AND ENTRAPMENT

During extrications it is essential that the roles of the fire and rescue personnel are clearly established, in particular which individual is leading on the technical aspects of the extrication and who is in overall charge. These should be two different roles. The Joint Emergency Services Interoperability Programme (JESIP) principles should be followed (Figure 3.7). Clinical findings will need to be conveyed to the leader of the extrication in order to determine the method and speed of the process.

Establishing whether a patient is trapped, and why, is essential. Entrapments may be *physical* (when the patient cannot get out irrespective of their clinical state because the structure of the vehicle impedes their removal) or *clinical* (relative) where analgesia and minimal manipulation will allow extrication. An example of the latter might be a fractured ankle 'trapped' by the pedals in the footwell of the car.

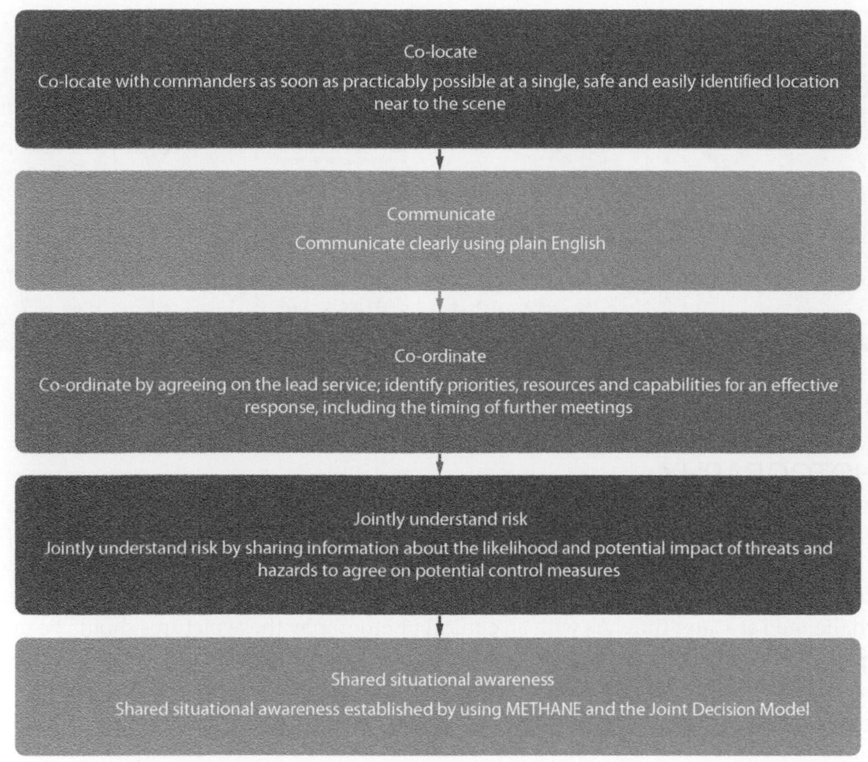

Co-locate
Co-locate with commanders as soon as practicably possible at a single, safe and easily identified location near to the scene
Communicate
Communicate clearly using plain English
Co-ordinate
Co-ordinate by agreeing on the lead service; identify priorities, resources and capabilities for an effective response, including the timing of further meetings
Jointly understand risk
Jointly understand risk by sharing information about the likelihood and potential impact of threats and hazards to agree on potential control measures
Shared situational awareness
Shared situational awareness established by using METHANE and the Joint Decision Model

Figure 3.7 The five principles of effective joint working.

Different mechanisms of injury produce different injury patterns. Frontal impact RTCs such as that in Figure 3.8 may be associated with injuries to the head and spine through contact with the windscreen or steering wheel or the deceleration forces themselves. As the torso loads the seat belt, injuries to the chest and abdomen can occur. Contact of the lower limbs on the dashboard can produce fractures to the knees, femurs or pelvic bones. Dislocation of the hip may also occur. In incidents where the energy transfer is so great there is deformation of the passenger cell, lower leg injuries may occur from crumpling of the footwell and pedals.

Side impacts (Figure 3.9) may be of greater clinical significance, as the crumple zone is smaller than in front or rear collisions. Injuries to the head can occur as the head impacts the side windscreen or bonnet of the other car or other roadside furniture. Forced lateral flexion of the neck may produce cervical spine injuries. As the torso makes contact with the intruding door, injuries to the chest and abdomen can occur, along with injuries to the limbs. Compression fractures of the pelvis and injuries to the acetabulum are also possible.

The police will undertake a detailed investigation of the scene if there have been fatalities, if a patient's life is threatened or there are life-changing injuries. This investigation will take time and result in the road being closed for a protracted time. Due consideration should therefore be given to the consequences when affirming an event is life threatening.

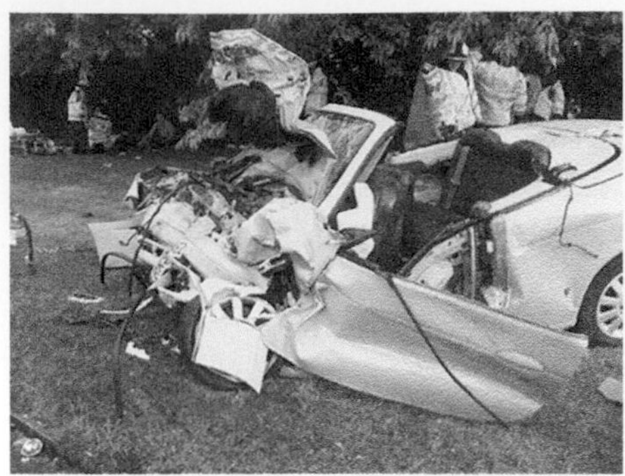

Figure 3.8 A front impact RTC.

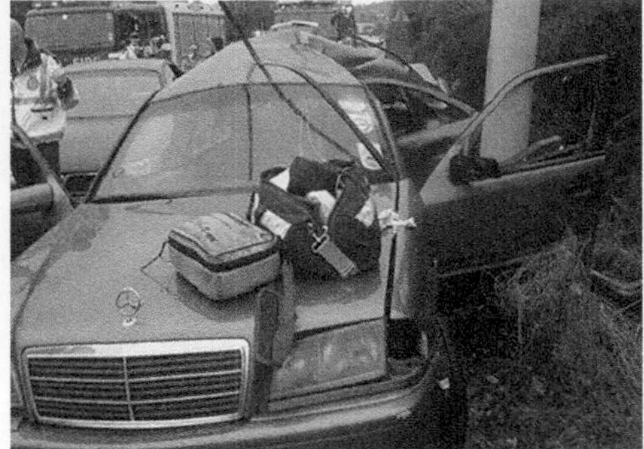

Figure 3.9 A side impact RTC.

PHOTOGRAPHY

The importance of understanding the mechanism of injury has been alluded to. Photographs of car wreckage may help convey some of this to hospital-based clinicians. When amputation is being considered, a photograph of the entrapment may prove useful if the decision to amputate is challenged at a later time. As with all clinical photography these pictures should be processed as part of the patient's record and the necessary consents established where practicable and possible. A dedicated clinical camera should be used for this purpose and not ad hoc use of a personal phone camera.

EGRESS AND TRIAGE

On occasion, access to the patient and egress *for* the patient may be difficult. It is important that there is clear allocation of clinical and non-clinical tasks. Two clinicians troubleshooting the same problem is inefficient. It is important therefore to be clear who is addressing clinical issues and who is working with other emergency personnel in defining the egress from the scene.

Establishing the most appropriate hospital for the patient will depend on the patient's injuries and local facilities. Most trauma networks will have guidance documents to help decision-making, however a consensus should be established from all involved especially the clinician first on scene.

Debriefing following an incident is an important process. It is useful to communicate with the leads from the other emergency services on scene to enquire if any issues have arisen and if a quick or a more formal debrief is required. For the clinical teams, a debrief should take place following handover at hospital after every significant incident. Having a structured debrief form or checklist ensures that all aspects of a mission are covered.

EN ROUTE TO HOSPITAL

The chosen hospital must be made aware of the patient's impending arrival. If the patient requires special resources or skills on arrival at hospital this must be made clear. If the patient needs a general trauma team or a specific specialty response (for example, a cardiothoracic surgeon), then this should be clearly stated. Many centres employ special code names for differing types of hospital responses such as *code red* for major haemorrhage.

CLINICAL NOTES

All patients should have a clinical record of their pre-hospital consultation and this should form part of the hospital record. All clinical notes must be made and kept in a way that is compliant with any relevant medical regulations. The notes convey important clinical information to hospital-based colleagues and should describe the mechanism of injury, the patient's physiology since the incident occurred, the injuries, relevant past medical history and all interventions undertaken. They should always include details from witnesses and other emergency services on scene before the arrival of the emergency services. The clinical notes are a reflection of the clinical care provided, and should be accurately, honestly and promptly completed.

SUMMARY

Managing the scene is an important part of patient care and one that requires practice. Establishing and maintaining good relationships with other responders will enhance patient care. Careful assessment of the scene (and questioning of witnesses) allows access to vital information which might otherwise be missed.

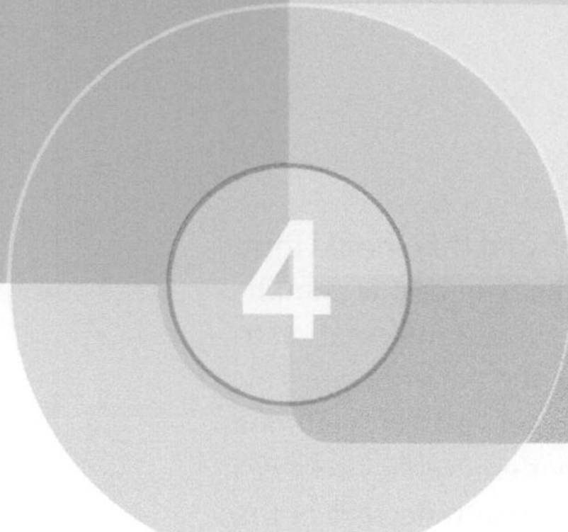

Communication in pre-hospital care

OBJECTIVES

After completing this chapter the reader will

- Understand the importance of communication in pre-hospital care
- Be able to pass important information effectively in order to ensure the patient receives the best pre-hospital care
- Understand the importance of on-scene communication with other agencies and the role of teamwork

INTRODUCTION

The pre-hospital management of patients who have suffered trauma starts from the moment the emergency services are contacted and ends when the patient arrives at the appropriate treatment centre and their care has been formally transferred to hospital staff. Throughout this process clinical care will only save the patient's life and ensure they reach the right hospital as quickly as possible, if on-scene communication between all the responding organisations is open, clear and timely. The importance of getting on-scene relationships right and ensuring effective communication has developed into a subject in its own right. A number of helicopter emergency medical services, BASICS schemes and ambulance services in the UK have now adopted *Crew Resource Management (CRM)* techniques to improve communication on scene by encouraging organisations to recognise the importance of how people work together most efficiently and constructively.

On-scene communication has for a number of years also been a source of concern at major incidents. In every one of the recent enquiries undertaken into these incidents, on-scene communication has been highlighted as a key issue requiring improvement. A report by Dr Kevin Pollock commissioned to review the lessons learnt relating to communications and interoperability from emergencies and major incidents since 1986 cites a number of lessons originating from shortcomings in inter-service communication. Out of the recommendations in this report and other work originated the national *Joint Emergency Services Interoperability Programme (JESIP)*.

COMMUNICATION AND RESPONDING TO THE TRAUMA CALL

In the UK access to the emergency services is gained by dialling 999 or 112. All calls to this number are directed to the service provider of the telephone (*BT emergency* or another service provider such as *Vodaphone, O2* or *Cable and Wireless*). The call is answered and then directed to the appropriate emergency service. In the case of patients who have suffered trauma, the ambulance service is obviously most commonly requested although the police and fire and rescue services may be required if there has been, for example, a road traffic collision. The call is directed to the ambulance service control room for the geographical area in which the calls originates. With the increasing number of calls being generated from mobile phones this can mean the call is not always routed to the geographically appropriate emergency service especially close to area boundaries or across areas of water (Box 4.1).

Once the call is passed to the ambulance service they have a target of ensuring that 95% of emergency calls are answered within 5 seconds of being routed to them. To speed up the essential information being taken, technology such as *Caller Line Identification (CLI)* is used by all ambulance services. This computer system allows the address, if the call is originating from a landline phone, to be automatically populated in the ambulance service call-taking screen. Mobile (cellular) phone location identification software is rapidly developing but in most cases exact locations cannot yet be reliably obtained.

BOX 4.1: Effective Messaging

Any effective communication should be:

- Intelligible
- Accurate
- Timely
- Clear
- As short as possible (concise)

All emergency calls in ambulance control rooms are recorded on a *computer aided dispatch* system (*CAD*). The *CAD* has an integrated mapping system which is linked to an address database to provide a map reference for the site at which the incident has occurred. Once the location details are obtained the caller is taken through a set of questions to determine the priority of the response required. Currently in the UK two triage systems are licenced to be used for prioritising calls: *Medical Priority Dispatch System (AMPDS)* and *NHS Pathways*. Where a call is identified as immediately life threatening (*Red 1 or 2*) the call has a resource dispatched. In most cases as soon as the address and type of incident are established the call is automatically passed by the computer system for dispatch. The rest of the questions can then be asked without slowing the response and the responding vehicle can then be updated as required with the relevant information.

All ambulances and single response vehicles are tracked through integrated satellite navigation systems, these are located in the vehicle and in most cases the Airwave handset. This enables the ambulance control centre to assign the closest resource to the call. All relevant call details are passed by mobile data systems enabling the vehicle mapping system to be automatically updated and reducing the time it takes the resource to locate the incident. Apart from the location, the clinician responding to a trauma call will require: the number of patients, a brief description of the main injuries and, in the case of a road traffic collision, details of whether any patients are trapped, how many vehicles are involved and the nature of any hazards. In many cases this information will not be immediately available but a substantial number of ambulance services now have critical care or incident desks manned by experienced staff who listen to calls and will then phone the caller back to obtain the necessary information so that the responding team can be informed and additional specialist assets assigned prior to the arrival of the first resource at the incident.

PRACTICE POINT

It is essential that as much information about the scene and the patient is obtained so that the appropriate resources can be dispatched to a trauma call.

COMMUNICATION ON ARRIVAL AT A SCENE

Once the pre-hospital care response is on scene, no further support will be sent unless it is asked for. It is therefore of fundamental importance that the ambulance control room is updated at regular intervals. Whilst this may seem obvious, delays waiting for assets which have not been requested are not uncommon. Forethought will enable additional assets to be sent including air ambulances, BASICS doctors or other dedicated resources to support patient and scene management.

Whilst information can be gathered en route to the scene from those already there, it is important that information is shared with ambulance control on arrival at the scene, and once an initial assessment has been made as well as at regular intervals whilst on scene. This information is relevant to both the patient's condition and also the scene in general and is especially important if the incident involves multiple patients or is a major incident.

Some ambulances services have introduced the *windscreen report* as a tool to communicate from the scene what is happening as visualized from the cab (through the windscreen) of their vehicle. This initial snap shot will provide useful information about the scene so that additional support from managers and extra resources can be organised. The windscreen report tells staff to describe what they see using the METHANE sequence.

INITIAL COMMUNICATION ON SCENE

All the emergency services through *JESIP* have adopted a common way of passing, information between emergency responders and control rooms in the initial stages of an incident. The mnemonic *METHANE* (Box 4.2) allows the establishment of a shared situational awareness of the scene and is as valid at smaller incidents as at major ones. It contains essential and detailed information about the scene providing an initial oversight of what is happening at that moment.

BOX 4.2: Approved Way of Passing Initial Information at the Scene of a Major Incident

M	Major incident declared or standby (may not be used)
E	Exact location
T	Type of incident e.g. explosion, transport incident
H	Hazards present, actual or potential
A	Access routes that are safe
N	Number, type and severity of patients
E	Emergency services now present and those required

On arrival at a trauma scene, initial communication should be with the first ambulance resource on scene or the ambulance manager who is leading and running the scene, or failing this with the senior officer of whichever emergency service is present. Where the practitioner is the first person on scene the first point of contact will obviously be with the patient *once the scene has been assessed to be safe*. In this situation it is essential that a METHANE (or similar) update is provided so that ambulance control can ensure the despatch of additional support including the best means of evacuation for the patient.

PRACTICE POINT

The use of METHANE as a mnemonic to provide an update to control rooms will ensure a common situational awareness is obtained.

RADIO VOICE PROCEDURE

Effective use of the radio to transmit clear and unambiguous messages to other emergency services personnel and others is an essential skill for all pre-hospital responders and one which must be practised until it is fluent. The phonetic alphabet must be mastered (Box 4.3) as well as the standard expressions used in transmitting messages (Box 4.4). Phonetic numbers are useful but less commonly used (Box 4.5).

When speaking on the radio (or the telephone) in order to pass important information, every care must be taken to ensure that the message is as clear as possible. This may mean writing down and briefly rehearsing the message first. Speech should be clear and consciously slower than in normal conversation. Women's voices tend to be clearer due to their higher pitch, and where

BOX 4.3: The Phonetic Alphabet

A	Alpha	N	November
B	Bravo	O	Oscar
C	Charlie	P	Papa
D	Delta	Q	Quebec
E	Echo	R	Romeo
F	Foxtrot	S	Sierra
G	Golf	T	Tango
H	Hotel	U	Uniform
I	India	V	Victor
J	Juliet	W	Whisky
K	Kilo	X	X-ray
L	Lima	Y	Yankee
M	Mike	Z	Zulu

BOX 4.4: Commonly Used Expressions in Passing Messages

Over	Start talking
Go ahead/Send	I am ready to receive your message
Understood/OK	I have understood your message
Say again	Repeat (*say again all after/say again all before*)
Spell	Indicates that what follows will be spelt out using the phonetic alphabet, or as *please spell* is used to request the spelling of a difficult or unclear word
Numbers	Indicates that a list of numbers is about to be transmitted such as a map reference or telephone number
Out	Indicates that the exchange is finished
Wait	I am unable to speak to you for a few seconds, please wait (occasionally the term *wait one*, meaning wait one minute, is used)
Wait out	I am unable to speak to you but will contact you very shortly
Wrong	Indicates an error and is followed by the correct version
Standby	Standby for further information
Acknowledge	Please confirm that you have received my message

BOX 4.5: Phonetic Numbers

1	Wun	6	Six
2	Too	7	Seven
3	Thuree	8	Ate
4	Fower	9	Niner
5	Fiyiv	0	Zero

possible strong regional accents are best avoided if the listeners are likely to be unfamiliar with them.

At the beginning of each radio transmission, the caller should state the call sign being called, give their own call sign, pass the message and terminate the message with *over.* Some services use the convention of giving their own call sign alone at the beginning of each transmission.

The term *over and out* is self-contradictory and should not be used. Once the call sign of the caller and the recipient have been exchanged, *go ahead* or *send* are used to indicate readiness to receive the reply, *over* means please speak in response. If the message transmitted was not clear, then *say again all after, say again all before,* or *say again* or alternatively *please spell* may be used to clarify. *Understood* and *OK* confirm that the message has been understood. *Spell* indicates that the following word or phrase will be spelt out using the phonetic alphabet and is most often used for names. *Numbers* should be used to indicate that a series of numbers such as a map reference or telephone number is to be given. The use of a*cknowledge* at the end of a message means that confirmation of receipt and understanding are required. When an error is made, this is acknowledged by *wrong* (spoken) followed by the correct version. *Difficult* implies a message which can be understood but is not clear, *broken* when only parts of a message can be heard and *unworkable* when only fragments can be heard or interference is so severe that the message is undecipherable. *Nothing heard* is self-explanatory (Box 4.6).

BOX 4.6: The Radio Check

Performing a Radio Check

A radio check begins with the call signs of the stations being called followed by the caller's own call sign and then by *radio check, over* ('Yankee 1, Yankee 2, Yankee 3 from Yankee 4, radio check over'). Once all the call signs have checked in, the initiator ends the call with *OK, Out* (i.e. 'Yankee 4 OK, out').

THE USE OF CREW RESOURCE MANAGEMENT (CRM) AND ON-SCENE COMMUNICATION

At the end of a message *out* is used. The phrase *call sign X out to you* can be used if communication is concluded with one or more call signs in a network, but further communication with other call signs is needed. If for any reason a speaker is unable to continue with a message, *wait* should be used, but only to cover a few seconds and it should not be repeated more than once. If a longer pause is necessary, *wait out* is the correct term and the communication is temporarily ended. The communication can then be restarted at a convenient time. *Standby* informs the listener that they must be alert for further messages which will follow shortly.

WHAT IS CRM?

CRM initially came from the commercial airline sector and over the last 10 years has been increasingly adopted in civilian pre-hospital care practice. The concepts of CRM include open and honest communication, the immediate analysis of alternate probabilities, and a reliance on the strengths of individuals and what they bring to the team. The implementation of CRM, which includes open and respectful feedback as well as a focus on collective awareness of the larger situation, can provide a much safer environment on scene and will result in better patient care being delivered.

CRM has rapidly become a standard operating model for all air ambulance operations in the UK along with other organisations that provide pre-hospital care such as BASICS. The essential principles of CRM are listed in Box 4.7.

BOX 4.7: The Principles of Crew Resource Management

- Working with an open and enquiring mind
- Being respectful to team members and patients
- Communicating effectively
- Thinking before speaking
- Being honest and admitting weaknesses or mistakes
- Working towards high reliability through continual learning

CONCEPTS OF CRM

For practitioners to understand how CRM can be used effectively in the delivery of pre-hospital care, it is necessary to understand a number of concepts. A key principle is that there is a need to understand and acknowledge that the team dealing with the incident extends out beyond its immediate members. In practice this means that all the responders on the scene are part of the team, not only the obvious agencies (personnel from the ambulance service for example). By taking an approach that values the expertise of all on scene and demonstrates trust and respect as well as flexibility, the team will have greater cohesion and be more effective. The key element in communication is practising proper forms of interpersonal engagement and showing appropriate respect. Greater value also comes from the concept that no one individual is as effective as the team they are working in. As a consequence, the team needs to have open and honest communication. Open communication allows continuing situational awareness which is one of the principles behind JESIP (see later).

Research from the United States has shown that maintaining situational awareness within a culture of CRM improves the safety of high risk, low frequency events. For example a pre-hospital emergency anaesthesia (PHEA) task standard has been developed using the CRM concepts of task allocation, open communication, clarification of the task and collective situational awareness. Checklists are used to train staff with the aim of standardising the skill and reducing error. This has been mirrored in all PHEA standard operating procedures (SOPs) in the UK. In these models, task standards divide the responsibilities among the individuals in the team. This facilitates effective and safe completion. In most UK models the team undertaking PHEA consists of at least two people: the team leader and an assistant. In addition up to two other people are needed especially when providing *manual in-line spine immobilisation (MILS).* The communication element of the task is maximisation of situational awareness to ensure nothing has been missed. All the people in the team must know what the patient's oxygenation level is and how the intubation by the team leader is progressing.

In tasks that do not adhere to CRM one of the common errors leading to loss of situational awareness is the tendency of individuals in the team to ignore or disregard information that maybe given out of context or whilst they are otherwise occupied. There are a number of cited examples of clinicians saying to the person undertaking an intubation that the patient was bradycardic or that they had been in the airway for longer then 30 seconds but who were consciously ignored or not heard due to the person being fixated on the critical component of the task of passing the tube. As a consequence of effective CRM, important signs which may be missed by the task-focussed team leader will be identified by the other team members and communicated so that appropriate action can be taken. Successful intubation is the responsibility of the team, not just the team leader.

PRACTICE POINT

CRM will ensure that the patient gets the best care by using open communication and common situational awareness, reducing the risks to patient safety.

METHODS OF COMMUNICATING ON SCENE

In today's society the number of methods of communication grown considerably. Whereas 15 years ago communication methods on scene at a pre-hospital care call were limited to voice, either face to face or via a limited range VHF/UHF radio and possibly the use of a pager, today there are mobile phone technology, social media, Airwave radio, e-mail and video conferencing. More reliable equipment allows real-time updates both visually and through speech. Nevertheless, the best method of communication on scene remains face to face where possible. In larger incidents, however, the commanders may not be able to do this so other methods will need to be employed.

AIRWAVE

The current national Airwave radio network is used by all the emergency services. Whilst all individual organisations have their own talk groups as well as inter-service channels, the facility exists for there to be multi-agency talk groups, especially in cases of major or serious incidents. The Airwave network is resilient, secure and recordable. Whilst there are a number of licenced hardware items that services can use, the functionality of them is broadly the same (Figure 4.1).

Practitioners should be familiar with the handset their organisation uses and understand how to change talk groups and make contact with the ambulance control centre.

The concept of using Airwave is the same as for two-way radio. The facility normally operates on the press-to-talk model. There are no range restrictions on the handsets, as they use the digital radio/phone network rather than radio waves. The network is secure and communication is instant on a controlled network. Airwave can be used in most tunnels as well as on the underground networks and there is national coverage over 99% of the UK. Application to use Airwave is through Ofcom.

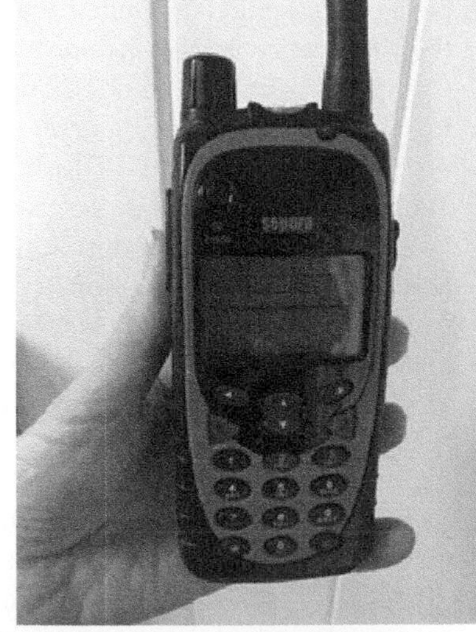

Figure 4.1 An Airwave handset.

MOBILE TELEPHONES

In most cases on-scene communication in pre-hospital care will be undertaken by mobile phone. It is important to realise that mobile phone coverage can be difficult in remote areas and cannot be relied upon, especially when passing clinical information to receiving hospitals. The conversations are not normally recorded and this may make audit difficult. Mobile phones are used because they are easy and do not rely on others for availability as most people have one. They provide a direct one-to-one communication method but are insecure, with a network that can easily be overloaded, for example on New Year's Eve at midnight. Wrong numbers can be dialled and misdirects can occur as can delays in connection. Although radio voice procedure is not necessary, the phonetic alphabet should be used where necessary to ensure clarity.

COMMUNICATING CARE ON SCENE

Whilst on scene with a trauma patient, especially one with multi-system injuries, providing ambulance control with updates regarding what has been found and what has been done will allow additional support to be dispatched if required. Providing updates to the receiving hospital will also ensure that they are ready for the patient with the required specialists and equipment ready and waiting, and blood available for immediate administration. In addition, operating theatres may be prepared and protocols activated. An early call through the co-ordination centre of the major trauma network will allow discussion with receiving hospitals regarding the patient and the options for transport and final destination, for example direct to a burns unit. This ensures that centres are not overloaded with a high number of patients when they do not have the capacity to manage them and facilitates the most appropriate care. The essential information regarding the patient can be best delivered based around the ATMIST mnemonic (Box 4.8) and must include specific details of any extra support required on arrival, such as mass transfusion capability or cardiothoracic surgery.

BOX 4.8: Essential Pre-Hospital Information

A	Age
T	Time of injury
M	Mechanism of injury
I	Injuries suspected or known
S	Signs as recorded
T	Treatment provided and its effect

COMMUNICATING EN ROUTE TO HOSPITAL

There may be occasions when the patient's condition changes en route to hospital. Where this occurs, an update to the receiving unit is essential, so that they are ready and have the right people in the resuscitation department. How this is done will depend on local protocols. Some areas use Airwave radio to speak directly with the receiving hospital while others use the telephone. It is essential to be familiar with local processes and to ensure that the correct numbers are stored in phones so that they can be easily accessed.

COMMUNICATION ON ARRIVAL AT THE RECEIVING UNIT

On arrival at the receiving hospital it is important that the handover is listened to by the trauma team who are not distracted by the patient's injuries and that the information is provided only once. Handover should occur once the patient has been transferred to the resuscitation trolley and no attempt should be made to remove a scoop stretcher at this stage. The person who has led the care of the patient in the pre-hospital part of their care should provide the handover using the ATMIST system. A structured handover should ensure that it is only necessary to give it once, although it is often helpful if pre-hospital personnel are able to wait before they leave so that other questions arising during the initial assessment can be answered. The handover should be given to the whole team, although it remains the team leader who must ensure that they at least have a clear overview of the patient and the history of the trauma.

AFTER AN INCIDENT

After the patient has been transported to the receiving unit, the final part of the management in pre-hospital care is a post-incident review and debrief. This element is often missed due to demands on clinicians' time but should occur as soon as possible after the call. The carrying out of a post-incident analysis is the final part of CRM but also provides the opportunity for learning and discussion regarding how the patient was managed, as well as reviewing what went well and what could be improved upon next time.

Non-learning teams are those that will only want to review calls that did not go well so blame can be placed or incompetence exposed. Learning teams, on the other hand, and those with good CRM will recognise the opportunity to critique and improve performance in a positive environment and to offer support in challenging circumstances.

A number of models are used to carry out the debriefing process and each individual should use the model with which they are familiar. Whichever model is used, *'What went well?' 'What could be improved next time?', 'What has been learnt?',* and *'What will be repeated the next time a similar scenario occurs?',* offer suitable headings under which a constructive discussion can be organised. Pre-hospital care is challenging and every situation is unique. Feeling that a situation could have been better managed, occasionally exacerbated by ill-considered criticism from hospital clinicians, is common, and constructive support which allows areas for improvement to be identified in a supportive way, and gives credit where it is due, is essential for the optimal mental health of clinicians.

JOINT EMERGENCY SERVICES INTEROPERABILITY PROGRAMME (JESIP)

The JESIP programme was set up at the Home Secretary's request following a number of public enquiries which found that better joint working between the three emergency services would enhance the collective ability to save lives and reduce harm. JESIP recognises that whilst major or complex incidents do not occur regularly, when they do there is a need to ensure efficient, effective and joined up responses. The programme is nationally recognised and staffed from the three emergency services. The process had full sign-up from the chief officers of all three blue light services as well as the Home Office, Cabinet Office, Department for Communities and Local Government, and the Department of Health. The programme provides courses at operational, tactical and strategic levels. JESIP principles of joint working are based on five key elements (Figure 4.2).

Throughout the programme the emphasis on shared situational awareness and open communication are essential for ensuring the objectives of JESIP are met. Of course the same principles exist with CRM and therefore it is vital that on-scene communication is open and that all the information is shared between the team to enhance the delivery of the care to the trauma patient.

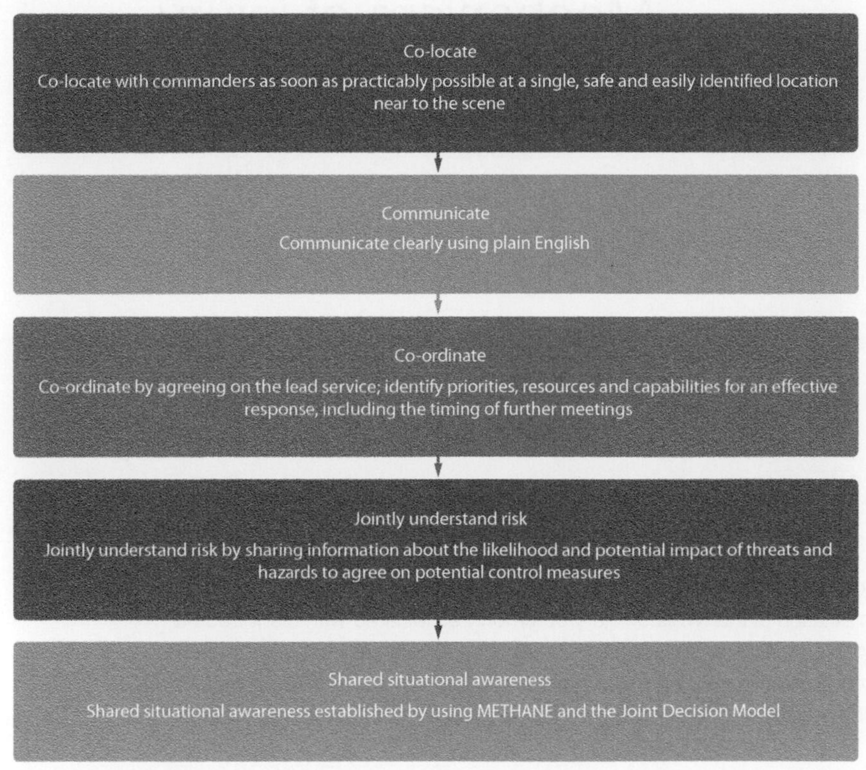
Co-locate
Co-locate with commanders as soon as practicably possible at a single, safe and easily identified location near to the scene
Communicate
Communicate clearly using plain English
Co-ordinate
Co-ordinate by agreeing on the lead service; identify priorities, resources and capabilities for an effective response, including the timing of further meetings
Jointly understand risk
Jointly understand risk by sharing information about the likelihood and potential impact of threats and hazards to agree on potential control measures
Shared situational awareness
Shared situational awareness established by using METHANE and the Joint Decision Model

Figure 4.2 JESIP principles.

SUMMARY

Effective and timely communication is key to pre-hospital care. Effective team working (crew resource management) is a skill that must be learnt and practised. In the UK joint working is enhanced by the Joint Emergency Service Interoperability Programme.

FURTHER READING

Joint Emergency Services Interoperability Programme Training. College of Policing, 2013.

Le Sage P, Dyar JT, Evans B. *Crew Resource Management: Principles and Practice.* Jones and Bartlett, 2011.

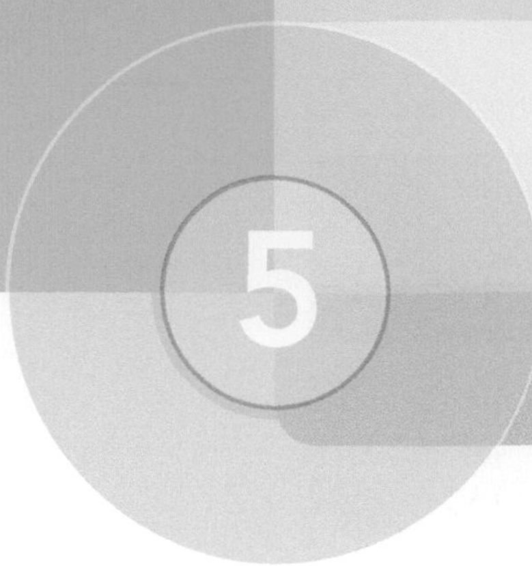

Mechanism of injury

OBJECTIVES

After completing this chapter the reader will

- Understand the scientific principles underlying energy transfer and the resulting injuries
- Have a broad appreciation of the types of injury commonly associated with blunt trauma (road traffic collisions and falls from a height), blast and penetrating trauma
- Understand the importance of mechanism of injury in terms of its relevance to individual patient care and the prediction of cohort injuries for the purposes of triage and research

INTRODUCTION

Mechanism of injury might be defined as the totality of the physical circumstances in which an injury arises. Analysis of mechanism of injury is frequently used to assist clinical decision-making in the care of the individual trauma patient throughout the continuum of care. In the pre-hospital phase, the mechanism of injury will be a key part of the information influencing decisions regarding the patient's hospital destination and means of evacuation. In the hospital phase, the mechanism of injury may determine the organisation of trauma team resources, with a view to actively excluding predictable and occult injuries.

Despite some evidence to the contrary (1), there is a growing body of evidence that both general and specific mechanisms of injury can be used to independently predict morbidity and mortality at a population level (2). This has led to mechanism of injury becoming an important factor in triage systems, trauma system evaluation and research. Nevertheless, caution must be sounded that mechanism of injury assessment *must not* result in clinicians missing injuries that are not predicted by the mechanism, but are nevertheless present, or cause them simply to assess the patient only to confirm their potentially incorrect assumptions.

PRACTICE POINT

Assessment of mechanism should not lead to incomplete clinical assessment designed to confirm preconceived but incorrect injury patterns.

PATHOPHYSIOLOGY

Before attempting to understand why human tissue behaves in a specific way depending on the insult it sustains, it is necessary to understand the characteristics of insults in terms of causation and the type and magnitude of the energy involved.

Insults cause injury as a result of *energy transfer* which exceeds the level at which tissue damage occurs. Thus the severity of injury can be determined by studying the physics of the energy transfer (which indicate the magnitude of transferred energy), and the anatomic and material characteristics of the tissue to which it is transferred. This chapter will focus on the most common energy transfers and how specific tissues are affected by these transfers.

Energy can be transferred to tissue in a variety of forms (Box 5.1). Injuries relating to *thermal energy* and *electrical energy* will be dealt with in the chapter on thermal injury (Chapter 19). Nuclear energy is not discussed further in this manual.

BOX 5.1: Types of Energy Capable of Causing Injury

- Kinetic Energy
- Chemical Energy
- Nuclear Energy
- Thermal Energy
- Electrical Energy

The energy possessed by a moving object is called *kinetic energy (KE)*, defined by the following equation:

$$\text{Kinetic energy} = \tfrac{1}{2}\ \text{Mass} \times (\text{Velocity})^2 \ \text{or}\ \text{KE} = \tfrac{1}{2}mv^2$$

This chapter will concentrate on the transfer of kinetic energy, which is the most common form of injurious energy transfer. The resulting injury can be broadly divided into that caused by interaction between tissue and either a *blunt or a penetrating object.*

The transfer of kinetic energy in blunt trauma takes place most commonly in road traffic collisions and falls from a height, and these will be considered later in some detail, followed by a brief review of blast injury and penetrating trauma which are discussed in more detail in Chapters 20 and 21.

THE PHYSICS OF ENERGY TRANSFER

When considering transfer of kinetic energy, it is useful to first revisit *Newton's 2nd Law of Motion,* and the relationship between velocity, energy and work done. In summary Newton's Second Law indicates that

$$\text{Force} = \text{Mass} \times \text{Acceleration or } F = ma$$

So force applied over a period of time will cause a change in momentum, and produce acceleration or deceleration. The concept of duration of time is critical, since it determines acceleration or deceleration.

Force (F) exerted over a period of time (t) results in an impulse (Ft), which brings about a change in the momentum (Mass × Velocity) of the object to which it is applied.

$$Ft = \text{Change in momentum}$$

$$Ft = m \times \text{Change in velocity}$$

$$F = m \times (\text{Change in velocity})/t$$

However, Change in velocity/t = Acceleration, and therefore F = ma.

Energy and *'work done'* are interchangeable.

Acceleration or deceleration (rate of change of velocity) of the tissue will determine the force acting on it (assuming mass is constant). A gradual change in velocity will subject tissue to far less force (for example an aircraft landing) than a sudden change in velocity (such as a car crashing into a tree).

Since the energy possessed by a moving object (kinetic energy) is defined as ½mass × $(\text{velocity})^2$ or ½mv^2, the kinetic energy of a moving object depends on its velocity – the faster it moves, the greater its kinetic energy.

Acceleration or deceleration brings about a change in velocity, and therefore a change in kinetic energy. When the kinetic energy of a moving object increases, work is being done on the object by an external force to increase its speed. When kinetic energy decreases, work is done by the object on itself and its environment. In a collision, for example, when a moving object stops moving, its kinetic energy is transferred or converted to *'work done'* in deformation, injury, sound, heat and friction. So force applied, change in velocity, and conversion of kinetic energy to work done all form part of the process we call energy transfer as it relates to injury in trauma.

KINETIC ENERGY AND BLUNT TRAUMA

A collision between an object and tissue can be thought of as *fully elastic* if all the kinetic energy is conserved as kinetic energy. Usually collisions are inelastic, and some or all of the available kinetic energy is converted into 'work done' (see earlier).

It is worth noting that in collisions between two freely moving objects, some kinetic energy may be retained if the two objects rebound from each other, or one passes through the other, and so not all kinetic energy is converted to work done. In collisions between a moving object and a fixed object (for example the ground) only the moving object can properly rebound, and so less energy may be retained, allowing more of the kinetic energy to be converted into work done, or damage.

The *direction* and *type* of collision are important, as they can have a major impact on the remaining kinetic energy after the collision (Figure 5.1). For example, in a head-on collision between two vehicles, in which the vehicles become 'locked' together and stop immediately, the resultant 'object' has no kinetic energy. All the kinetic energy has been used to produce deformation and injury. This can be contrasted with a front-to-side impact of two vehicles (a *T-bone*–type collision), in which the resultant 'object' continues to move. Since some kinetic energy remains, not all has been converted into work done.

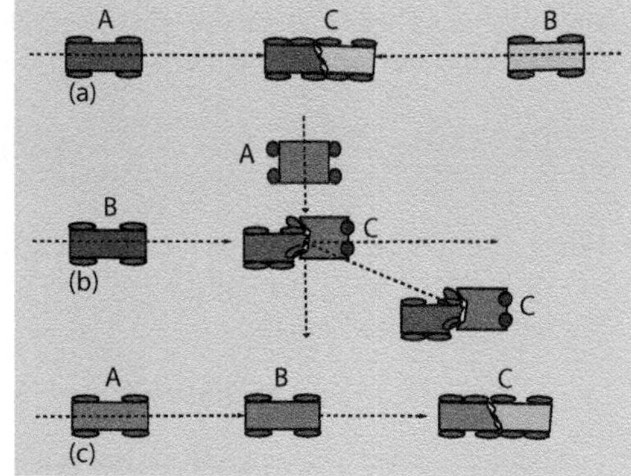

Figure 5.1 Energy and momentum available in various motor vehicle collisions. (a) Frontal collision with maximum change in momentum over the shortest period of time and hence the highest force generated. (b) T-bone collision: when cars A and B collide their resultant momentum directs them to their final position C. The individual momentums in the x and y axes are dissipated over a greater time resulting in smaller forces than scenario A. (c) Rear-end collision: since these vehicles are moving in the same direction, the changes in momentum and resultant forces are smaller.

The detailed effect of collisions on the occupants of a vehicle in a collision, who are likely to continue to move after the vehicle stops, will be considered later.

When a force is applied to tissue as a result of energy transfer (work done), how the tissue reacts depends on its material characteristics (which are in turn related to the tissue's micro- and macroscopic anatomy). *Stress* can be defined as load or force per unit area and is responsible for tissue deformation. *Strain* can be defined as the distance of this deformation relative to the original length of the material. If stress and strain are plotted, the results show an initial elastic component whereby deformation is reversible (the absorbed energy is released), followed by a *plastic* part where the deformation is permanent. Higher density structures (such as solid organs like liver) are generally less able to perform elastically and therefore absorb more energy with a consequent increase in damage.

It is also important to recognise that injuries often result from multiple interactions between tissue and the injuring object. For example, during one 'overall' collision, a vehicle occupant can sustain injuries that are directly affected by several separate collisions. The *first* collision is between the vehicle and some external object. In this collision some of the kinetic energy of the vehicle is converted into work done deforming the vehicle. The *second* collision is between the occupant (who is travelling at the same velocity as the vehicle) and the internal structure of the vehicle. The kinetic energy of the occupant is converted into work done, injuring the occupant where he meets the internal surface of the vehicle. (If the occupant is wearing a seat belt, the second collision is between the occupant and the seat belt, which is designed to absorb some of this kinetic energy without causing major injury, and which will slow the occupant's forward motion, resulting in less injurious subsequent collisions.) The *third* collision is where the internal organs of the occupant (still moving forward) meet his now stationary inner body cavity surfaces. Again the kinetic energy of the organs is converted into work done injuring the same. Finally, a *fourth* collision can occur where loose objects in the vehicle make contact with the now stationary occupant. Again, the kinetic energy of these objects will be converted into work done in injuring the occupant.

TYPES OF INCIDENT

Road traffic collision as an injury mechanism can be further subdivided into collisions involving vehicle occupants and those involving pedestrians.

VEHICLE OCCUPANT COLLISIONS

In vehicle collisions, it is possible to predict the likely injuries sustained, alongside the probable morbidity and mortality, by examining the collision type (for example, *head-on*, *side impact*, *rear impact*, *rollover* and *ejection*).

In a *head-on collision* (Figure 5.2), the driver may slide forward below the steering wheel or up and over the steering wheel. With the former, the first point of contact is between the knee and the dashboard, possibly giving rise to a posterior dislocation and vascular injury. Next, the upper abdomen and chest make contact with the steering wheel, where compression may give rise to rib fractures, cardiac contusions and pneumothoraces. Continuous forward motion of solid organs causes shear stresses and may give rise to rupture of the thoracic aorta. With the *up and over the steering wheel* motion, the initial contact of the occupant is of their head with the windscreen, causing head and brain injury. Once the head has stopped moving, the cervical spine is then the location bearing the brunt of the energy transfer, resulting in vertebral and

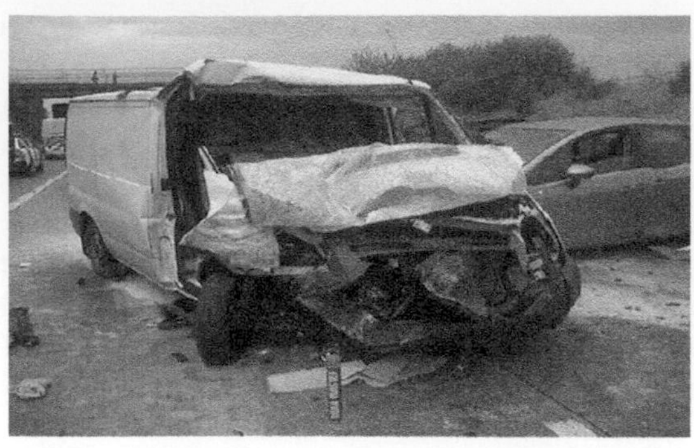

Figure 5.2 A head-on collision.

spinal cord injury. Following this, the chest and upper abdomen impact with the steering wheel with the possible injuries already noted. Alternatively, the driver may simply be crushed between steering wheel and seat. Similar but usually less severe injuries will be found in front seat *passengers.*

In *side impacts,* chest and abdominal injuries are more common than in head-on collisions (3). It is interesting to note that although there is a marked reduction in space between the occupant and the side of the vehicle compared with head-on impacts, the overall mortality is still much lower. As previously remarked, the vehicles involved in this type of impact generally continue to move for some distance, so that the deceleration is slower, the force experienced by the vehicle and occupant is smaller, and transfer of kinetic energy to work done takes place more gradually, resulting in less severe injury.

Rear impacts classically give rise to neck injuries and have the lowest overall mortality. This is possibly because the majority of them are at low velocity, but also because both vehicles generally continue to move, so that some kinetic energy remains and not all has been converted into work done.

A *rollover* scenario carries a mortality in between that of rear impacts and other types of collision (3). The reason for this may be that despite the dramatic appearance of these impacts, the deceleration experienced can occur in many directions, and not all deceleration is in a direction that directly involves the occupant, who is partially restrained by his seat belt as the car rolls. So the occupant may 'lose' his kinetic energy randomly and not as a result of a single direct forward motion such as might be experienced in a head-on collision. As a consequence of this, injury patterns are much more difficult to predict. For these reasons and somewhat contentiously, rollover has been removed from some algorithms as a predictor of serious injury (4).

Last, *ejection*, compared with other mechanisms of injury, is associated with significantly worse outcomes, with a fivefold increase in injury severity score and mortality, a fourfold increase in admissions to critical care and a threefold increase in the incidence of severe traumatic brain injury (5). This is thought to be due to the fact that the occupant has the same initial velocity as the vehicle when he collides with an immovable object (the ground), so that on impact most if not all kinetic energy is immediately converted to work done in producing devastating injury. The occupant also impacts the ground without any of the inherent protection of being a car occupant.

PEDESTRIAN COLLISIONS

The vast majority of *pedestrian road traffic collisions* involve being struck by the front of a vehicle (6). This usually results in a fairly predictable pattern of events and their consequent injuries.

The *wrap* is the commonest pattern, with an initial bumper strike to the leg (the exact position is determined by the vehicle size and configuration and the height of the pedestrian) causing injury and rotating the head and torso, which are then injured by contact with the bonnet, windscreen and its surround (the *secondary impact*). The pedestrian is now travelling at the same speed as the vehicle, but the vehicle usually brakes and therefore slows down faster than the pedestrian, who then slides off the front of the bonnet, impacting the road surface (the *tertiary impact*).

Forward projection is the next most common pattern, often involving a large flat-fronted vehicle and a small child. The pedestrian is thrown forwards instead of upwards, increasing their risk of subsequently being run over.

A *wing top* collision describes the situation in which the pedestrian impacts with the front corner of the vehicle, is carried over the wing and then impacts with the ground, whereas *rooftop* and *somersault* describe situations in which the vehicle is travelling at high speed or when the vehicle fails to brake. As the name implies, in the former the pedestrian slides up and over the roof after the bonnet impact, whereas in the latter the speeds are such that there is no further impact after the initial bumper impact until the pedestrian impacts with the ground.

FALLS FROM A HEIGHT

The kinetic energy gained by a falling person is determined by the velocity reached as a result of the acceleration due to gravity and the height fallen. Impact with the ground is not elastic, and almost all of the kinetic energy gained will be converted to work done in deformation and injury. The other major factors determining the injuries sustained are the position of the person on impact and to a lesser extent the surface of impact. So called *fall-specific mechanisms* of injury are thought to be related to factors including sudden deceleration, direct impact and a possible hydraulic ram effect from sudden compression of the abdomen. A study of 603 patients falling from heights over 3 m showed that 88% of fatalities were due to multiple injuries. The most frequently injured areas were thorax (98%), head (82%) and abdomen and pelvis (79%) (7).

Thoracic aortic injuries were found in 51% of fatalities (complete transaction in 70% cases and full thickness rupture in 30%). The most common site for tearing in traumatic aortic rupture is the proximal descending aorta, near where the left subclavian artery leaves it. Tethering by the ligamentum arteriosum makes this site prone to shearing forces. Cardiac injuries are common, with lacerations (predominantly right sided) found in up to 48% of fatalities. It has been suggested that the hydraulic ram effect mentioned above may contribute to this. Cardiac and thoracic aortic injuries occur together in 75% of fatalities. Lung injuries and rib fractures are also common (80% of fatalities). It is thought that the hydraulic ram effect (increasing intrathoracic pressure) may contribute to lung injury when rib fractures are absent.

In the aforementioned study, traumatic brain injury was present in 37% of fatalities, with 20% of these being massive disruption of the brain and head consistent with a primary impact. Feet-first impacts are associated with ring fractures to the base of skull and brainstem injuries. All types of brain injury are possible, although subarachnoid haemorrhage is the most common on post-mortem.

Injuries to the abdomen are predominantly to the solid organs, as would be expected due to the main mechanism of injury being rapid deceleration. The most frequently damaged is the liver, followed by the spleen and kidney. Fractures of the pelvis are found in 50% of fatalities, with the vertical shear fracture (and its accompanying catastrophic haemorrhage) being almost exclusively associated with significant falls.

In one study of patients from a relatively low fall height (of <6 m), fractures were found in 75% of patients, with spinal fractures occurring in 19% to 22% (36% of all fatalities). These are predominantly in the thoracic area and may be associated with the vertical transmission of deceleration forces up the axial skeleton (8).

BLUNT INJURIES BY REGION

Having detailed some of the specifics of energy transfer and the resultant injuries related to road traffic collisions and significant falls, it is also useful to review specific anatomical areas of the body and how the forces applied in blunt trauma cause damage.

Traumatic brain injury is extremely important, as it is the single most important factor contributing to death and disability after trauma (9). The internal collision previously described between the brain and the inner surface of the skull results in a direct compressive strain on the surface of the brain (the *coup* injury) and a corresponding tensile strain on the opposite surface (often damaging bridging veins). The brain then rebounds, giving rise to another compressive strain on the opposite surface (the *contre-coup*). Damage to deeper brain structures (with or without surface damage) may be due to the so-called stereotactic phenomenon where the concavity of the skull reflects multiple pressure waves and focuses them on areas deep in the brain causing injury. This phenomenon is also thought to be responsible for traumatic loss of consciousness when waves are focused on the reticular activating system.

Thoracic injury is a result of directly applied external compressive strain and is due to differential deceleration between fixed and mobile structures. As with other fractures, ribs fracture as a result of direct compressive strain on the outer cortex, with tensile strain on the inner cortex. There can also be fractures remote to the point of impact, such as at the lateral and posterior rib angles where forces are focused. As with injury to the deeper brain structures, stress waves can penetrate deep into the chest with distortion and shearing forces especially at areas of significant pressure differential (air-filled alveoli and lung tissue). This results in pulmonary contusions.

The classic areas of injury due to the continued movement of mobile structures which are attached to solid structures are the thoracic aorta (fixed at the ligamentum arteriosum connected to the mobile heart) (10) and the bronchial tree (fixed at the hilum connected to the mobile lungs).

Abdominal injuries are somewhat different to those of the thoracic cavity, in part due to the lack of protection afforded by the rib cage. However, they also result from direct compressive strain and points of attachment causing differential movement. The latter can be responsible for injuries at splenic and renal points of attachment, and of the free pancreatic tail. Shear forces in the liver can cause injury around the falciform ligament anteriorly and the hepatic vein posteriorly. Perforation of hollow structures is comparatively rare with blunt trauma (11) and is related to shear strains and overpressures (forming a temporary closed loop). The latter mechanism can also be responsible for diaphragmatic rupture.

Musculoskeletal injuries are less likely to be fatal than the injuries just described, but are potentially very costly to society in terms of repair, rehabilitation and permanent disability.

Vertebral fractures are important due to the potential for associated spinal cord injury. There are three main mechanisms of primary cord injury: *impact with persistent or transient compression, distraction* and *laceration or transection*. The first is the most common and may occur with retropulsed bone fragments compressing the cord. Distraction, such as from vertebral dislocation, can cause a shearing force on the spinal cord and its blood supply, and is the predominant mechanism when there is no radiological abnormality (12).

BLAST INJURY

Blast injury is covered in detail in Chapter 21 and only an overview is given here. Tissue damage due to blast injury combines blunt trauma (from kinetic energy transfer) and penetrating injury from fragments. Conventional explosions involve a solid or liquid undergoing a chemical reaction, generating gaseous by-products and releasing a large amount of stored energy. It must be remembered that the majority of explosions are caused not by bombs, but by chemical reactions and release of flammable materials in an industrial or domestic context. The release of energy compresses the surrounding air, producing a spherical wave of compressed gas known as the blast wave (with increased temperature, pressure and density). The movement of the air and explosive products produce the blast wind. The *blast overpressure* is defined as the difference between the wave front pressure and atmospheric pressure. It is related to the amount of energy released in the blast and the distance from the blast (falling away exponentially with increasing distance). Following this overpressure is a small period of negative pressure. When the blast wave hits an object, kinetic energy is converted to work done causing deformation and injury. Tissue damage as a result of blast can be divided into *primary, secondary, tertiary* and *other effects* (13). This classification is summarised in Box 5.2.

BOX 5.2: A Classification of Blast Injury

- Primary injury is as a result of tissue interaction with the over pressure (blast wave).
- Secondary injury is a result of the explosion transferring kinetic energy to objects (which are either part of the device or close by it), which then become projectiles.
- Tertiary injuries are caused by the blast wind.
- Other injuries include burns, crush injuries, psychological effects, and the effects of toxins and bacteria or viruses.
- Radiation effects may result from a bomb contaminated with radioactive material.

In *primary blast injury* air-filled organs (such as the ears, lung or gastrointestinal tract) are at the greatest risk of injury (usually contusion or perforation), which is more severe in confined spaces where overpressure waves are reflected from walls or other surfaces (14). Secondary injuries are the result of the impact of energised fragments and are almost invariably multiple. Primary fragments are components of the explosive device, and secondary fragments arise from the environment and include debris and body parts. Secondary injury is more common than primary as these projectiles travel over a much greater distance than the original blast wave.

Tertiary injuries are caused by the blast wind. Victims may be projected considerable distances, suffer traumatic amputation, or when very close to the point of detonation suffer whole-body disruption.

Radiation effects may result from a bomb contaminated with radioactive material (a so-called *dirty bomb*) or theoretically from a *nuclear detonation*. Other injuries include burns, crush injuries, psychological effects, and the effects of toxins and bacteria or viruses (sometimes transferred by the impact of body parts or a deliberate contaminant of an explosive device).

KINETIC INJURY AND PENETRATING TRAUMA

Many of the principles already mentioned are equally relevant to penetrating trauma. *Ballistics* is the study of projectiles, usually from firearms, which are an increasingly common cause of penetrating trauma. Ballistics is discussed in detail in Chapter 20 and only a brief overview is given here.

The kinetic energy of the projectile can be transferred in a number of ways, namely heat, sound, deformation of the projectile, and work required to move tissue out of the way radially and to crush it frontally. The latter two result in the phenomena of cavitation, which may be permanent or temporary. The temporary cavitation is important as the transiently subatmospheric pressure that cavitation generates will result in contaminants being sucked into the wound.

The amount of energy transferred is the difference between the kinetic energy of the projectile as it enters and that as it exits the tissue – clearly, if it does not exit, all the energy has been transferred to the tissue in the form of tissue damage. Projectiles have various characteristics that may increase this transfer of energy and tissue damage. First, the kinetic energy of the projectile as it reaches the tissue is partly determined by the energy imparted to it by the firearm, via the muzzle velocity ($KE = \frac{1}{2}mv^2$). Second, characteristics which increase the surface area of the contact between the projectile and tissue, will increase the energy transfer. These characteristics are yaw, tumble, deformation and fragmentation (15).

NON-PROJECTILE PENETRATING INJURY

Non-projectile penetrating injury (stab injury) is generally at low velocity, and tissue injury severity is principally related to damage to vital structures.

USE OF MECHANISM OF INJURY

As well as the drawing the attention of the clinician to critical injury patterns associated with a particular mechanism, mechanism of injury information has been extensively used to inform triage decisions (Figure 5.3)

In 1987 the American College of Surgeons Committee on Trauma produced the *field triage criteria* (4), which included mechanism of injury as well as physiological and anatomical factors. These criteria have been used worldwide, both on an individual patient and population level, and have been regularly revised and updated.

Since the 1980s, studies into the validity of mechanism of injury in predicting injury patterns, have shown varying results, with wide variations in sensitivity and specificity. These wide variations depend on the different specific mechanisms of injury studied. The data in these studies can often be compared using the concept of over- and under-triage. *Over-triage* happens when patients are triaged as more severely injured than they actually are (this is safer but has a severe impact on available resources), and *under-triage* when patients are categorised as less severely injured than they actually are (this is less safe but allows more efficient resource utilisation). The American College of Surgeons Committee on Trauma has deemed an under-triage rate of 5% to 10% to be acceptable, with a corresponding over-triage rate of 30% to 50%. For example, a systematic review of triage criteria to inform deployment of advanced trauma care by helicopter services identified 4982 patients in 5 studies (15). In these patients the positive predictive value of mechanism of injury for a major trauma level Injury Severity Score (15 or greater) varied from 27% (general mechanism of injury) to 59% (for ejection specific mechanism of injury).

This study and others have concluded that the best positive predictive value is achieved by combining mechanism of injury with physiological and anatomical factors, and that mechanism of injury is important. Another study of 515,464 trauma patients showed that mechanism

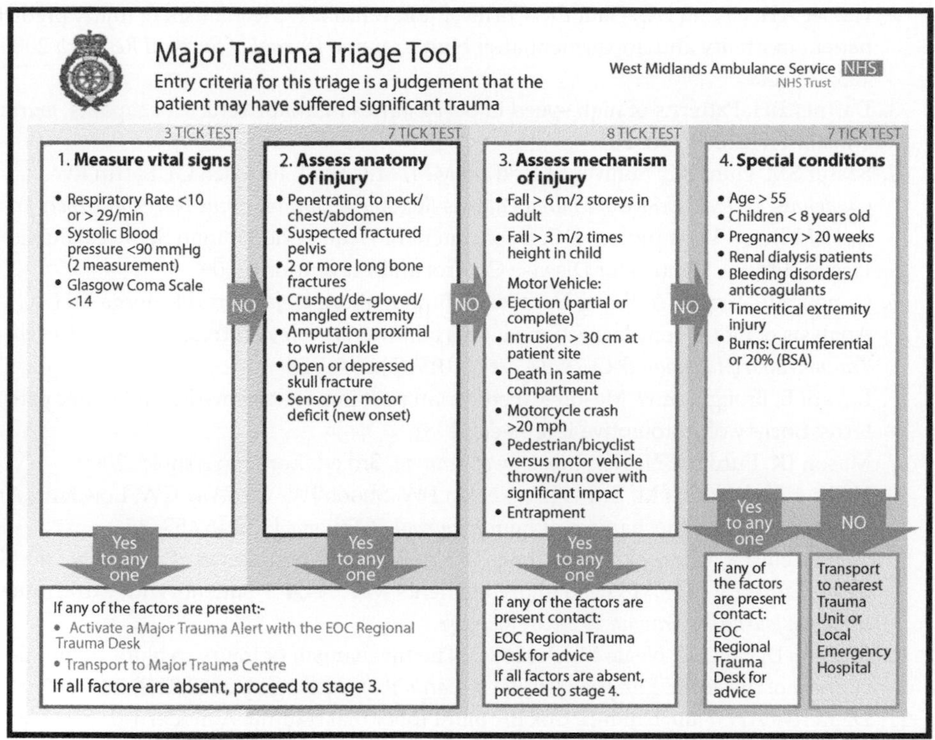

Figure 5.3 The major trauma triage tool.

of injury was an independent predictor of mortality and long-term functional impairment (2). The Committee on Trauma field guidelines are reviewed on a regular basis and amended when required (for example regarding the relevance of vehicle damage with specific velocities, as safety engineering improves).

SUMMARY

Injury is caused by energy transfer (usually of kinetic energy) to tissue. The amount of energy transferred is determined by the specific situation, and it is helpful to analyse this by reference to the physics of energy transfer in different situations. By reviewing the specific situations in turn, it is possible to determine possible injury patterns and to examine how the energy transfer has caused these injuries. The utility of being able to predict injuries based on knowledge of the mechanism has been well validated and is emphasised by its continued status as an important component of field triage algorithms.

REFERENCES

1. Santaniello JM, Esposito TJ, Luchette FA, Atkian DK, Davis KA, Gamelli RL. Mechanism of injury does not predict acuity or level of service need: Field triage criteria revisited. *Surgery* 2003;134(4):698–703.

2. Haider AH, Chang DC, Haut ER, Cornwell EE, Efron DT. Mechanism of injury predicts patient mortality and impairment after blunt trauma. *Journal of Surgical Research* 2009; 153:138–142.
3. Daffner RH. Patterns of high speed impact injuries in motor vehicle occupants. *Journal of Trauma* 1988;28(4):498–501.
4. Sasser SM, Hunt RC, Sullivent EE, Wald MM, Mitchko J, Jurovich GJ, Sattin RW. *Guidelines for Field Triage of Injured Patients: Recommendations of the National Expert Panel on Field Triage.* Washington, DC: Department of Health and Human Services, Public Health Service, Centers for Disease Control and Prevention, 2009.
5. Góngora E, Acosta JA, Wang Dennis SY, Brandenburg K, Jablonski K, Jorda MH. Analysis of motor vehicle ejection victims admitted to a level I trauma center. *Journal of Trauma-Injury Infection & Critical Care* 2001;51(5):854–859.
6. Ravani B, Brougham D, Mason R. Pedestrian post impact kinematics and injury patterns. Society of Automotive Engineers, 1982.
7. Mason JK, Purdue BN. *The Pathology of Trauma*. 3rd ed. London: Arnold, 2000.
8. Helling TS, Watkins M, Evans LL, Nelson PW, Shook JW, Van Way CW. Low falls: An underappreciated mechanism of injury. *Journal of Trauma* 1999;46:453–456.
9. Gennarelli TA, Champion HR, Copes WS, Sacco WJ. Comparison of mortality, morbidity and severity of 59,713 head injured patients with 114,447 patients with extracranial injuries. *Journal of Trauma* 1994;37:962–968.
10. Richens D, Field M, Neale M, Oakley C. The mechanism of injury in blunt traumatic rupture of the aorta. *European Journal of Cardiothoracic Surgery* 2002;21(2):288–293.
11. Dauterive AH, Flancbaum L, Cox EF. Blunt intestinal trauma: A modern-day review. *Annals of Surgery* 1985;201(2):198–203.
12. Dumont RJ, Okonkwo DO, Verma S, Hurlbert RJ, Boulos PT, Ellegala DB, Dumont AS. Acute spinal cord injury, part I: Pathophysiologic mechanisms. *Clinical Neuropharmacology* 2001;24(5):254–264.
13. Medical Research for Prevention, Mitigation and Treatment of Blast Injuries. Department of Defence Directive 2006. July 2006. http://www.dtic.mil/whs/directives/corres/html/602521.htm. Accessed January 22, 2015.
14. Ritenour AE, Baskin TW. Primary blast injury: Update on diagnosis and treatment. *Critical Care Medicine* 2008;36(7):S311–S317.
15. Ringburg AN, de Ronde G, Thomas SH, van Lieshout EM, Patka P, Schipper IB. Validity of helicopter emergency medical services dispatch criteria for traumatic injuries: A systematic review. *Prehospital Emergency Care* 2009;13(1):28–36.

6 The primary survey

OBJECTIVES

After completing this chapter the reader will

- Understand the aims of the primary survey in the pre-hospital environment
- Understand the structure of the primary survey
- Be able to prioritise the management of immediately life-threatening injuries

INTRODUCTION

This chapter is an overview of the *primary survey*. Each section is also covered in detail in the relevant chapter. The primary survey of a trauma patient is the initial assessment of the patient conducted in order to identify and manage any immediately life-threatening injuries and to determine the urgency and means by which the patient will be best evacuated to hospital. With the establishment of trauma networks and centres, it is information gathered during the primary survey which will determine the level of facility most appropriate for the patient. The primary survey begins on the approach to the patient when information can be gathered from the scene and environment, from bystanders and relatives and from other health professionals and members of the emergency services (Box 6.1).

As life-threatening problems are identified, they are immediately managed. Life-threatening problems which can only be managed in hospital mandate rapid completion of the primary survey and expedited transfer to hospital. The desired end state is a patient *in whom all immediately life-threatening problems have been detected and those amenable to pre-hospital intervention have been managed.* As part of the process, other, less time-critical problems are likely to be identified. These can be managed either on scene, if no life-threatening injuries are present, or after lifesaving treatment in hospital.

BOX 6.1: Sources of Information at an Incident

- The scene
- Bystanders
- The patient
- Relatives
- The emergency services

The primary survey should be conducted at the first safe opportunity. The immediate pre-hospital priority is always to ensure the safety of the rescuers, other persons present and the patient. If the initial environment is non-permissive, the primary survey may be abbreviated or delayed to allow rapid evacuation or securing of the area. If so, it should be repeated or completed as soon as possible. It should also be repeated if the patient's condition alters significantly and at handovers of care. The term *golden hour* was an important one, designed to emphasise the importance of the trauma victim reaching definitive care within 60 minutes of injury. However, it is best avoided, as it risks introducing a degree of complacency into the assessment and evacuation process. The aim must be to evacuate the seriously or critically injured patient to the care they need to provide the best chance of survival at the earliest opportunity. The aim of the primary survey is to identify these patients and ensure that there is no unnecessary delay on scene, interventions being restricted to those needed immediately to save life.

PRACTICE POINT

Saving minutes saves lives and reduces the long-term effects of injury.

THE INITIAL APPROACH

The following is a suggested sequence, based on the principles of the British Armed Forces *Battlefield Advanced Trauma Life Support (BATLS)* (1) course endorsed by the Ministry of Defence. This protocol incorporates changes based on recent civilian and military experience.

The separate stages of the primary survey are listed, in order, in Box 6.2.

BOX 6.2: The Sequence of the Primary Survey

<C>	Catastrophic external haemorrhage
A	Airway, with Cervical Spine control
B	Breathing
C	Circulation
D	Disability
E	Exposure and environment

Given that the numbers of personnel are normally limited in the pre-hospital environment, these activities will normally be conducted in sequence, but if additional personnel are available, a parallel approach may be taken. This requires excellent communication and co-ordination to ensure that the entire sequence has been completed.

As the patient is approached, the first thing that must be assessed is the patient's level of response, as this guides the next steps and gives a good global assessment of the patient's status. A patient who can speak and answer questions sensibly and without difficulty is likely to have a patent airway, reasonable cerebral function and adequate respiratory function.

<C> – CATASTROPHIC HAEMORRHAGE

The first stage of the primary survey (<C>) is identification of *external catastrophic haemorrhage. Internal bleeding* is identified during the C component, which is when a pelvic binder, if appropriate, should be applied. Only life-threatening bleeding requires action during this stage; other minor bleeding is ignored. Massive external haemorrhage is particularly common in casualties with penetrating or blast injuries. Although civilian and military experience is not directly comparable, evidence has shown that the majority of battlefield casualties who die prior to hospital do so because of uncontrolled bleeding (2,3). It is logical therefore that where such haemorrhage is found, simple and rapid steps are immediately taken to arrest it.

PRACTICE POINT

<C> is an initial rapid assessment, asking, 'Does this patient have exsanguinating external bleeding?'

If such bleeding is identified, the initial intervention should be the application of direct pressure, by gloved hand if necessary, or with the use of a suitable haemostatic dressing. If the bleeding is from a limb, the injured limb should be elevated. In limb trauma, if pressure fails to stem the bleeding, it may be necessary to apply a tourniquet to gain control, especially if the limb damage is extensive. In mangled amputations, immediate application of an arterial tourniquet may be needed to stem very heavy bleeding (4). If a tourniquet is used, the time of application should be documented, on the patient's body if necessary. Clinicians should also note that effective tourniquets are very painful, and that good analgesia will be needed as soon as the primary survey is complete (5). In some cases, application of a second tourniquet may be required.

In junctional areas, such as the groin and axilla, tourniquet application will not be possible and direct pressure should be applied and maintained, for example by pressure from a fist onto an applied dressing (6). Novel haemostatic agents have a role in the management of this type of bleeding, although the choice of agent and method of use will be determined locally.

A – AIRWAY (WITH CERVICAL SPINE CONTROL)

If there are no signs of massive external bleeding, attention should move to management of the airway. Particularly in head-injured patients, any reduction in level of consciousness may lead to obstruction of the airway, either from debris such as blood or vomit, or from posterior movement of oropharyngeal tissues. The aim during the primary survey is to ensure that the patient has a patent airway in order to allow oxygenation. At this stage of the resuscitation, airway management may not involve definitive airway intervention, although this may be necessary. In many cases, the primary survey will continue whilst the drugs and equipment for intubation are prepared.

The assessment has already begun if the patient is talking or able to answer questions. Failing this, the next stage is to establish whether the patient is breathing, and if so, is the breathing normal? If it is, the airway can be assumed to be adequate at least initially. Assessment can then move on to B. If the patient can count to 10 in a single breath without distress, the airway is patent. Signs suggesting a partially obstructed airway include snoring, gurgling or paradoxical respiration. Strategies for managing the airway must follow a set sequence beginning with simple techniques and progressing to more complex manoeuvres if simple ones are inadequate to establish and maintain airway patency. Any obvious obstructing foreign body should be removed if possible, using fingers, Magill forceps or suction. Movement of the cervical spine should be minimised, and hence the *jaw thrust* is the preferred *simple airway-opening manoeuvre*.

Airway adjuncts should be used if needed and if tolerated. Care should be taken with nasopharyngeal airways in significant facial trauma, as there is a small risk of insertion through a fracture into the cranial cavity. However, there is no convincing evidence to suggest any significant risk in head injury, providing the correct insertional technique is used. If an oropharyngeal airway is placed, and tolerated, the patient is not able to protect his airway and is likely to require a definitive airway. If *pre-hospital emergency anaesthesia (PHEA)* is available, it should be considered as soon as possible and performed as expeditiously as is safe.

As soon as the airway is patent, high-flow oxygen should be administered, at 15 L/min by facemask with reservoir. Care should be taken with the use of oxygen in confined spaces if there is a possibility of fire (7).

During this phase, an assessment of the likelihood of cervical spine injury should be made. Routine *reflex* immobilisation of the cervical spine is inappropriate and may significantly compromise outcome in patients with head injury as well as making airway management more difficult. A brief but careful examination of the neck should be carried out at this stage if a collar and immobilisation are applied, otherwise it will wait until B.

In some cases, it will be impossible to clear the cervical spine at the scene, due to the presence of distracting injuries and reduced conscious level. Nevertheless, if the components of a validated clinical clearance pathway can be met, the spine can be cleared, and immobilisation may not be required (8,9). If immobilisation is needed, a three-point restraint with collar, blocks and tape should be used. If a spinal board is used for extrication, the patient should then be transferred to a scoop stretcher or other appropriate device and immobilised. It should be noted that an ambulance trolley with a firm mattress will conform better to a patient's natural contours and reduce pressure effects while providing good spinal immobilisation. If possible, the patient should be placed on the trolley using a scoop stretcher, then secured with the scoop stretcher in place. Under no circumstances should the patient be secured by the head and neck alone. In the head-injured patient, the use of a tight-fitting collar risks increased intracranial pressure and pressure sores, and so if the head can be adequately immobilised using blocks, the collar may be omitted (10–12). In some patients agitation can make immobilisation dangerous (13). The patient who is secured and struggling is likely to exert more pressure on their spine and may exacerbate an injury. Unless they can be safely sedated, immobilisation may not be practical in these patients. A collar alone may be used, or manual in-line stabilisation may be all that is possible.

B – BREATHING

Examination of *breathing* should start at the neck and work down. As part of the airway assessment, therefore, the neck should be briefly but carefully examined. This is partly to check for local injuries and partly to check for signs of significant thoracic injury. The neck should be examined in the following sequence using the mnemonic TWELVE (Table 6.1):

The B component of the primary survey is designed to examine the chest for life-threatening thoracic injuries. These may or may not be amenable to treatment pre-hospital, but their detection should trigger expedited evacuation (14). The injuries being sought are listed in Box 6.3.

Table 6.1 Features of neck examination and potential clinical significance

Feature	Significance
Tracheal deviation	This is a late sign of tension pneumothorax.
Wounds	
Surgical **E**mphysema	Suggests disruption to airway or chest wall, likely pneumothorax.
Larynx	Crepitus may indicate fracture and associated airway compromise.
Veins	Suggests raised intrathoracic pressure, although unreliable in hypovolaemic shock.
Exposure	Ensure collars are loosened to allow proper examination.

BOX 6.3: Potentially Life-Threatening Chest Injuries

A Airway obstruction
T Tension pneumothorax
O Open pneumothorax
M Massive haemothorax
F Flail chest
C Cardiac tamponade

Some of those conditions can and must be managed rapidly at scene. These are

- Airway obstruction
- Tension pneumothorax
- Open pneumothorax

A logical and effective system for the management of the airway is described in Chapter 8. The best initial management of tension pneumothorax in the ventilated patient is thoracostomy; otherwise a needle decompression is appropriate. An open chest wound should be sealed with a commercial one-way valve dressing.

If massive haemothorax is identified in the pre-hospital environment, the management is immediate evacuation to hospital. Major flail segments are best managed by intubation and ventilation. Cardiac tamponade is difficult to diagnose outside hospital and unless a thoracotomy can be performed, immediate transport to hospital is the most prudent course. Chest injuries and their immediate management are the subject of Chapter 9.

When examining the chest, full exposure is essential; otherwise subtle injuries will be missed. Like all examinations, B must follow a structure and begin with inspection. The conventional sequence look – feel – percuss – auscultate is followed.

PRACTICE POINT

The chest should be fully exposed in order to assess for injury.

PRACTICE POINT

If anything changes or you become confused, always go back to <C>.

INSPECTION

The respiratory rate must be assessed or recognised to be normal. Bruising, deformity and asymmetry must be sought. Abnormal movements of the chest wall are best seen from low down looking tangentially across the chest or upwards from the feet. The amount of effort breathing requires should be noted, together with the use of accessory muscles. The front of the chest should be carefully assessed and wherever possible the back. In some cases this may not be possible, but if glass or other sharp objects can be excluded, at the very least a gentle palpation of the back should be carefully carried out in search of bleeding or wounds. If spinal injury is possible from the mechanism of injury, diaphragmatic breathing should be sought, which is suggestive of high spinal cord injury.

PALPATION

Thorough palpation should be performed for tenderness, crepitus and surgical emphysema. If it is unclear whether chest movement is symmetrical, the patient should be examined low down looking upwards from their feet.

PERCUSSION

Percussion is often of limited value in the pre-hospital environment due to the levels of ambient noise. Ideally a brief assessment for resonance or dullness should be carried out, identifying asymmetry of resonance. In practice hyper-resonance is difficult to demonstrate.

AUSCULTATION

Like percussion, auscultation is challenging in the presence of background noise. Where possible, an assessment should be made of air entry, and differences between the right and left sides identified.

It is essential to be absolutely clear about the aims of the primary survey in assessing the respiratory system. The information which can be gained by clinical examination of the neck and chest will almost inevitably be compromised by the environment and should be supplemented by monitoring, including oxygen saturation and end tidal carbon dioxide ($ETCO_2$). However, the aim of B is to immediately identify the life-threatening problems listed earlier, and in the absence of signs suggestive of these, or deteriorating respiratory function, the patient will be monitored whilst the primary survey continues, and the chest will be revisited if there is any sign of deterioration.

C – CIRCULATION

Exsanguinating external haemorrhage will have been identified and managed in <C>. The second C has three key objectives. First, an assessment of the adequacy of the patient's circulatory system must be made, with a view to ascertaining whether end organs are being adequately perfused. Second, an assessment should be made as to whether there is a suspicion of occult internal bleeding, and if so its site must be identified. Where appropriate, splints should be applied to reduce bleeding from the pelvis or long bones. Third, intravaneous or intraosseous access must be obtained with judicious administration of intravenous fluid to maintain end organ perfusion.

The adequacy of circulation has already been partly assessed by talking to the patient. A lucid patient is by definition perfusing their brain adequately. Note should also be made of the patient's skin colour and temperature, as sympathetic activation in response to hypovolaemia will reduce skin perfusion. The skin may be cold, clammy and pale. The hypovolaemic patient may complain of feeling cold, regardless of the external temperature, anxious and may also be nauseated. The radial pulse should be felt, and the rate noted. Along with the rate, they clinician should take note of whether the pulse is full or weak. If possible, blood pressure should be measured. A poor oxygen saturation trace may indicate poor peripheral circulation. Single measurements of vital signs in isolation mean little, but serial observation may indicate deterioration or improvement. Regular recording of respiratory rate, O_2 saturations, pulse and blood pressure should therefore take place.

When assessing blood loss, the mnemonic 'blood on the floor, and four more' is useful. Box 6.4 lists the potential sites for occult blood loss. Significant amounts of *blood on the floor* should already have been addressed under <C>. The other potential sites should now be considered.

BOX 6.4: Potential Sites for Blood Loss

- External
- Chest
- Abdomen
- Pelvis
- Femurs

Palpation of the abdomen is of limited value in assessing injury to internal organs, but the presence of bruising may lead to increased suspicion (15). No attempt should be made to elicit pelvic instability or pain as such attempts may precipitate or exacerbate haemorrhage and in any case are insufficiently sensitive to indicate significant injury with any relaibility. The pelvis should be immobilised based on mechanism of injury, symptoms (usually pain), or signs such as bruising, open wounds or blood at the urinary meatus. A simple pelvic splint must be applied and should remain in place until appropriate imaging has been performed (16). If fractures of the femurs are noted, reduction and splintage will reduce pain and bleeding. If there is no concern regarding pelvic fracture, a traction splint may be used. Where there is the potential for the co-existence of a pelvic fracture, a traction splint which does not apply pressure to the pelvis is appropriate.

Any other significant but non-life-threatening external bleeding should be identified and managed by covering with dressings. Other fractures should be splinted, and if open, dressed. Distal circulation should be examined, and recorded both before and after any manipulation, which should be restricted to that required for the application of splintage or where limb circulation is threatened and evacuation may be delayed. Evacuation of the critically injured, however, must under no circumstance be delayed for unnecessary practical procedures.

Venous access should be gained at this stage, if possible. A large bore cannula should be placed in a large vein and secured. It may be, however, that intravenous access is impractical and that intraosseous (IO) is the only viable option. Time should not be wasted in multiple attempts at intravenous access. Either an IO needle should be inserted or immediate evacuation should be carried out. The choice of location for access depends on the injuries and equipment available. The tibia is usually the first option, followed by the sternum or humeral head, although the iliac crest may also be utilised. Care should be taken in obese or muscular patients, especially when using the humeral head, as standard adult needles may not be long enough to enter the marrow cavity.

The administration of intravenous fluids is a matter of some debate, with regard to the ideal fluid and time of administration. Clearly, if the patient is on the verge of circulatory collapse, fluid should be given immediately. Studies demonstrate that patients who receive limited crystalloid resuscitation in the early phase of their injury have better outcomes than those who receive aggressive volumes (17,18). Although this initially led to the suggestion that casualties should be resuscitated to below normal blood pressure (*hypotensive resuscitation*), animal models of haemorrhage have shown that prolonged hypotension leads to acidosis and coagulopathy. A consensus, therefore, has emerged that the target blood pressure for the first hour after injury should be 90 mmHg (or a radial pulse if measurement is impossible), but that thereafter normal physiology should be the target (19).

The choice of fluid to administer has likewise been the matter of much debate. There is now overwhelming evidence that blood product resuscitation produces better outcomes, with blood and fresh frozen plasma being given in a 1:1 ratio (20). The logistical difficulties of providing blood supplies forward of hospital are considerable, and at present this capability is confined to services which see very high volumes of major trauma, mainly air ambulances (21). There is no evidence of benefit from treatment with colloids, and given their cost and increased risk of allergic reactions, when blood products are not available, volume resuscitation, if required, should be with crystalloids.

D – DISABILITY

After the circulatory assessment, the patient's neurological status should be determined. During the primary survey, the aim is to immediately identify life-threatening problems; hence a full neurological examination will be delayed until the patient arrives in hospital. The assessment should therefore be rapid and focussed on significant injuries to the central nervous system.

PRACTICE POINT

Every so often do a 'Where are we up to check' out loud
For example:

'So that's:
<C> No severe external haemorrhage
A Airway patent and talking
B Respiratory rate 24, breath sounds equal and normal, expansion equal and normal, seat belt bruising to left side of chest
OK, let's carry on ...'

BOX 6.5: Primary Survey Part D

Is the patient:
- **A**lert — **A**
- Responsive to **V**oice — **V**
- Responsive to **P**ain — **P**
- **U**nresponsive — **U**

Head and face
- For signs of head and facial injury

Pupils
- Size, equality, reaction

Limbs
- Movement and weakness
- Abnormal movements or posturing

The first assessment is of the patient's level of consciousness, although this will of course have started the moment the patient is approached. At this stage, the AVPU assessment should be used (Box 6.5) together with examination of the pupils for size equality and reactivity. If possible, the eyes should be examined before the administration of any drugs, as pupils are affected by opiates and muscle relaxants. The size and responsiveness of the pupils should be documented prominently, especially if anaesthesia is contemplated, as neurological assessment of sedated patients is challenging.

A gross assessment of limb movement and weakness should be performed. If involuntary limb movements or abnormal posturing are seen, this should be documented. Other signs of spinal injury should be looked for, such as lower limb vasodilation and priapism, but these are unreliable, and their absence does not exclude injury.

In addition, when there is time, without causing delay in evacuation (for example during transfer), the patient's *Glasgow Coma Scale* (GCS) score should be calculated, and documented, to allow changes to be clearly identified. This scale is divided into three segments, and the best score in each category is used to calculate the overall score out of 15. Table 6.2 shows the components of the GCS and the corresponding scores.

Table 6.2 The Glasgow Coma Scale

Motor response	Verbal response	Eye opening
Obeys commands (6)	Oriented (5)	Spontaneous (4)
Localises pain (5)	Confused speech (4)	To voice (3)
Withdraws from pain (4)	Inappropriate words (3)	To pain (2)
Abnormal flexion (3)	Moans (2)	No eye opening (1)
Abnormal extension (2)	No verbal response (1)	
No Motor Response (1)		

The patient should also be assessed for external head injury. Lacerations and contusions to the scalp should be noted and the patient examined for signs of underlying fracture. Examination should be made for signs of basal skull fracture, looking for periorbital bruising, blood or cerebrospinal fluid draining from nose or ears. Battle's sign (bruising to the mastoid process) suggests fracture if present, but may take some hours to become apparent.

In any patient with reduced conscious level, it is essential to check the blood sugar and treat hypoglycaemia immediately with 1 mL/kg of 10% glucose intravenously. Particular care should be taken with known diabetics, young children, the elderly and alcoholics, but any patient can become hypoglyaemic when stressed.

E – EXPOSURE AND ENVIRONMENT

Whilst every effort must be made to safeguard the patient's modesty, exposure must be sufficient to ensure effective inspection. The patient must also be kept warm using conventional blankets or active warming blankets. Wet clothes must be removed. Wrapping a patient wearing cold wet clothes in a silver foil blanket will likely only lead to the development of hypothermia. Temperature control has a key role in the maintenance of haemostasis, and so normothermia must be maintained (22,23). Hypovolaemia can cause hypothermia even in hot climates. If the patient has a temperature of less than 35°C, they should be actively rewarmed.

TIMELINES

In this section, examination must ensure that all significant or serious injuries are identified. This is not the time to search for, identify and document every single injury, however minor. That is what the secondary survey is for. Following this assessment, the patient must be packaged for transfer.

If hospital is nearby or life-threatening injuries have been identified, it may be that it is more appropriate to transfer the patient and complete the examination in a more conducive environment. On the other hand, if the transfer is likely to be prolonged, a more thorough examination may be desirable.

SUMMARY

By the end of the primary survey, the clinician must have identified the patient's life-threatening injuries and should be aware of other significant injuries. Where immediate lifesaving intervention is possible, it should have been performed. Where no intervention is possible, but urgent treatment is needed to save life or prevent serious deterioration, this should provide impetus to the process of urgent evacuation and the time spent on the primary survey may decrease. The emphasis of the primary survey is treatment of what can be treated immediately to save life and identification of those injuries that need treatment in hospital. Decisions must be made about any further on-scene interventions which may be needed, and how and when safe transfer to hospital may be effected. If at any point the patient deteriorates significantly, the primary survey should be repeated and any new problems attended to.

REFERENCES

1. *Battlefield Advanced Trauma Life Support*. 3rd ed. Defence Medical Services Department, 2005.
2. Champion HR, Bellamy RF, Roberts CP, Leppaniemi A. A profile of combat injury. *Journal of Trauma* 2003;54(5):S13–S19.
3. Holcomb JB, McMullin NR, Pearse L, Caruso J, Wade CE, Oetjen-Gerdes L, Champion HR et al. Causes of death in U.S. Special Operations Forces in the Global War on Terrorism: 2001–2004. *Annals of Surgery* 2007;245(6):986–991.
4. Parker P, Clasper J. The military tourniquet. *Journal of the Royal Army Medical Corps* 2007;153(1):10–12.
5. Lakstein D, Blumenfeld A, Sokolov T, Lin G, Bssorai R, Lynn M, Ben-Abraham R. Tourniquets for hemorrhage control on the battlefield: A 4-year accumulated experience. *Journal of Trauma* 2003;54(5):S221–S225.
6. Englehart MS, Cho SD, Tieu BH, Morris MS, Underwood SJ, Karahan A, Muller PJ, Differding JA, Farrell DH, Schreiber MA. A novel highly porous silica and chitosan-based hemostatic dressing is superior to HemCon and gauze sponges. *Journal of Trauma* 2008;65(4):884–892.
7. Calland V. *Safety at Scene*. London: Mosby, 2000.
8. Hoffman JR, Mower WR, Wolfson AB, Todd KH, Zucker MI. Validity of a set of clinical criteria to rule out injury to the cervical spine in patients with blunt trauma. *New England Journal of Medicine* 2013 Jan 6;343(2):94–99.
9. Vaillancourt C, Stiell IG, Beaudoin T, Maloney J, Anton AR, Bradford P, Cain E et al. The Out-of-Hospital Validation of the Canadian C-Spine Rule by Paramedics. *Annals of Emergency Medicine* 2009;54(5):663–671.
10. Harrison P, Cairns C. Clearing the cervical spine in the unconscious patient. *Continuing Education in Anaesthesia, Critical Care & Pain* 2008;8(4):117–120.
11. Chendrasekhar A, Moorman DW, Timberlake GA, Printen K. An evaluation of the effects of semirigid cervical collars in patients with severe closed head injury. *The American Surgeon* 1998;64(7):604–606.
12. Hunt K, Hallworth S, Smith M. The effects of rigid collar placement on intracranial and cerebral perfusion pressures. *Anaesthesia* 2001;56(6):511–513.
13. Greaves I, Porter K, Garner J, editors. *Trauma Care Manual*. 2nd ed. Edward Arnold, 2009.
14. Willett KM. The future of trauma care in the UK. *British Journal of Hospital Medicine* 2009;70(11):612–613.
15. Michetti CP, Sakran JV, Grabowski JG, Thompson EV, Bennett K, Fakhry SM. Physical examination is a poor screening test for abdominal-pelvic injury in adult blunt trauma patients. *Journal of Surgical Research* 2010;159(1):456–461.
16. Lee C, Porter K. The prehospital management of pelvic fractures. *Emergency Medicine Journal* 2007;24(2):130–133.
17. Bickell WH, Wall MJ, Pepe PE, Martin RR, Ginger VF, Allen MK, Mattox KL. Immediate versus delayed fluid resuscitation for hypotensive patients with penetrating torso injuries. *New England Journal of Medicine* 1994;331(17):1105–1109.
18. Bickell WH, Bruttig SP, Millnamow GA, O'Benar J, Wade CE. The detrimental effects of intravenous crystalloid after aortotomy in swine. *Surgery* 1991;110(3):529–536.

19. Consensus Working Group on Pre-Hospital Fluids. Fluid resuscitation in prehospital trauma care: A consensus view. *Journal of the Royal Army Medical Corps* 2001;147:147–152.
20. Joint Doctrine Publication 4–03.1: Clinical Guidelines for Operations. Ministry of Defence, 2011.
21. Greer SE, Rhynhart KK, Gupta R, Corwin HL. New developments in massive transfusion in trauma. *Current Opinion in Anaesthesiology* 2010;23(2):246–250.
22. Jurkovich GJ, Greiser WB, Luterman A, Curreri PW. Hypothermia in trauma victims: An ominous predictor of survival. *Journal of Trauma* 1987;27(9):1019–1024.
23. Beilman G, Nelson T, Nathens A, Moore F, Rhee P, Puyana J, Moore E, Cohn S. Early hypothermia in severely injured trauma patients is a significant risk factor for multiple organ dysfunction syndrome but not mortality. *Critical Care* 2007;11(Suppl 2): P345.

7 Catastrophic haemorrhage

OBJECTIVES

After completing this chapter the reader will

- Understand why catastrophic haemorrhage requires immediate management
- Be aware of the methods available for the control of catastrophic haemorrhage
- Be able to rapidly and effectively control catastrophic junctional or extremity haemorrhage

INTRODUCTION

Catastrophic haemorrhage is defined as severe and sustained bleeding which if left untreated would lead to rapid exsanguination and death. It is the leading cause of early preventable death following traumatic injury both on the battlefield and in civilian trauma (1,2). Catastrophic haemorrhage may be divided into internal and external bleeding, external haemorrhage being identified and controlled during part <C> of the *primary survey,* and internal haemorrhage during C. Internal sources of haemorrhage include injury to the great vessels (for example, the aorta or vena cava) or their major branches supplying the chest, abdomen, retroperitoneum, or pelvis. External sources include injury to the vessels within the upper and lower limbs (extremities) and the junctional zones of the axilla, neck, groin, perineum and buttocks (Figure 7.1).

The elastic content of arteries makes them highly resistant to blunt injury, but susceptible to incision or ballistic fragment penetration. Catastrophic extremity or junctional haemorrhage is therefore relatively rare following blunt trauma, with early deaths usually resulting from central vascular deceleration injuries or traumatic brain injury (3). In contrast, the superficial location of blood vessels within the extremities and across junctional zones makes them particularly vulnerable to penetrating injury at these sites (4). Traumatic amputation is a common cause of catastrophic haemorrhage following blast injury on the battlefield (5) but uncommon in civilian practice where it occasionally follows farming and industrial accidents or accidental explosions. However, the rise in terrorist activity over the last decade means such injuries are likely to become increasingly common in civilian practice, too.

The recognition that catastrophic bleeding requires immediate management has led to the widespread adoption of the <C>ABCDE paradigm across military and civilian pre-hospital care, where <C> represents immediate control of catastrophic haemorrhage.

CONTROL OF BLEEDING

A number of methods are now available for the control of catastrophic external haemorrhage. Many of these have been informed by developments in tactical combat casualty care during the recent wars in Iraq and Afghanistan. These are listed in Box 7.1.

The anatomical site of the bleeding and the environment in which care is to be delivered will determine the method and order in which these techniques are employed. In a low-threat environment the continued application of direct pressure may be sufficient to control catastrophic limb haemorrhage. Conversely, in a high-threat environment (for example, where there is a risk of building collapse or a secondary terrorist explosive device), rapid haemorrhage control with a tourniquet and extraction to a safer environment would be a more appropriate immediate action.

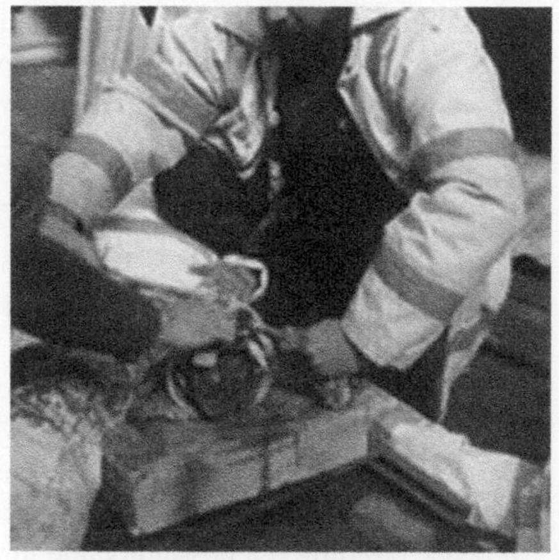

Figure 7.1 Massive external haemorrhage from a limb wound.

BOX 7.1: Methods of Control of Catastrophic Haemorrhage

- Direct pressure with elevation
- Haemostatic dressings
- Extremity tourniquets
- Truncal and junctional tourniquets
- Tissue clamps

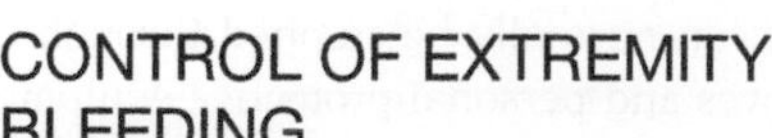

CONTROL OF EXTREMITY BLEEDING

Critical extremity and junctional external bleeding are controlled in the <C> component of the primary survey. In most circumstances extremity bleeding can be controlled by the stepwise application of basic haemorrhage control techniques. Direct pressure through a dressing in combination with limb elevation (above the level of the heart) will be sufficient to manage most cases. Where bleeding cannot be controlled by these measures, or the environmental threat precludes their use, the early application of a tourniquet, haemostatic dressing or indirect pressure device should be considered.

CONTROL OF JUNCTIONAL BLEEDING

Due to the proximal location and involvement of large vessels, junctional injuries can be challenging to manage. Early consideration should be given to the use of haemostatic dressings (see later). Direct pressure through a dressing should be applied immediately to the region of the bleeding vessel while the haemostatic dressing is made ready. The haemostatic dressing is then packed into the wound cavity and pressure re-applied. Pressure may need to be continued until proximal surgical control can be gained in an operating theatre. Application of direct pressure can be complicated by the presence of important adjacent structures such as the trachea in the neck. In these cases early definitive airway management may be required before effective haemorrhage control can be achieved. Although junctional injuries are not amenable to standard limb tourniquets, specific junctional tourniquets are now available for use in the axilla and groin, although their role is not yet clearly established. Other novel techniques such as balloon tamponade (6), wound clamping and truncal tourniquets may be useful alternatives, but currently evidence is limited. Blind clamping of vessels in deep wounds is time-consuming, frequently ineffective and is discouraged.

CONTROL OF INTERNAL BLEEDING

The optimal management for non-compressible internal haemorrhage within the thoracic or abdominal cavity is rapid and definitive operative haemostasis or interventional radiology. Early recognition and rapid evacuation to a major trauma centre is therefore critical to patient survival. A clear appreciation of the mechanism of injury, pattern of physical injury and temporal changes in physiology will allow the pre-hospital practitioner to rapidly identify those patients at risk. At the current time there are few other management options available to the pre-hospital practitioner other than appropriate fluid replacement, application of a pelvic sling if pelvic bleeding is a possibility and limb elevation. Experimental work looking at pre-hospital resuscitative endovascular balloon occlusion of the aorta (REBOA) (7,8), intraperitoneal injection of self-expanding polyurethane polymer (9) and suspended animation (10) may offer potential options for this group of patients by providing a bridge to life-saving surgery.

HAEMORRHAGE CONTROL TECHNIQUES

DIRECT PRESSURE

Haemorrhage from the extremity or junctional zones can normally be stopped through the effective application of direct pressure. Disposable gloves and personal protective equipment (including eye protection) should always be worn due to the risk of blood-borne virus transmission. Traditionally, pressure is applied through gauze swabs or dressings using the rescuer's fingers, palm or fist. Cellulose fibres within the dressing activate the extrinsic clotting pathway and act as a matrix for subsequent clot formation. Care should be taken to ensure pressure is maximal over the bleeding vessel. Targeted, firm digital pressure through a single dressing over a bleeding vessel will often be more effective than diffuse pressure applied over a wad of bulky layered dressings. Some field dressings now incorporate a pressure bar or cap to focus direct pressure more effectively. If bleeding continues despite direct pressure, the addition of further dressings on top is rarely beneficial, as these serve only to distribute the applied force over a wider area. Similarly the requirement for ongoing pressure not only prevents the rescuer undertaking further interventions but also becomes less effective over time as the rescuer tires. In such circumstances, alternative haemorrhage control techniques should be considered. There is no role for the use of compression over proximal 'pressure points' in significant external bleeding.

New Ideas

The *XSTAT™* (Revolutionary Medical Technologies™, Wilsonville, Oregon, United States) is an alternative device for packing a bleeding wound and uses multiple small sponges that are injected into the wound cavity using an applicator. The sponges expand and swell rapidly to fill the wound cavity within 20 seconds of contact with blood. This rapid expansion not only packs the wound cavity but also applies pressure to bleeding vessels negating the need for external direct pressure. Each sponge contains an X-ray detectable marker to aid in surgical removal. It is currently undergoing trials (11).

HAEMOSTATIC DRESSINGS

Haemostatic dressings possess active haemorrhage control properties and come in a variety of presentations (for example impregnated gauzes, pads, powders and granules). They are particularly useful for controlling bleeding from junctional zones but must be used in combination with a standard dressing and direct pressure. Haemostatic agents in current usage work by three main mechanisms to promote clotting:

- Factor concentrators
- Procoagulant supplementers
- Mucoadhesive agents

FACTOR CONCENTRATORS

These agents promote clot formation by concentrating clotting factors at the site of injury through the adsorption of water from plasma. They rely on the patient's intrinsic clotting mechanism for clot formation and are therefore less effective when clotting is impaired due to hypothermia or anticoagulant drugs.

QuikClot® (Z-Medica®, Wallingford, Connecticut, United States) is a factor concentrator based on a naturally occurring volcanic mineral called zeolite. When zeolite comes into contact with blood it rapidly adsorbs water in an exothermic reaction concentrating clotting factors and large protein components on its surface. It also provides calcium ions and causes platelet activation as further adjuncts to coagulation.

Zeolite is biologically inert but needs physical removal following use due to the risk of delayed granuloma or abscess formation (12). In the first generation of Quikclot, granular zeolite was designed to be poured into a wound cavity. Whilst effective as a haemostatic agent, it had a number of disadvantages including thermal injury to surrounding skin as a result of the exothermic reaction, and the practical limitation of only being able to pour downwards into wounds. There was also a risk of the material being blown into the eyes of those treating the casualty. This drove the development of second-generation dressings such as the *Quikclot Advanced Clotting Sponge* (Quikclot ACS) and the *Quikclot Advanced Clotting Sponge Plus* (Quikclot ACS+) in which zeolite beads are packaged within a mesh bag. The mesh bag permits application to wounds at any orientation and minimises the risk of thermal burns to surrounding skin by containing the product within the wound. Quikclot ACS+ uses a re-engineered formula that is less exothermic and has interior baffles within the dressing to ensure equal distribution of the beads. It also has the addition of a silicon rod within the bag for ease of location on wound radiographs. All Quikclot products require the application of direct pressure over the wound for a minimum of 3 minutes following application of the dressing.

New Ideas

Self-Expanding Haemostatic Polymer (Payload Systems Inc, Cambridge, Massachusetts, United States) consists of a highly absorbent polymer with a wicking binder contained within a microporous nylon bag that stretches as the polymer expands. It swells in the wound providing tamponade without the need for direct pressure, whilst also acting as a factor concentrator. It has shown promise in animal trials and has the advantage of being non-exothermic (13). Further comparative studies are required to gauge its effectiveness against other agents in common use.

PROCOAGULANT SUPPLEMENTERS

These agents function by delivering procoagulant factors to the bleeding wound to promote blood clotting.

QuikClot Combat Gauze (Z-Medica, Wallingford, Connecticut, United States) is a non-woven surgical gauze coated in kaolin in use with the US military. Kaolin is a layered clay with the active ingredient aluminium silicate which activates factor XI and factor XII of the intrinsic coagulation pathway on contact with blood. It does not produce any exothermic reaction and despite relying on intrinsic coagulation pathways has been shown in animal studies to be effective in the presence of hypothermia and haemodilution (14). As a gauze roll, it is easy to handle and pack into cavity wounds. It is also easily removed at surgical debridement. Direct pressure must be applied over the wound for a minimum of 3 minutes following application of the haemostatic dressing.

The *Dry Fibrin Sealant Dressing* (American Red Cross Holland Laboratory, Rockville, Maryland, United States) incorporates highly purified human fibrinogen, thrombin, calcium and coagulation factor XIII onto a mesh that can be applied directly to the bleeding wound. This dressing enhances coagulation by providing a high local concentration of coagulation factors. Pre-hospital use is currently precluded by lack of dressing durability and high cost (£300–800) (15).

MUCOADHESIVE AGENTS

Mucoadhesive agents are chitosan-based dressings which adhere to and physically seal bleeding wounds. Chitosan is a naturally occurring biodegradable polysaccharide derived from the shells of marine arthropods such as shrimp. Being positively charged it rapidly cross-links with negatively charged red cells and adheres strongly to the wound surface. This process is independent of intrinsic clotting mechanisms and so is unaffected by hypothermia, anticoagulant drugs, antiplatelet agents or the acute coagulopathy of trauma. There are two main chitosan-based products available: *Celox*™ and *HemCon*®.

Celox (Sam Medical Products, Newport, Oregon, United States) is a mucoadhesive agent currently in use with UK armed forces (Figure 7.2). It is available as either granules or impregnated gauze. Celox granules are very high surface area flakes that can either be poured (Celox Granules) or injected into the wound cavity using an applicator (Celox-A™). Celox Gauze (Figure 7.2) is a high-density gauze, impregnated with Celox granules and available in either a 3 m roll or 1.5 m Z-folded pack. When Celox comes in contact with blood, the granules swell and stick together to make a gel-like clot that adheres to the wound. Direct pressure must be applied over the wound for a minimum of 3 minutes following application of the haemostatic dressing. The second-generation *Celox RAPID* employs an activated form of chitosan (Chito-RTM) bonded to gauze. Only 1 minute of direct pressure is required following

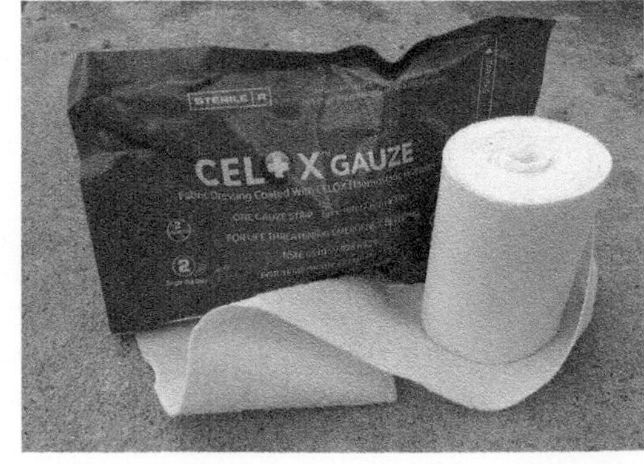

Figure 7.2 Celox™ Gauze. Celox is a mucoadhesive agent.

application of this dressing presenting some advantage in the pre-hospital setting. Celox products are removed by irrigating the wound with water or saline.

HemCon Medical Technologies (Portland, Oregon, United States) produces a range of chitosan-based products for catastrophic haemorrhage control. The HemCon bandage (HemCon Bandage PRO) combines deacetylated chitosan acetate with a sterile foam-backing pad to produce a wafer-like dressing that can be directly applied to bleeding vessels, organs or wounds. It is inflexible and has only one mucoadhesive side. Recognising these limitations, HemCon developed a flexible double-sided impregnated dressing (ChitoFlex® PRO) and an impregnated gauze (ChitoGauze® PRO) which are more suited to packing large wound cavities. Direct pressure must be applied over the wound for a minimum of 3 minutes following application of the haemostatic dressing.

TOURNIQUETS

Tourniquets are an effective means of arresting catastrophic extremity haemorrhage if used appropriately. The use of tourniquets was controversial, with the debate centring on the potential risk of limb loss due to prolonged ischaemia versus the ability to improve survival through control of haemorrhage. However, the high rate of extremity blast trauma seen in the recent Afghanistan conflict drove the widespread reintroduction of tourniquets to deployed military forces. Tourniquets can be rapidly self-applied by the casualty or applied by a bystander. Such has been their success in Afghanistan that their introduction led to a drop in mortality from extremity bleeding from 7.4% to 2.6% (2). A windlass-type tourniquet is recommended for routine inclusion in pre-hospital care equipment.

Their use is not restricted to the battlefield and there has been an increasing recognition of their value within the civilian setting. The rapidity of application makes them ideal for use in high-threat environments (for example, marauding terrorist firearms incident) or mass casualty incidents where only limited medical intervention is desirable. They also provide an alternate means of controlling limb haemorrhage where standard techniques have failed.

WINDLASS TOURNIQUETS

The *Combat Application Tourniquet* (CAT®, North American Rescue, South Carolina, United States) is the windlass tourniquet currently recommended for use by the UK Armed Forces. It is light, compact and simple to use. It has been shown to be effective in arresting haemorrhage, however, its relatively narrow band means higher arterial occlusion pressures are required than their wider competitors (16). Self-application of the CAT (Figure 7.3) is easy, but there have been anecdotal reports of plastic windlass failure and Velcro slippage particularly when wet or contaminated with mud or sand (17).

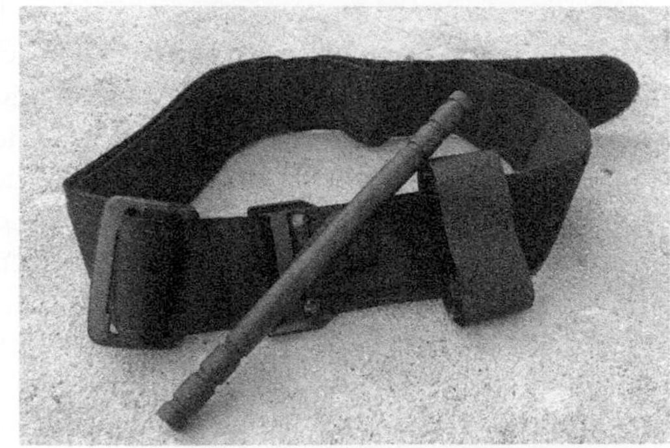

Figure 7.3 Combat Application Tourniquet (CAT®, North American Rescue, South Carolina, United States).

RATCHET TOURNIQUETS

The *Mechanical Advantage Tourniquet* (MAT®, Pyng Medical, Richmond, Canada) is a ratchet-style tourniquet that consists of a rigid collar that goes around the limb with a constricting strap that is tightened using a rotary turnkey. It is quicker and easier to apply than its windlass competitors (18), however, the size of the collar and ratchet mechanism makes the device less practical for carriage and storage.

ELASTICATED TOURNIQUETS

Attention has turned to the development of wider tourniquets that will occlude arterial flow at lower pressures thereby lessening pain and the risk of nerve and tissue damage. The *Stretch Wrap and Tuck Tourniquet* (SWAT-T™, TEMS Solutions, Abingdon, Virginia, United States) consists of a broad elasticated band that can be tightly wrapped around the affected limb to provide arterial occlusion. It is lightweight, can be self-applied and has the advantage over competitors that it can be used on any sized limb (including paediatric).

PNEUMATIC TOURNIQUETS

Pneumatic tourniquets are commonly used in surgery to safely establish a bloodless surgical field. The *Emergency & Military Tourniquet* (EMT, Delphi™ Medical, Vancouver, Canada) is a portable pneumatic tourniquet similar to a manual blood pressure cuff. Whilst effective at arresting haemorrhage, it is larger and more expensive than its competitors and being pneumatic carries the risk of puncture (19), making it less attractive for field use.

TOURNIQUET APPLICATION

Tourniquets should be placed as distally as possible on the affected limb and should be tightened until all bleeding ceases. In amputation due to blast, more proximal application may be necessary to control haemorrhage. Application over a joint should be avoided. Some oozing may continue even following correct tourniquet application due to bleeding from fractured bone ends, however, this is easily controlled with direct pressure. Tourniquet application is often more painful than the injury itself and so judicious use of intravenous analgesia should be considered. The commonest practical error is the failure to apply a tourniquet tight enough, often due to concern over pain. This practice can actually increase bleeding from distal soft tissue injuries if there is occlusion of venous outflow, but inadequate arterial occlusion (20). Proximal lower limb bleeding, for example from the thigh, may require the application of more than one tourniquet to achieve control. The time of application must be noted on either the tourniquet, patient or in the handover notes. Tourniquet times greater than 2 hours are associated with increased risk of complications including permanent nerve or vascular injury, rhabdomyolysis, compartment syndrome, skin necrosis and muscle contractures (16). Casualties with tourniquets applied should therefore be prioritised for urgent evacuation to a surgical facility. There is no evidence to support periodic reperfusion by loosening the tourniquet at intervals during evacuation and this practice may lead to incremental exsanguination (21). It is vital that tourniquets are reassessed regularly during both the resuscitation process and evacuation, as they may require adjustment if bleeding recurs as a result of muscle relaxation or blood pressure changes.

New Ideas

Truncal tourniquets. The ***Abdominal Aortic and Junctional Tourniquet*** (Compression Works, Birmingham, Alabama, United States) is designed to compress the infrarenal aorta above the level of the bifurcation in order to gain proximal control of catastrophic pelvic, junctional and lower extremity bleeding (Figure 7.4). The device consists of a circumferential abdominal strap with a windlass mechanism and inflatable wedge-shaped bladder for aortic compression. The device can be applied in less than a minute by a single responder and should not remain in place for more than 1 hour. The device has been shown to be 100% effective at flow reduction in healthy volunteers with 94% achieving complete occlusion of their common femoral artery on Doppler ultrasound (22). The device has also been used to arrest haemorrhage from the upper extremity by axillary application (23). It is contraindicated in pregnancy and patients with a known abdominal aortic aneurysm. Penetrating abdominal trauma is a relative contraindication and the device may be less effective with abdominal obesity. There is currently insufficient evidence to recommend its use in pre-hospital care.

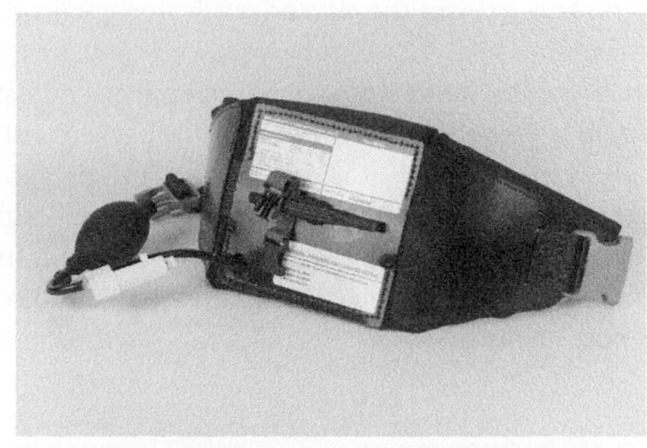

Figure 7.4 Abdominal Aortic and Junctional Tourniquet (Compression Works, Birmingham, Alabama, United States).

JUNCTIONAL TOURNIQUETS

A junctional tourniquet should be considered when direct pressure and haemostatic agents have failed to control a catastrophic junctional bleed. There are three currently in use: the Junctional Emergency Treatment Tool, Combat Ready Clamp and SAM® Junctional Tourniquet. These devices are not currently recommended for routine use.

The *Junctional Emergency Treatment Tool* (JETT™, North American Rescue, Greer, South Carolina, United States) consists of a pelvic binder assembly with bilateral trapezoid-shaped pressure pads attached to threaded T-handles which can be used to apply pressure onto the common femoral arteries either unilaterally or bilaterally. It can be used to apply direct pressure to junctional bleeds in the groin or to gain proximal control of lower extremity bleeding. The binder assembly also serves as a pelvic binder to stabilise the pelvis. The manufacturers recommend that application time should not exceed 4 hours.

The *Combat Ready Clamp* (CRoC™, Combat Medical Systems, Fayetteville, North Carolina, United States) is an aluminium C-clamp with an adjustable pressure disc designed to exert mechanical pressure over the groin or axilla in order to control junctional bleeding or gain proximal control of extremity haemorrhage (24). The device is bulky and assembly and application can take up to 1–2 minutes (25). There are reports of severe pain on application and concerns over dislodgement during patient transfer. Application time should not exceed 4 hours.

The *SAM® Junctional Tourniquet* (SAM Medical Products®, Wilsonville, Oregon, United States) consists of a belt with two inflatable bladders called Target Compression Devices (TCD).

The two TCD are moveable and can be positioned over a wound or the junctional vessels if proximal control is the aim. It can be applied in under 25 seconds. When applied to the inguinal region the belt can also be used as a pelvic binder. An auxiliary strap is required for application to the axilla. Tourniquet time should not exceed 4 hours.

WOUND CLAMPS

The *iTClamp*™ (Innovative Trauma Care, San Antonio, Texas, United States) is a temporary wound closure device designed for wounds with opposable edges. It consists of two pressure bars connected by a clutched hinge. Along each pressure bar there are four 21-gauge needles, which serve to evert the skin edges during application and fix the device in place once closed. The iTClamp seals the wound closed and creates a temporary pool of blood under pressure that then clots. The hinge has a clutch release mechanism that allows removal or repositioning of the device. Large wound cavities can be packed with gauze or haemostatic agent before application of the iTClamp. It is designed for use on the extremities and junctional zones but may also be used for wound closure on the trunk or scalp. The device is compact and well tolerated by patients. It has the potential advantage over tourniquets of preserving distal blood flow if the artery is not transected, although it has yet to convincingly demonstrate a role for itself in pre-hospital care.

SUMMARY

Catastrophic haemorrhage must be managed rapidly and aggressively. Most bleeding can be managed through the stepwise application of basic haemorrhage control techniques. Where this fails, haemostatic dressings and tourniquets should be used. We recommend that a windlass tourniquet is available to all pre-hospital practitioners, accepting that the occasions when it will be required are likely to be rare. As the range of haemostatic techniques increases, it is important that the pre-hospital practitioner remains abreast of these developments in order to maintain currency and to provide optimum patient care. However, we caution that practitioners should not be seduced by complex equipment that is likely to be infrequently used and for which a strong evidence base for appropriate effective pre-hospital use is not available.

REFERENCES

1. Kauvar DS, Wade CE. The epidemiology and modern management of traumatic hemorrhage: US and international perspectives. *Critical Care* 2005;9(5):S1–S9.
2. Eastridge BJ, Mabry RL, Seguin P, Cantrell J, Tops T, Uribe P, Mallett O et al. Death on the battlefield (2001–2011): Implications for the future of combat casualty care. *Journal of Trauma and Acute Care Surgery* 2012;73:S431–S437.
3. Chiara O, Scott JD, Cimbanassi S, Marini A, Zoia R, Rodriguez A, Scalea T, Milan Trauma Death Study Group. Trauma deaths in an Italian urban area: An audit of pre-hospital and in-hospital trauma care. *Injury* 2002;33(7):553–562.
4. Perkins ZB, De'Ath HD, Aylwin C, Brohi K, Walsh M, Tai NR. Epidemiology and outcome of vascular trauma at a British Major Trauma Centre. *European Journal of Vascular and Endovascular Surgery* 2012;44(2):203–209.

5. Morrison JJ, Hunt N, Midwinter M, Jansen J. Associated injuries in casualties with traumatic lower extremity amputations caused by improvised explosive devices. *British Journal of Surgery* 2012;99(3):362–366.
6. Navsaria P, Thoma M, Nicol A. Foley catheter balloon tamponade for life-threatening hemorrhage in penetrating neck trauma. *World Journal of Surgery* 2006;30(7):1265–1268.
7. Stannard A, Eliason JL, Rassmussen TE. Resuscitative endo-vascular balloon occlusion of the aorta (ReBoA) as an adjunct for hemorrhagic shock. *Journal of Trauma and Acute Care Surgery* 2011;71:1869–1872.
8. Andersen NG, Rehn M, Oropeza-Moe M, Oveland NP. Pre-hospital resuscitative endo-vascular balloon occlusion of the aorta. *Scandinavian Journal of Trauma, Resuscitation and Emergency Medicine* 2014; 22(1):19.
9. Rago AP, Duggan MJ, Beagle J, Peev MP, Marini J, Hwabejire JO, Hannett P et al. Self-expanding foam for prehospital treatment of intra-abdominal hemorrhage: 28-day survival and safety. *Journal of Trauma and Acute Care Surgery* 2014;77(3 Suppl 2):S127–S133.
10. Alam HB, Duggan M, Li Y, Spaniolas K, Liu B, Tabbara M, Demoya M et al. Putting life on hold-for how long? Profound hypothermic cardiopulmonary bypass in a swine model of complex vascular injuries. *Journal of Trauma and Acute Care Surgery* 2008;64:912–922.
11. Mueller GR, Pineda TJ, Xie HX, Teach JS, Barofsky AD, Schmid JR, Gregory KW. A novel sponge-based wound stasis dressing to treat lethal noncompressible hemorrhage. *Journal of Trauma and Acute Care Surgery* 2012;73(2 Suppl 1):S134–S139.
12. Wright FL, Hua HT, Velmahos G, Thoman D. Intracorporeal use of the hemostatic agent QuickClot in a coagulopathic patient with combined thoracoabdominal penetrating trauma. *Journal of Trauma and Acute Care Surgery* 2004;56:205–208.
13. Velmahos G, Tabbara M, Spaniolas K et al. Self-expanding hemostatic polymer for control of exsanguinating extremity bleeding. *Journal of Trauma and Acute Care Surgery* 2009;66:984–988.
14. Johnson D, Bates S, Nukalo S, Staub A, Hines A, Leishman T, Michel J, Sikes D, Gegel B, Burgert J. The effects of QuikClot Combat Gauze on hemorrhage control in the presence of hemodilution and hypothermia. *Annals of Medicine and Surgery* 2014;3:21–25.
15. Granville-Chapman J, Jacobs N, and Midwinter MJ. Pre-hospital haemostatic dressings: A systematic review. *Injury* 2011;42:447–459.
16. Wakai A, Winter DC, Street JT, Redmond PH. Pneumatic tourniquets in extremity surgery. *Journal of the American Academy of Orthopaedic Surgeons* 2001;9:345–351.
17. Childers R, Tolentino JC, Leasiolagi J, Wiley N, Liebhardt D, Barbabella S, Kragh JF Jr. Tourniquets exposed to the Afghanistan combat environment have decreased efficacy and increased breakage compared to unexposed tourniquets. *Military Medicine* 2011;176(12):1400–1403.
18. Ruterbusch VL, Swiergosz MJ, Montgomery LD, Hopper KW, Gerth WA. ONR/MAR- SYSCOM evaluation of self-applied tourniquets for combat applications. Navy Experimental Diving Unit Technical Report TR 05-15, November 2005.
19. Kragh JF, O'Neill ML, Walters TJ, Dubick MA, Baer DG, Wade CE, Holcomb JB, Blackbourne LH. The Military Emergency Tourniquet Program's lessons learned with devices and designs. *Military Medicine* 2011;176(10):1144–1152.
20. Starnes BW, Beekley AC, Sebesta JA, Andersen CA, Rusk RM Jr. Extremity vascular injuries on the battlefield: Tips for surgeons deploying to war. *Journal of Trauma and Acute Care Surgery* 2006;60:432–442.

21. Clifford CC. Treating traumatic bleeding in a combat setting. *Military Medicine* 2004;169(12 Suppl):8–10.
22. Taylor DM, Coleman M, Parker PJ. The evaluation of an abdominal aortic tourniquet for the control of pelvic and lower limb hemorrhage. *Military Medicine* 2013;178(11): 1196–1201.
23. Croushorn J, Thomas G, McCord SR. Abdominal aortic tourniquet controls junctional hemorrhage from a gunshot wound of the axilla. *Journal of Special Operations Medicine* 2013;13(3):1–4.
24. Kheirabadi BS, Terrazas IB, Hanson MA, Kragh JF Jr, Dubick MA, Blackbourne LH. In vivo assessment of the Combat Ready Clamp to control junctional hemorrhage in swine. *Journal of Trauma and Acute Care Surgery* 2013;74:1260–1265.
25. Kotwal RS, Butler FK, Gross KR, Kheirabadi BS, Baer DG, Dubick MA, Rasmussen TE, Weber MA, Bailey JA. Management of junctional hemorrhage in tactical combat casualty care: TCCC Guidelines? Proposed Change 13-03. *Journal of Special Operations Medicine* 2013;13(4):85–93.

8 Airway management

OBJECTIVES

After completing this chapter the reader will

- Be capable of recognising the obstructed or partially obstructed airway
- Understand the principles of stepped airway care
- Be able, by selecting the most appropriate method, to provide a patent airway for every trauma victim.

INTRODUCTION

It is fundamental that, with the rare exception of controlling catastrophic haemorrhage, management of the airway is the first priority when assessing and treating a trauma casualty (1–3). The principles are simple: to provide a reliable pathway to deliver oxygen to the lungs and to allow the ventilation of carbon dioxide from the body. It is of concern therefore that repeated reports continue to highlight poor or absent pre-hospital airway management in the hands of healthcare professionals as an ongoing cause of death and morbidity (4–6).

Complex interventions such as surgical cricothyroidotomy or pre-hospital anaesthesia with intubation are rare when compared to the number of trauma casualties requiring some form of airway support. Effective airway care is not, in the vast majority of cases, difficult, requiring the mastery only of a sequence of straightforward techniques. Therefore if the reports referred to are accurate, there must be a gap between what providers are learning in both basic and advanced courses, and what is being delivered to patients. The potential causes of such a gap are given in Box 8.1.

BOX 8.1: Potential Causes of Poor Airway Management

- Lack of recognition of an airway at risk
- Lack of theoretical knowledge
- Lack of practical skill
- Lack of confidence in delivering these skills

In addition, it should not be forgotten that overconfidence associated with unnecessarily complex interventions is also a cause of morbidity.

This chapter aims to describe the pathophysiology of airway trauma, explain the signs of an airway at risk and illustrate the possible interventions to maintain an airway.

CERVICAL SPINE CONSIDERATIONS

There is little evidence that patient outcomes are improved through meticulous spinal precautions when coupled with inadequate airway management. There is, however, plenty to suggest that good airway management saves lives and reduces morbidity. It is reasonable to suggest therefore that good airway management with associated provision of oxygenation and adequate ventilation should be the priority (7). As much care as possible should be taken to protect a potentially injured spine from further movement and damage, but not at the expense of managing an airway at risk.

THE AIRWAY

The airway starts at the lips and the nostrils, and terminates in the alveoli of the lungs. Every part of this network of passages is susceptible to damage or compromise as a result of trauma. However,

- If a pathway can be found that allows the movement of gas in and out of the lungs, then the airway is *open*.
- If this pathway is held open despite the natural tendency to occlude, the airway is *supported*.
- If this pathway is supported such that contamination and further disruption of the airway is impossible, the airway is *secured*.

A safe airway is open, supported and secure.

There are two reasons why it may be important to actively manage an airway in the prehospital environment.

The first and most obvious need is to provide enough oxygen to the lungs to meet the metabolic requirements of the casualty. Lack of oxygen will cause cellular malfunction within minutes and hypoxic brain injury with cardiac arrest will quickly follow.

Adequate oxygenation can theoretically be provided with a single breath of 100% oxygen per minute, but this does not address the second component of ventilation – the removal of carbon dioxide. This function requires substantially greater volumes of gas to be exchanged in order to allow the carbon dioxide produced through metabolism to be cleared from the bloodstream. Uncontrolled rises in carbon dioxide do not threaten life as quickly as uncontrolled drops in oxygen levels, but they do cause alterations in blood pH, intracranial pressure, function of the myocardium and coagulation pathways which may all increase secondary damage to the body (8–10). It is therefore important to differentiate *oxygenation* from *ventilation* and to realise that one can be achieved without the other: A patient with an open airway on supplemental oxygen can demonstrate normal pulse oximetry but still be hypo-ventilating, accumulating carbon dioxide and sustaining secondary injury. In contrast, adequate ventilation of carbon dioxide can be achieved in an oxygen poor environment, but hypoxia will occur.

THE PATHOPHYSIOLOGY OF AIRWAY TRAUMA

INDIRECT TRAUMA

Indirect trauma describes a traumatic injury that, whilst not disrupting the airway, may cause the airway to occlude. The most common cause of this type of injury is a traumatic brain injury with subsequent alteration or loss of consciousness. This usually manifests itself in one of two ways (Box 8.2).

BOX 8.2: Indirect Trauma to the Airway

Significant reduction in consciousness to the point that normal muscle tone is lost. This results in the collapse of the soft structures within the airway, especially if the patient is lying on their back. This may also include patients who following reduction in consciousness rest in a position where the neck is flexed forward occluding the airway (for example slumped forward in a car seat).

Alteration in consciousness to the point that the patient may appear agitated, combative and muscle tone is increased. This results in clenching of the jaw (trismus) and an inability to clear secretions or debris from the airway.

DIRECT TRAUMA

Physical damage to the airway may occur as a result of an impact to the head or the neck. Blows to the head may result in fractures of the facial bones with subsequent bleeding into the airway followed by swelling and occlusion of the nasal passages. Blows around the jaw may cause mandibular fractures and loss of teeth into the airways, as well as bleeding and swelling of the tongue. Direct force to the neck, especially the anterior neck, can disrupt the anatomy of the larynx causing collapse of the airway or the passage of gas into the surrounding tissues that can become swollen and distorted (surgical emphysema and expanding haematoma). Untreated, all of these can be rapidly life threatening and must be both identified and managed as early as possible.

THERMAL TRAUMA

Burns can be divided into two types with regard to the airway.

FLASH BURNS

A flash burn is commonly seen when a flammable material rapidly ignites and dissipates (for example when an accelerant is used to light a fire and causes a brief flare of heat). This type of burn will usually affect the skin and soft tissues of the neck and face, but if the casualty does not inhale the hot gases, the swelling is mainly confined to the external tissues and may be assessed in hospital regarding whether observation and conservative management in hospital is appropriate (11).

INHALATIONAL INJURIES

An inhalational injury is more often seen in a burn sustained in an enclosed area with an enduring source of heat (such as a house or vehicle fire). The inhalation of hot toxic gases in this situation is almost inevitable and will result in damage to the mucosa lining the airways, swelling of the tongue, oropharynx and vocal cords. In addition, deposition of carbonaceous and chemical soot within the airways causes further irritation and inflammation. This type of burn presents an immediate risk to the airway and must be recognised as a life-threatening emergency.

CONTAMINATION AS A RESULT OF TRAUMA

It is quite common following trauma for the airway to be open or supported, and for contamination to occur causing inhalation or blockage due to debris. This may take the form of blood or blood clots, liquid or particulate vomit, secretions or foreign material, all of which can be difficult to remove even with suction. This cause of airway obstruction can be more difficult to recognise as there may be no external signs of injury. By way of example, there have been several cases of young children found unresponsive and not breathing whilst securely fastened into an appropriate child seat in a relatively undamaged car following a minor collision. There has been no apparent explanation for their respiratory arrest until a small sweet was identified lodged in their larynx, inhaled at the point of impact.

ASSESSMENT OF THE AIRWAY

The assessment of the airway must be conducted in a simple and methodical fashion and any finding that is not entirely normal should raise concern. As with many examinations in medicine, the system of *look, listen and feel* will identify all but the most subtle of signs.

LOOK

The casualty's chest should be exposed to view the umbilicus to the neck, and both chest walls to the armpits. On general observation (*wide view*) cyanosis, and signs of obstructed or partially obstructed respiration must be identified, as must respiration that is inadequate. Examining the chest more closely (*close view*) must identify the signs of specific trauma to the face and neck as well as assessing mouth opening. See Box 8.3.

BOX 8.3: The Airway: *Look*

Wide view

- Cyanosis
- Obstruction or partial obstruction
- Ineffective respiration

Close view

- Specific injury to the face and neck
- Mouth opening

WIDE VIEW

Cyanosis

It may be readily apparent that a patient is suffering from global hypoxia from their skin colour. This is, however, not reliable in those who are cold, in poor or very bright light conditions (12), or those with heavily pigmented skin. By the time cyanosis is visible, however, cerebral function is often disturbed with the patient becoming agitated, confused or obtunded.

Obstructed Respiration

Respiratory effort in the presence of an occluded airway manifests as *paradoxical* or *see-saw* movements of the chest and abdomen. In normal respiration, the chest wall and abdomen rise and fall together but in occluded respiration the abdomen will recess as the chest rises, and vice versa creating a see-saw effect. This is a sign of impending respiratory arrest and must be acted upon immediately. Partially obstructed respiration as indicated by use of accessory muscles, in-drawing of the abdominal wall and gasping are all indicative of an increased effort of breathing, which in trauma can suggest compromise of the patent airway at some point along its path.

Ineffective Respiration

Within a few seconds it should be apparent whether the rate or depth of respiration is abnormal. Occasional sighing breaths (referred to as *agonal*) commonly precede a respiratory arrest. Very rapid shallow breaths are both ineffective and quickly tiring. Note should be made of the rate and depth of breathing as subsequent deterioration or improvements can then be recorded and acted upon.

CLOSE VIEW

Signs of direct trauma, bleeding or swelling around the face and neck, should be noted. These are likely to suggest disruption or potential swelling to the normal airway anatomy and may require early and definitive intervention.

Mouth opening should be assessed to determine muscle tone of the airway and access to the airway. A slack jaw that opens easily suggests that when supine the mandible is likely to drop backwards causing the tongue to fill the oropharynx and cause noisy or occluded respiration. A clenched jaw suggests a degree of cerebral irritation and any airway intervention is likely to be difficult without careful sedation. If the mouth can be opened, a visual inspection for vomit, blood, saliva or foreign objects will determine whether suction is required immediately.

LISTEN

Whilst at the patient's head examining the mouth, listening should provide a very easy indication of the state of the airway. Normal respiratory effort through an open airway will sound like normal breathing. Any other sound is therefore abnormal (13) (see Box 8.4).

BOX 8.4: The Airway: Listen for Added Sounds

- **Snoring** is the sound of gas passing between the collapsed soft tissues of the upper airway. It is usually amenable to simple airway manoeuvres.
- **Bubbling or gurgling** sounds are caused by liquid within the upper airways. This may be saliva, blood or vomit. Air exiting the lungs bubbles through this liquid. As air is drawn back into the lungs it will inevitably bring some of this fluid with it causing contamination of the airways and secondary damage.
- **Groaning or straining** noises come from the muscular contraction of the vocal cords and indicate that there is a reduced level of consciousness that may deteriorate further, requiring airway support.
- **Stridor** is a very specific noise which may be inspiratory, expiratory or both. It arises from the vocal cords being almost, but not completely closed causing production of a moderately high-pitched sound as gas passes through the larynx. This is usually due to swelling or oedema of the cords and surrounding structures, and is a clear indication that total airway occlusion is imminent, even in a conscious patient. It must not be ignored.
- **Wheeze** may be audible and indicates narrowing of the airways below the larynx. This may be medical in origin such as asthma or anaphylaxis, trauma related such as inhalational burns, or caused by airway irritation due to contamination with a chemical irritant such as vomit.

FEEL

A gentle bilateral palpation starting at the angle of the mandible and running forward to the chin may identify any step or swelling associated with a mandibular fracture, before running down the front and sides of the neck feeling for surgical emphysema or swelling that might impact on the airway. Finally, a brief assessment of the area around the cricothyroid membrane is useful so that if the need for a needle or surgical airway arises, there is already some familiarity with the area.

AIRWAY MANAGEMENT

Having taken into account the mechanism of injury and conducted a brief but methodical assessment of the airway, it may be that some intervention is required to restore an open supported and secure airway. It is obvious that different healthcare providers have varying levels of skill and equipment available, but this in no way suggests that good basic first aid is of less value than advanced interventions. Indeed, often it is the basic principles performed well that allow the patient to survive until advanced interventions are possible. Airway management should always start simple!

PRACTICE POINT

Airway management should always start simple!

This part of the chapter will address possible airway interventions in turn, starting with simple manoeuvres, and although later interventions may be outside the skill set of some practitioners, it is useful for all providers to be aware of what steps may follow if required.

BASIC AIRWAY MANOEUVRES

MANUAL MANOEUVRES

Jaw thrust (Figure 8.1) *and chin lift* (Figure 8.2) are the basic foundations of every first aid course and are remarkably effective in the majority of patients. The airway from the larynx to the mouth is in effect a simple tube. With the head tilted forward this tube is bent, and with the pressure of the jaw falling rearward, it is then easily occluded by the tongue.

By lifting the chin, the airway is straightened out, and the tissues around the neck and jaw pulled into some tension that may be enough to open the airway.

Placing a finger underneath each angle of the jaw and lifting the jaw forward will bring the jaw and the base of the tongue forward at the same time, further creating space in the oropharynx and allowing free passage of air. When there is a suspicion of a cervical spine injury, a jaw thrust will cause less movement than a chin lift and is preferable, but if a combined jaw thrust and chin lift are the only means by which the airway can be opened, the airway takes priority.

The benefit of these simple manoeuvres is that they require someone to remain engaged and physically in contact with the airway so changes or deteriorations are immediately noticed; equally this is labour intensive and reduces the number of available hands to assist with other tasks.

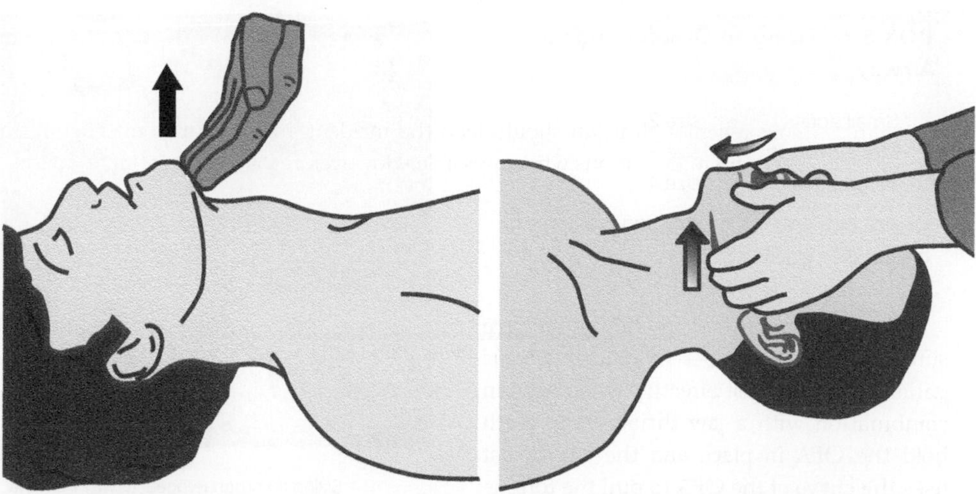

Figure 8.1 The jaw thrust manoeuvre.

Figure 8.2 The chin lift manoeuvre.

NASOPHARYNGEAL AIRWAY (NPA)

A nasopharyngeal airway (NPA) is a simple and effective device that can help bypass the base of the tongue in a similar fashion to a jaw thrust. If a jaw thrust proves effective but on release returns to a partially occluded state, a nasopharyngeal airway is likely to be effective.

Once sized correctly (see Box 8.5), the NPA should be lubricated and passed into either nostril aimed directly towards the back of the head rather than upward. There is no real evidence to suggest that the bevel should lie away from or against the midline. In adults, gentle rotation will aid insertion.

BOX 8.5: Sizing a Nasopharyngeal Airway

Adult female: 6.0–7.0 mm (internal diameter)
Adult male: 7.0–8.0 mm (internal diameter)
Or use an airway the size of the patient's nostril.

Once fully inserted, air should pass freely and audibly through the tube. If this does not work, the tube should be left in situ as further manoeuvres may render it effective, and any bleeding that may have been caused will be compressed and partially controlled by the presence of the tube.

The use of an NPA is recommended in the semi-conscious casualty as once in situ it is well tolerated and unlikely to cause gagging. There is a frequently expressed concern that any suspicion of a base of skull fracture is a contraindication to use of a nasopharyngeal airway. This is based upon very limited evidence involving two individual case reports (14,15) in which an NPA penetrated the skull vault through a base of skull fracture and has resulted in many patients being denied appropriate airway management. Current guidance (16) suggests that the risks from misplacement of an NPA are outweighed by the both the potential benefit in airway compromise and by the risk of vomiting caused by use of an oropharyngeal airway in the semi-conscious patient.

OROPHARYNGEAL AIRWAY (OPA)

The oropharyngeal airway (OPA) is another simple device used to elevate the base of the tongue away from the posterior wall of the oropharynx. Once sized appropriately (Box 8.6), the mouth should be opened, the OPA inserted curved upwards, and rotated 180° as it is advanced. This allows the end to rotate around the rear of the tongue rather than pushing it backwards.

BOX 8.6: Sizing an Oropharyngeal Airway

Small adult:	size 2
Medium adult:	size 3
Large adult:	size 4

Or size between the incisors and the angle of the jaw (see Figure 8.3).

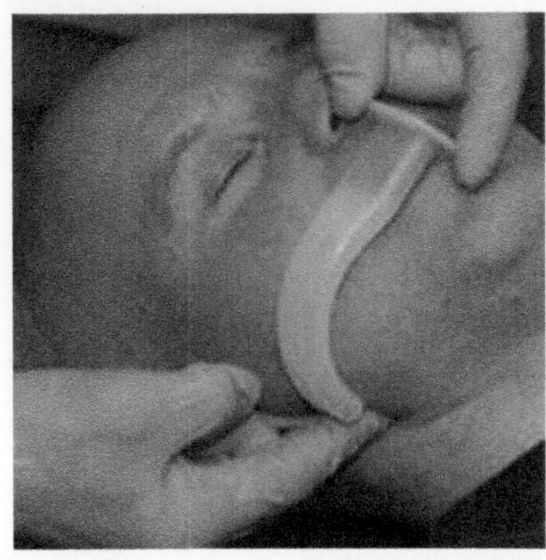

Figure 8.3 Sizing an oropharyngeal airway from the incisor teeth to the angle of the jaw.

Often the presence of an OPA will relieve simple airway obstruction in an unconscious patient, but it is most effective when used in combination with a jaw thrust – the teeth hold the OPA in place and the jaw thrust uses the curve of the OPA to pull the tongue forward. The use of an appropriate OPA does not relieve the provider of having to provide continuing close observation and ongoing support of an airway that by definition is at risk.

The main risk of using an OPA is that it may induce a gag reflex and vomiting in a conscious or semi-conscious patient. It should only be considered in the obtunded patient, and if any resistance occurs it should be withdrawn and an NPA considered.

BAG–VALVE–MASK

The *bag–valve–mask (BVM)* is a simple and efficient means of providing assisted or complete ventilation of the lungs through an open or supported airway. With the use of a jaw thrust and NPA/OPA as required, the mask can be applied over the face (see Figure 8.4) and positive pressure applied by squeezing the bag until the chest is observed to rise. Unless experienced in its use, a two-handed technique is recommended with a second operator tasked with squeezing the bag. The pressure required to inflate the lungs is not great so assertive squeezing of the bag will only serve to force gas into the oesophagus, inflate the stomach and cause vomiting. Failure of the chest to rise with gentle squeezing of the bag should instead be addressed by reassessing the patency of the airway.

Ventilation should consist of a single-handed squeeze of the bag at a rate of 10 to 12 squeezes per minute. The natural tendency is to overventilate.

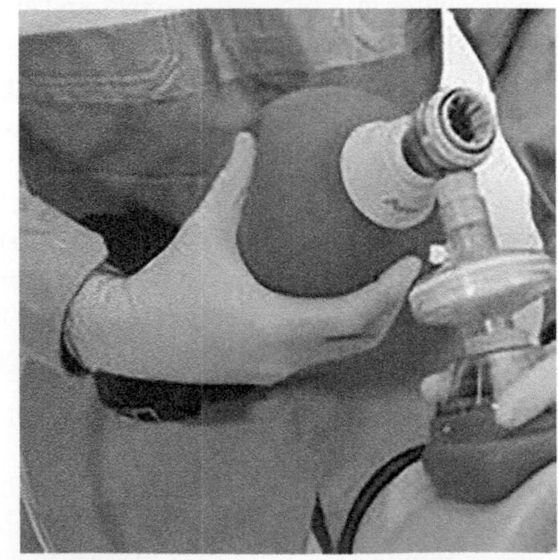

Figure 8.4 Bag–valve–mask ventilation.

INTERMEDIATE AIRWAY MANOEUVRES

The airway interventions that follow should be accompanied by monitoring of exhaled carbon dioxide (capnography). This demonstrates the presence of alveolar gas and therefore a patent airway.

THE LARYNGEAL MASK AIRWAY

Also known as a *supraglottic airway device (SAD)* and of varying designs, the laryngeal mask airway (LMA) is quite literally a mask that is applied directly over the laryngeal inlet with an attached tube that extends out of the mouth to allow active ventilation.

There are two common designs: with an inflatable cuff and with a solid gel cuff, both of which conform to the shape of the laryngeal inlet. Insertion in both types is similar and simple, that is the mouth is opened and the lubricated device passed backwards over the tongue base into the oropharynx. Once it is in position and will advance no further, the cuff is inflated (if applicable).

The laryngeal mask has evolved since it was first designed and second-generation devices incorporate moderate degrees of protection from aspiration of stomach contents, the facility for easy and rapid insertion (17), and the ability to generate relatively high airway pressures without bypassing the cuff and causing inflation of the oesophagus and stomach (18). As such, these newer devices are now widely considered to be first-line airways in many patients including those in cardiac arrest and in unconsciousness. Early insertion in an unconscious patient requiring assisted ventilation has demonstrated reduced incidence of regurgitation (19).

ADVANCED AIRWAY MANOEUVRES

ENDOTRACHEAL INTUBATION

Endotracheal intubation is regarded as the definitive or 'gold standard' airway for the following reasons:

- There is an uninterrupted connection from the ventilator source to the trachea.
- An inflatable cuff effectively seals the trachea from the oropharynx.
- The presence of the cuff renders further contamination of the airway unlikely and allows positive pressure ventilation with no chance of gastric insufflation.
- Exhaled gas can be sampled and analysed.

However, prolonged attempts at intubation coupled with a high chance of misplacing an endotracheal tube, the opportunity to damage teeth with risks of aspiration, and the possibility of causing vomiting or laryngospasm in the semi-conscious patient all are associated with significant potential for morbidity or death.

PRACTICE POINT

There are two broad circumstances in which endotracheal intubation may be possible:

- In a patient who is deeply unconscious or in cardiac arrest
- In a patient who has been sedated and paralysed (pre-hospital emergency anaesthesia)

Therefore, intubation should not be undertaken lightly. The essential requirements are given in Box 8.7 and the risks and benefits in Table 8.1.

With appropriate training and in the right pre-hospital operational environment, endotracheal intubation can be an effective, safe and reliable way of offering early and definitive airway management to trauma patients (20). Without investment in equipment, training and governance, patients can suffer worse outcomes than with simple airway manoeuvres alone (21). A strong and effective clinical governance system is essential for any service which provides pre-hospital anaesthesia. Standards of care must be effectively the same as those provided in the resuscitation room and the system must be able to identify and manage cases where analysis reveals unnecessary and potentially harmful interventions.

PRE-HOSPITAL EMERGENCY ANAESTHESIA

The most advanced airway intervention is to administer potent and potentially fatal anaesthetic drugs to a conscious patient and commit the attending team to securing a definitive airway and taking complete control of the ventilation and oxygenation of that patient (Table 8.2). This decision and process is clearly a critical sequence of steps any of which may cause the patient harm if performed incorrectly.

BOX 8.7: Minimum Requirements for Tracheal Intubation

The minimum equipment required for intubation consists of

- Two personnel (one intubator, one assistant)
- Powered suction
- Laryngoscope with illuminated blade (with spares)
- Selection of endotracheal tubes
- 10 mL syringe to inflate cuff
- Stethoscope
- Oxygen
- Tube holder or tie to secure tube
- Bougie
- The facility to monitor exhaled carbon dioxide (capnography)

CRICOID PRESSURE VERSUS BURP

There are two actions that the airway assistant may be asked to perform during attempts at endotracheal intubation that are frequently confused.

As shown in Figure 8.5, there are three surface landmarks that can be felt at the front of the neck:

- The thyroid cartilage (Adam's apple)
- The cricoid cartilage – the thin ring of cartilage below the thyroid cartilage
- The cricothyroid membrane – the small depression between the two aforementioned cartilages

Cricoid pressure is designed to occlude the oesophagus through firm pressure applied rearwards on the cricoid cartilage which encircles the trachea. This pressure is transmitted through

Table 8.1 Risks and benefits of intubation

Benefit	Risk
• Prevention of further aspiration of vomit or blood once tube placed • Ability to effectively ventilate with positive pressures/PEEP • Ability to measure exhaled carbon dioxide • Ability to accurately control ventilation to normalise gas exchange • Ability to provide continuous ventilation during patient transfers • Freeing up attending staff to perform other tasks	• Aspiration during intubation attempts • Failure to correctly site tube (into oesophagus or bronchus) • Hypoxia during intubation attempts • Hypotension due to anaesthetic drugs administered to a shocked patient • Progression of an undiagnosed pneumothorax • Adverse reaction to anaesthetic drugs (e.g. anaphylaxis)

Table 8.2 Rapid pre-hospital emergency anaesthesia

Decision	Indication	Airway obstruction
		Anticipated airway problem during transport
		Risk of aspiration
		Oxygenation/ventilation failure
		Reduced consciousness
		Severe shock/injury
		Major burns
		Planned surgical intervention
	Location	Out of adverse weather (wind, rain, cold, direct sun)
		Away from onlookers
		Safe (from traffic, violence, flowing water, hazards)
		360 degree access to patient
		Well lit, adequate space
	Attending team	Competent and trained
		At least one pre-hospital doctor
		At least one assistant trained in RSI (rapid sequence induction of anaesthesia)
		Working to agreed standard operating procedure
	Equipment	Airway equipment as listed in standard operating procedure
		Monitoring (ECG, oximetry, blood pressure, capnography)
		Powered suction
Procedure	Preparation	Pre-oxygenation
		Two free-running points of vascular access (iv/io)
		Equipment checked and tested
		Drugs drawn up, checked and doses agreed
		Roles of team agreed and confirmed
		Suitable pre-induction checklist performed
	Successful attempt	Drugs administered
		Ongoing oxygenation
		Cricoid pressure if required
		Intubation
		Confirmation of tube position
		Tube secured
	Failed attempt	30-second drills
		Failed intubation algorithm
		Surgical airway
Subsequent care	Safety	Ensuring tube secured
		Taping eyes to prevent corneal drying/damage
		Ensuring pressure points protected
		Maintenance of core temperature
		Splinting of limbs and dressing of open wounds
	Maintenance	Provision of anaesthesia/sedation
		Mechanical ventilation
	Monitoring	Ongoing monitoring with ECG, BP, SpO2 and ETCO2
		Assessment for depth of sedation
		Close observation for adverse events

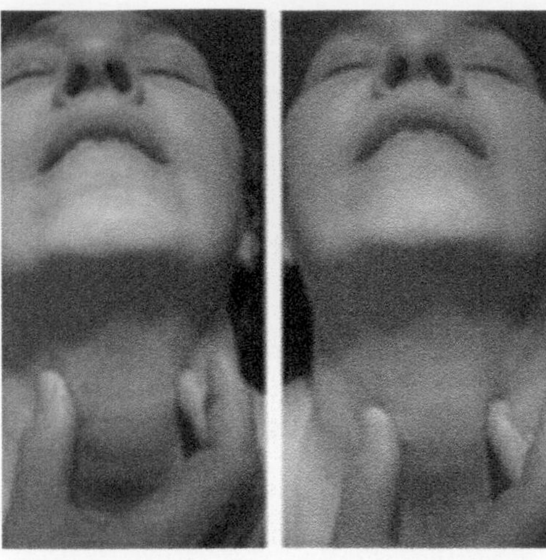

Figure 8.5 Anatomical landmarks on the front of the neck.

the cartilage ring and compresses the oesophagus lying behind it. The suggestion is that this will reduce passive regurgitation of stomach contents into the oropharynx. The evidence for this being effective is very limited (22) and when performed correctly it may make laryngoscopy and intubation more difficult (23). There is worldwide variation in the use of cricoid pressure with little if any difference in aspiration rates (24). The use of cricoid pressure remains common practice in some areas and may still be asked for but is no longer routinely recommended. If, however, the application of cricoid pressure is impeding laryngoscopy, the pressure should be released (25).

During laryngoscopy, the blade of the laryngoscope may force the larynx anteriorly (forwards), caudally (downwards) and leftwards. This may make direct vision of the larynx difficult. The assistant may be asked for a BURP manoeuvre which counters this forward–downward–leftward displacement by placing the fingers on the thyroid cartilage and applying *backward–upward–rightward pressure (BURP)*. This can improve the view and make intubation substantially easier (26).

Cricoid pressure and BURP are applied in different places, for different reasons and have different effects on intubation and it is important to differentiate between them.

DIFFICULT OR FAILED AIRWAY

All pre-hospital airway management should be approached as potentially difficult. When compared with in-hospital intubation, trauma patients in the pre-hospital environment present as a very challenging group – unstarved, unprepared, often shocked with some degree of respiratory failure, and without the benefit of pre-anaesthetic investigations, a dedicated well lit and warm area with a tilting trolley at optimum height and the ability to perform a full chin-lift/head tilt.

As a result, a robust protocol to minimise risk and optimise the conditions that exist is required. The first look at laryngoscopy requires strong muscle relaxation, a laryngoscope blade which offers the best opportunity to visualise the larynx (often a size 4 Macintosh blade is used), routine use of a bougie and support from an assistant skilled both in pre-hospital emergency anaesthesia and in working in this environment.

If, after 30 seconds, tube placement has not been successful the assistant should be empowered to stop further attempts to allow re-oxygenation to occur.

A second look with any further optimisation possible follows and if unsuccessful within 30 seconds, the protocol in Table 8.3 should be followed. Multiple unsuccessful attempts simply increase the risk of airway damage, swelling, aspiration and hypoxia, all of which worsen an already serious situation.

Following failure to intubate, if it is not possible to ventilate with airway adjuncts and a two-person bag–valve–mask technique, then an immediate move to plan B must occur. A supraglottic airway should be placed. If this works well, it may be satisfactory to leave the supraglottic

Table 8.3 Timings for emergency anaesthesia

0 sec	Induction of anaesthesia	
45 sec	First attempt at laryngoscopy	If tube placement successful, end of pathway If unsuccessful within 30 seconds continue
1 m 15 sec	Re-oxygenate for 30 seconds	Reposition self, reposition patient as able, suction
1 m 45 sec	Second attempt	Consider reducing cricoid in favour of BURP
2 m 15 sec	Re-oxygenate for 30 seconds	Change operator
2 m 45 sec	Final attempt	
3 m 15 sec	Re-oxygenate for 30 seconds	Prepare failed airway equipment
3 m 45 sec	Insert supraglottic airway	Remove cricoid pressure if required

airway in situ. If it is not possible to ventilate or ventilation is inadequate with the supraglottic airway, then a rapid decision must be made to perform a surgical airway. If BVM ventilation is possible but no further changes can be made to improve the chances of successful intubation, then the options are to place a supraglottic airway or to consider a surgical airway if the supraglottic airway is not functioning well.

Rarely, consideration should be given to allowing a patient to wake and spontaneously breathe during transfer. Cautious sedation with midazolam may be required to maintain control of the situation.

CRICOTHYROIDOTOMY

Pre-hospital cricothyroidotomy is performed for two reasons:

- To secure an airway in an emergency when other airway manoeuvres are impossible (for example a driver trapped in a vehicle with reduced consciousness, torrential facial bleeding and impending airway compromise)
- To secure an airway when other airway manoeuvres have failed (for example following an airway burn with glottic oedema where intubation is impossible and a laryngeal mask device will not create an effective seal)

The method of providing a cricothyroidotomy varies according to skill, equipment and circumstance. The process must be exhaustively practised if it is to be successful when used for real.

Needle cricothyroidotomy involves placing a large bore needle through the cricothyroid membrane and delivering relatively small volumes of 100% oxygen. It is impossible to adequately ventilate a patient by this method, but the delivery of oxygen can be life saving until a definitive airway is established.

Surgical cricothyroidotomy creates an incision through the cricothyroid membrane to allow passage of a cuffed endotracheal or tracheostomy tube through which the airway can be secured and properly ventilated.

SUMMARY

Management of the airway in trauma often generates considerable anxiety amongst healthcare providers of all levels of experience. It is however amenable to a methodical and simple assessment which should direct the provider towards the appropriate treatment. If that treatment is beyond the scope of practice of the provider, simple manoeuvres performed with confidence can provide the patient with life-saving oxygen until such time as definitive treatment is available.

REFERENCES

1. Nolan, Jerry P., ed. *2010 European Resuscitation Council Guidelines*. Elsevier, 2010.
2. American College of Surgeons, Committee on Trauma. *ATLS, Advanced trauma life support for doctors: Student course manual*. American College of Surgeons, 2012.
3. First aid manual, 9th edition. St John Ambulance, St. Andrew's Ambulance Association, British Red Cross Dorling Kindersley.
4. National Confidential Enquiry into Patient Outcome and Death (NCEPOD). Trauma: Who cares: http://www.ncepod.org.uk/2007report2/Downloads/SIP_report.pdf.
5. JRCALC Airway Working Group. A critical reassessment of ambulance service airway management in prehospital care. Recommendation for Future Airway Management Pre Hospital. Nottingham: JRCALC, 2008.
6. Lockey DJ, Healey BA, Weaver AE, Chalk G, Davies GE. Is there a requirement for advanced airway management for trauma patients in the pre-hospital phase of care? *Scandinavian Journal of Trauma, Resuscitation and Emergency Medicine* 2014;22 (suppl. 1): P8.
7. Kwan I, Bunn F, Roberts IG. Spinal immobilisation for trauma patients. *Cochrane Database of Systematic Reviews* 2001; Issue 2: art. no. CD002803.
8. Engström M, Schött U, Romner B, Reinstrup P. Acidosis impairs the coagulation: A thromboelastic study. *Journal of Trauma-Injury, Infection & Critical Care* 2006;61(3):624–628.
9. Bruce DA, Langfitt TW, Miller JD, Schutz H, Vapalahti MP, Stanek A, Goldberg HI. Regional cerebral blood flow, intracranial pressure, and brain metabolism in comatose patients. *Journal of Neurosurgery* 1973;38:131–144.
10. Werner C, Engelhard K. Pathophysiology of traumatic brain injury. British *Journal of Anaesthesia* 2007;99(1):4–9.
11. Oscier C, Emerson B, Handy JM. New perspectives on airway management in acutely burned patients. *Anaesthesia* 2014;69:105–110.
12. Medd WE, French EB, Wyllie VM. Cyanosis as a guide to arterial oxygen desaturation. *Thorax* 1959;14(3):247–250.
13. Rathlev NK, Medzon R, Bracken ME. Evaluation and management of neck trauma. *Emergency Medicine Clinics of North America* 2007;25(3):679–694.
14. Muzzi DA, Losasso TJ, Cucchiara RF. Complication from a nasopharyngeal airway in a patient with a basilar skull fracture. *Anaesthesiology* 1991;74:366–368.
15. Schade K, Borzotta A, Michaels A. Intracranial malposition of nasopharyngeal airway. *Journal of Trauma* 2000;49(5):967–968.
16. Roberts K, Whalley H, Bleetman A. The nasopharyngeal airway: Dispelling myths and establishing the facts. *Emergency Medicine Journal* 2005;22(6):394–396.
17. Castle N, Owen R, Hann M, Naidoo R, Reeves D. Assessment of the speed and ease of insertion of three supraglottic airway devices by paramedics: A manikin study. *Emergency Medicine Journal* 2010;27(11):860–863.
18. Uppal V, Fletcher G, Kinsella J. Comparison of the i-gel with the cuffed tracheal tube during pressure-controlled ventilation. *British Journal of Anaesthesia* 2009;102(2): 264–268.
19. Stone BJ, Chantler PJ, Baskett PJF. The incidence of regurgitation during cardiopulmonary resuscitation: A comparison between the bag valve mask and laryngeal mask airway. *Resuscitation* 1998;38(1):3–6.

20. McQueen C, Crombie N, Hulme J, Cormack S, Hussain N, Ludwig F, Wheaton S. Prehospital anaesthesia performed by physician/critical care paramedic teams in a major trauma network in the UK: A 12 month review of practice. *Emergency Medicine Journal* 2015;32(1):65–69.
21. Davis DP, Hoyt DB, Ochs M, Fortlage D, Holbrook T, Marshall LK, Rosen P. The effect of paramedic rapid sequence intubation on outcome in patients with severe traumatic brain injury. *Journal of Trauma and Acute Care Surgery* 2003;54(3):444–453.
22. Sellick BA. Cricoid pressure to control regurgitation of stomach contents during induction of anaesthesia. *The Lancet* 1961;278(7199):404–406.
23. Haslam N, Parker L, Duggan JE., Effect of cricoid pressure on the view at laryngoscopy. *Anaesthesia* 2005;60:41–47.
24. Benhamou D. Cricoid pressure is unnecessary in obstetric general anaesthesia. *International Journal of Obstetric Anesthesia* 1995;4(1):30–31.
25. Ellis DY, Harris T, Zideman D. Cricoid pressure in emergency department rapid sequence tracheal intubations: A risk-benefit analysis. *Annals of Emergency Medicine* 2007;50(6):653–665.
26. Knill RL. Difficult laryngoscopy made easy with a "BURP". *Canadian Journal of Anaesthesia* 1993;40(3):279–282.

9 Chest injuries

OBJECTIVES

After completing this chapter the reader will

- Be able to recognise the clinical features of critical chest injuries
- Understand the significance of critical decision making in managing chest trauma
- Understand the indications for life-saving interventions in critical chest injuries

INTRODUCTION

Thoracic injuries are a cause of significant morbidity and mortality with blunt chest trauma causing 25% of all trauma deaths and being a major contributor in another 50% of deaths (1). Although many deaths occur at time of injury (for example massive aortic disruption), some can be avoided through effective use of simple interventions (Box 9.1). Only 10% of these patients require formal surgery (2), although those that do are often critically unstable.

BOX 9.1: Simple Interventions in Chest Trauma

- Oxygen
- One-way valve dressing
- Needle thoracocentesis
- Analgesia
- Critical decision-making regarding evacuation location and urgency

Further deaths can be avoided by the use of a range of more complex interventions which will be discussed later. The key to the management of these challenging injuries is effective prompt and correct decision-making, especially with regard to interventions that should be performed on scene and when, how and where to evacuate for further intervention.

POSSIBLE THORACIC INJURIES

IMMEDIATELY LIFE-THREATENING CHEST INJURIES

Immediately life-threatening injuries can be remembered using the mnemonic ATOM FC (Box 9.2). There are a number of other injuries, however, which may progress to become life threatening, but which in general do so less rapidly than those in ATOM FC. There is, inevitably, some overlap between the two groups. These potentially life-threatening injuries include aortic (and other great vessel) injury, tracheal injury, oesophageal injury, myocardial contusion, pulmonary contusion and diaphragmatic injury.

BOX 9.2: Immediately Life-Threatening Injuries

- **A** Airway obstruction
- **T** Tension pneumothorax
- **O** Open pneumothorax
- **M** Massive haemothorax/mediastinal traversing injury
- **F** Flail chest
- **C** Cardiac tamponade

MECHANISMS OF INJURY

BLUNT TRAUMA

Although road traffic collisions are the commonest cause of blunt trauma, similar injuries may result from other causes such as falls from height or assault with a blunt object. The legal requirement to wear a seatbelt and the introduction of airbags have resulted in a major reduction in the incidence of severe chest injury with those driving commercial vehicles who are not compelled to wear a seat belt remaining at greatest risk. Blunt trauma is usually associated with external evidence of injury such as bruising, abrasions, fracture crepitus or subcutaneous emphysema. In severe blunt trauma the most important injuries to consider are tension pneumothorax, flail chest, pulmonary contusion and massive haemothorax.

Cardiac tamponade has a 99% mortality rate in blunt trauma patients who are in arrest and 98% in those who have not yet suffered a cardio-respiratory arrest (3). Myocardial contusion occurs but is rarely severe and hypotension must always be assumed to be from blood loss (4). Tracheal and oesophageal injury may produce subcutaneous emphysema (as may a pneumothorax with a significant leak).

PENETRATING TRAUMA

Internal haemorrhage is more likely to be uncontrolled in penetrating than in blunt trauma. Flail chest, myocardial contusion and pulmonary contusion do not occur to the same extent in penetrating trauma.

Penetrating trauma can be divided into low-energy trauma such as knife wounds and impalement (Figure 9.1) and high-energy trauma from gunshot wounds. Knife crime is the most common isolated penetrating mechanism in the UK. Impalement by fencing or other objects occasionally occurs at road traffic collisions, falls or industrial accidents where it may co-exist with blunt injury. Although gun crime is on the rise, it is much less common than in the United States.

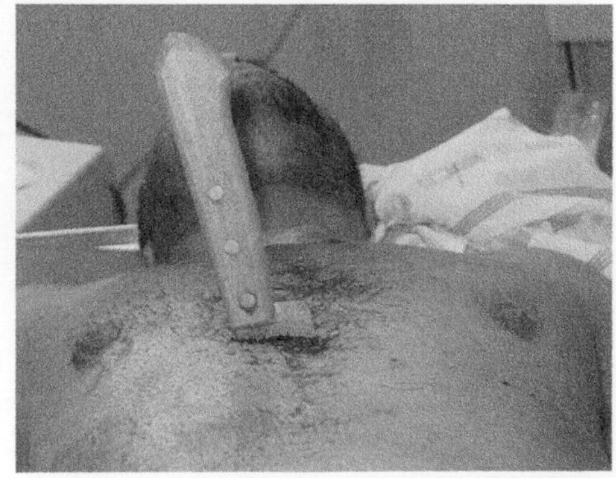

Figure 9.1 Low-energy penetrating trauma.

An appreciation of the anatomy of the chest cavity is pertinent to the expected injuries in penetrating trauma. The site and size of the external wound bears no relationship to the degree of internal damage. Wounds around

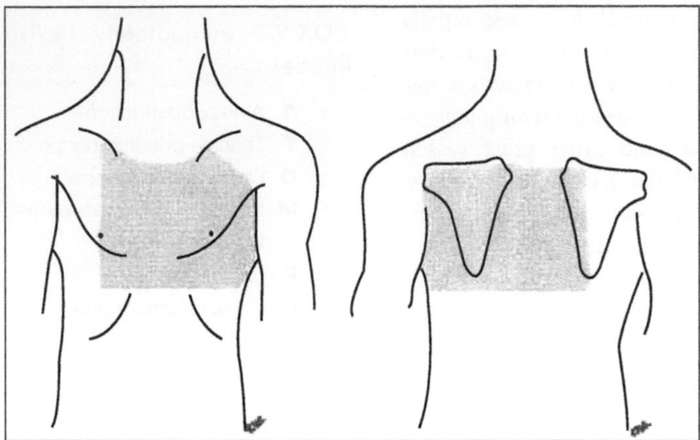

Figure 9.2 The cardiac box.

the neck or upper part of the chest risk involving both areas, whilst wounds lower than the nipples risk involving the abdominal cavity. Likewise wounds in the abdominal cavity risk involving the chest. Any wounds in the 'cardiac box' (see Figure 9.2) risk involving the heart.

PRACTICE POINT

Penetrating 'thoracic' trauma can involve any structures in the chest, neck and abdomen.

BLAST TRAUMA

Blast injuries are considered in detail in Chapter 21. It is essential to remember that both blunt and penetrating injuries may be present in blast victims. Blunt injury occurs if the patient is thrown against a hard object or from a height by the explosion, or is hit by a large object. Penetrating injury occurs due to fragments energised by the explosion.

PATHOPHYSIOLOGY OF THORACIC TRAUMA

The end stage of severe thoracic trauma will be cardio-respiratory arrest if blood oxygenation fails in the normotensive patient, or if the primary problem is obstruction or hypovolaemia. The different pathophysiologies are discussed next.

HYPOXAEMIA

Hypoxaemia leading to tissue hypoxia is the cardinal feature of most severe thoracic trauma. It is caused by either damage to the chest wall or by 'ventilation–perfusion mismatch'.

CHEST WALL

Loss of mechanical function of the chest wall (muscles, ribs, diaphragm, parietal pleura) causes hypoxaemia in *flail chest* and *open pneumothorax.* The chest wall may also be damaged in soft tissue injury, simple pneumothorax and isolated rib fracture, but these injuries will not usually cause hypoxaemia. However, minor chest wall injuries in the elderly may prove fatal due to respiratory function compromise.

VENTILATION–PERFUSION MISMATCH

Ventilation–perfusion mismatch is a cause of hypoxaemia in pulmonary contusion and tension pneumothorax. In pulmonary contusion, de-oxygenated blood passes through injured alveoli that themselves are full of blood and oedema instead of air. This prevents oxygenation of this blood, which even when combined with the oxygenated blood that has passed through un-injured lung will profoundly lower the average oxygenation level of the blood returning to the left-hand side of the heart. Blood passing through the lung on the side of tension pneumothorax is poorly oxygenated leading to a ventilation–perfusion mismatch. This hypoxaemia worsens and may turn into a vicious circle when the respiratory centre in the brainstem, intercostal muscles, diaphragm and myocardium themselves become hypoxic (5).

HYPOTENSION

Hypotension will cause tissue hypoxia due to vasoconstriction. The commonest causes of hypotension in severe thoracic trauma are listed in Box 9.3.

BOX 9.3: Causes of Hypotension in Thoracic Trauma

Hypovolaemia caused by:

- Massive haemothorax (blunt or penetrating)
- Aortic (and other great vessel) injury
- Penetrating cardiac injury (without tamponade)
- Cardiac tamponade (constrictive/obstructive shock)
- Myocardial contusion (myocardial/'pump' failure)
- Tension pneumothorax (more likely to occur earlier in the artificially ventilated patient)

ASSESSMENT

INITIAL ASSESSMENT

In thoracic trauma as in other types of injury, *time* is the patient's greatest enemy. Unnecessary delay increases time to definitive care and risks hypothermia along with coagulopathy. In trapped patients it may be necessary to do a brief assessment before extrication, then a more detailed assessment in the ambulance. In the case of chest trauma, examination should follow the sequence outlined in Box 9.4 look, feel, percuss, ausculate.

BOX 9.4: Initial Assessment of the Chest

Questions to Ask in Suspected Thoracic Trauma

- Is there an open pneumothorax that needs dressing?
- Is there a tension pneumothorax to decompress?
- Is there a hypoxaemic injury that requires intervention?
- Is there penetrating trauma?
- What is the quickest way to access this care?
  - Pre-hospital team
  - Emergency department (local)
  - Major trauma/cardiothoracic centre
- Is RSI required?
- Is finger thoracostomy required?
- Is blood required?
- Is thoracotomy required?

LOOK

A consistently raised or increasing respiratory rate (tachypnoea) is the hallmark of severe chest injury causing hypoxaemia. However, many patients have a high respiratory rate by virtue of anxiety, fear and pain, which may settle with reassurance.

New Ideas

Chest injury screening test in blunt trauma

In blunt trauma, a brief assessment of respiratory status combined with the presence or absence of pleuritic pain as a 'chest injury screening tool' is all that is required initially. If this is normal, more detailed assessment can wait. It is especially useful if access to the chest is restricted or there is a noisy environment.

The *chest injury screening test* is normal in blunt trauma if the patient has

- Breathing that 'feels' normal
- No respiratory distress
- Normal respiratory rate
- No pleuritic pain (on cough and deep breath)
- Normal SpO_2 on air

Note: A patient with an isolated hypotensive pathophysiology from a very low velocity penetrating trauma (such as knife stabbing) may pass this screening test. It does not rule out significant penetrating trauma.

Severe respiratory distress is indicated by

- Inability to count to 10 or speak a sentence in one breath
- A respiratory rate consistently >30–40 per minute
- Cyanosis
- SpO_2<92% on air

A low respiratory rate may be due to head injury, drugs (particularly opiates) or hypothermia.

A consistently raised and increasing respiratory rate is the hallmark of severe chest injury causing hypoxaemia.

PRACTICE POINT

Assessment of respiratory distress:

- Count the respiratory rate as the first observation.
- Reassure the tachypnoeic patient, then reassess respiratory rate.
- *Consistent* tachypnoea is an early feature of significant chest injury.
- Consider anxiety, pain and fear as causes of *intermittent* tachypnoea.

General observation will also reveal whether the skin is clammy, cold and sweaty. In the absence of head injury or shock, confusion and agitation indicate probable cerebral hypoxia secondary to thoracic trauma.

A brief examination of the neck is essential before a collar is applied. The things to examine for can be remembered by the mnemonic TWELVE (Table 9.1).

Evidence of chest injury includes wounds, bleeding, abrasions and bruising. The patient has a back and sides (including the axillae), all of which must be examined. It may be sufficient to run hands under the patient's back to feel for wounds, but especially in penetrating trauma

Table 9.1 A system for examining the neck

Feature	Significance
Tracheal deviation	This is a late sign of tension pneumothorax.
Wounds	
Surgical Emphysema	Suggests disruption to airway or chest, likely pneumothorax.
Larynx	Crepitus may indicate fracture and associated airway compromise.
Veins	Suggests raised intrathoracic pressure, although unreliable in hypovolaemic.
Exposure	Ensure collars are loosened to allow proper examination.

a more formal examination of the back is required (Figure 9.3).

The chest must be inspected for movement and symmetry. Deliberate inspection along the line of the chest (low tangential inspection) is vital (6). Causes of immobility and hypoventilation include pain, rib fractures including flail segment, pneumothorax, haemothorax and pulmonary contusion. Both hypomobility and hyperinflation occur in tension pneumothorax of which the combination is pathognomonic.

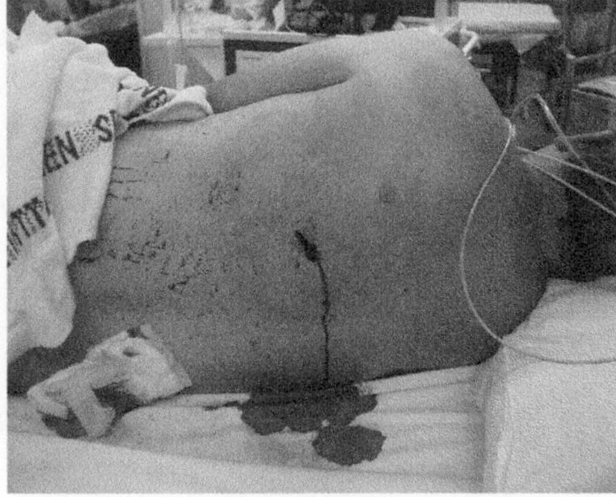

Figure 9.3 This significant wound could easily be missed if the back was not adequately assessed.

FEEL

As mentioned earlier, a brief 'hand sweep' down the back of the patient may identify a source of bleeding. Palpation may also identify crepitus and pain from rib fractures, sternal fractures or surgical emphysema. Surgical emphysema infers pneumothorax in 75% of cases. and major airway injury or oesophageal injury in the remaining 25% (7).

LISTEN

The chest should be carefully auscultated for reduced, absent or altered breath sounds. Axillary auscultation is less likely to pick up transmitted sounds.

> In a noisy environment looking and feeling are more useful than listening.

New Ideas

Portable ultrasound may have a role in the immediate pre-hospital environment in the diagnosis of pneumothorax, haemothorax and cardiac injury by bringing an imaging modality forward from the resuscitation room. This capability is operator dependent and relies on appropriate training and regular refreshing of skills.

IMMEDIATELY LIFE-THREATENING INJURIES

TENSION PNEUMOTHORAX

Tension pneumothorax is rare (in the Vietnam War it was thought to have caused 0.3% of the deaths in the pre-hospital environment) (8–10). However, it is also easily treatable and hence one of the most important immediately life-threatening injuries. Tension pneumothorax occurs when pleural damage allows more air into the pleural space during inspiration than escapes during expiration. This leads to a build up of air in the pleural space with an increase in intra-thoracic pressure. As a result there is further collapse of the lung and pushing of the diaphragm down, ribs outwards and mediastinum across to the other hemithorax. Tension pneumothorax occurs in both blunt and penetrating trauma.

If the glottic opening is closed, air trapped in the alveoli or airways may rupture the visceral pleura if the chest is subjected to blunt trauma. In the awake self-ventilating patient, tension pneumothorax does not usually kill immediately and many will compensate for some significant time. Final decompensation presents as worsening respiratory status with respiratory arrest preceding cardiac arrest. Hypotension is late and results from decreased venous return to the right side of the heart along with a hypoxic myocardium. In contrast, ventilated patients declare themselves at the time of decompensation in as little as 5 minutes from onset.

CLINICAL FEATURES

Table 9.2 lists the presenting features of tension pneumothorax.

MANAGEMENT

In the spontaneously ventilating patient, needle thoracocentesis is a useful temporising measure. In the ventilated patient, the definitive pre-hospital treatment for tension pneumothorax is finger thoracostomy. This is usually done in the 4th intercostal space, and in the UK is only performed by a medical practitioner or critical care paramedic. A chest seal may then be applied. The most effective chest seal currently available is probably the Russell® chest seal. Both the Asherman® and Bolin® are prone to blockage by blood (11).

Finger thoracostomy avoids some of the complications associated with drain insertion and allows repeat intra-pleural finger sweeps to check that the patient is not re-tensioning. This is particularly useful in the ventilated patient who drops their SpO_2 or blood pressure whilst en route to hospital.

Reasons for failure of needle thoracocentesis include a chest wall too thick for the needle, blockage with blood or tissue, and kinking. In one series chest walls were thicker than 3 cm in 50% of patients but thicker than 4.5 cm in only 5% (12,13). Therefore, the needle should

Table 9.2 Features of tension pneumothorax

- Respiratory distress
- Low oxygen saturation on air
- Ipsilateral hyperexpansion and reduced movement
- Absent breath sounds
- Tachycardia
- Hyporesonance
- Tracheal deviation (late – not present if tension is bilateral)
- High inflation pressures
- Distended neck veins if the patient is not hypovolaemic

be longer than 4.5 cm. Needle thoracocentesis should initially be performed in the 2nd intercostal space mid-clavicular line, but if this is unsuccessful it should be repeated in the 4th or 5th intercostal space mid-axillary line (the usual site for trauma chest tube placement). Following this a chest tube will usually need to be placed whether or not a tension truly existed, although this should normally wait until arrival in hospital. So whatever the outcome of needle thoracocentesis, the cannula should be left in place until the patient reaches hospital, as this will be a visual reminder of the need to critically assess the chest to determine whether a chest tube is necessary.

There may not be a rush of air on finger thoracostomy or needle thoracocentesis, however, an immediate improvement in vital signs, especially SpO_2 but also respiratory rate, heart rate and less commonly blood pressure, confirms the diagnosis.

In the spontaneously breathing patient, decompression should be performed when the diagnosis is suspected and examination of the chest reveals supporting signs. Although the maxim 'if in doubt decompress' is valid, decompression should be a considered decision. It may be made over a period of observation and re-observation. Care is essential as needle decompression is undoubtedly overused and frequently undertaken because of perceived decreased air entry (often associated with lung contusion, which is not a pre-hospital diagnosis) not because of the signs of tension.

In the ventilated patient, the decision to decompress should be made rapidly as they present at the point of decompensation. If the SpO_2 or blood pressure of the ventilated patient with thoracic trauma suddenly drops and there is no other apparent and immediately correctable cause, they should be assumed to have a tension pneumothorax. Finger thoracostomy (unilateral if good lateralising signs of tension or bilateral if this is not the case) should be performed immediately.

OPEN PNEUMOTHORAX

When a penetrating chest wall injury creates a direct communication between the thoracic cavity and the external environment, an *open pneumothorax exists* (Figure 9.4). Smaller defects (for example from stab wounds) usually seal off, although air may be seen bubbling around the edge of the wound. Either way, these are at risk of tensioning. Larger defects (most commonly seen with shotgun wounds in the civilian sector) cause a 'communicating pneumothorax'. In these patients there is immediate equilibration between the atmospheric pressure and the intrapleural pressure. If the defect is sufficiently large, air preferentially flows through the hole in the chest wall which may be called a *sucking chest wound*. The loss of chest wall integrity causes the lung to paradoxically collapse (completely) on inspiration and expand slightly on expiration – forcing air in and out of the wound. This results in a significant ventilation–perfusion mismatch and profound hypoxaemia.

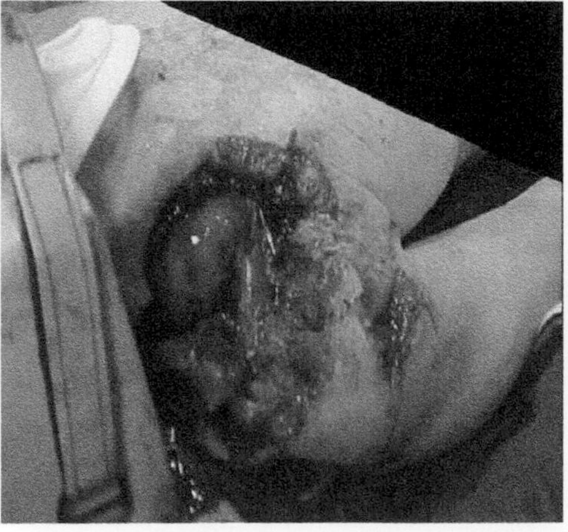

Figure 9.4 A large open pneumothorax to the apex of the right lung.

CLINICAL FEATURES

The clinical features of an open pneumothorax are listed in Box 9.5.

BOX 9.5: Clinical Features of an Open Pneumothorax

- Chest pain
- Respiratory distress
- Low SpO_2
- Cyanosis
- Confusion/agitation
- Visible open wound
- Ipsilateral chest signs (hypomobility, hypoinflation, reduced breath sounds, hyperresonance)
- Tachycardia

MANAGEMENT

The definitive treatment of the respiratory distress associated with a large open pneumothorax is mechanical ventilation (with chest drain insertion and wound dressing). A temporising, but potentially life-saving, treatment is the application of a one-way valve type dressing.

The one-way valve dressing should be a proprietary dressing. There is no evidence to suggest that the often described 'dressing sealed on three sides' acts as anything other than a simple dressing. If the wound is larger than the chosen chest seal only part of it needs to be covered with this. The remainder of the wound can be dressed with a completely occlusive dressing. Likewise, if there is more than one wound, only one per hemithorax needs a one-way valve dressing and the others can be sealed. If circumstances, skills and experience permit, the defect may be sealed with an occlusive dressing and the patient carefully watched to ensure there is no deterioration due to development of a tension pneumothorax.

MASSIVE HAEMOTHORAX

Massive haemothorax is defined as >1500 mL of blood in the hemithorax which represents about 30% of the average blood volume. Its incidence is higher in penetrating than blunt trauma (14). Most (small) haemothoraces are the result of rib fractures, lung parenchymal injury and minor venous injuries. They tend to be self-limiting due to the compressive effect of the haemothorax, the high local concentration of thromboplastin and low pulmonary artery pressure, which combine to produce early clotting and haemostasis (Box 9.6).

BOX 9.6: Clinical Features of Massive Haemothorax

- Haemorrhagic shock (tachycardia and hypotension)
- Ipsilateral chest signs
  - Hypomobility
  - Hypoinflation
  - Reduced breath sounds
  - Dullness to percussion
- Respiratory distress (may be mild)

Less commonly, there is an arterial injury or major vein injury, or there are multiple injuries to the intercostal vessels, which may produce massive haemothorax. The incidence of haemopneumothorax (and mortality) increases with multiple rib fractures and ranges from 6.7% with no rib fractures to 81.4% with more than three rib fractures (7).

Although massive haemothorax is a 'B' injury and can cause hypoxaemia due to ventilation–perfusion mismatch, the hypotensive component may manifest itself before there is significant respiratory compromise.

MANAGEMENT

The definitive treatment for massive haemothorax is chest drain insertion, sometimes followed by formal thoracotomy by a trauma or cardiothoracic surgeon. Pre-hospital interventions should expedite this. There are few if any indications for drainage of a massive haemothorax in the pre-hospital environment. Massive haemothorax may occasionally be discovered when performing finger thoracostomy on a ventilated patient. The pre-hospital team should initiate blood transfusion as soon as possible if massive haemothorax is 'discovered' in this way and blood products are available.

PRACTICE POINT

Draining a massive haemothorax is hazardous and should be avoided in the pre-hospital environment.

FLAIL CHEST

Flail chest is exclusively a disease of blunt trauma. It occurs when adjacent ribs are fractured in multiple places. This separates a segment, so that part of the chest wall moves in the opposite direction (paradoxically) to the rest of the chest wall. This is the *flail segment.* Counter-intuitively, large, especially symmetrical flail segments involving the sternum, can on occasion be more difficult to detect than smaller flails.

The number of ribs that must be broken varies by differing definitions: some sources say at least two adjacent ribs are broken in at least two places, some require three or more ribs in two or more places (15). Mortality rises with an increasing number of rib fractures: 0.2% with no fractures, 4.7% with three or more and 17% if a flail segment is present (7). Other work has shown mortality up to 50% when severe flail chest is present (16). In another study the number of rib fractures beyond which mortality was found to increase dramatically was four (from 2.5% to 19%) (17).

The associated pulmonary contusion with its ventilation–perfusion mismatch is primarily responsible for the severe hypoxaemia that occurs with flail chest, although the paradoxical movement also plays a part if the minute volume can not be maintained. The multiple rib fractures may result in significant blood loss causing haemothorax (sometimes 'massive'), whilst the pleural injury can lead to tension pneumothorax, especially after ventilation of severe flail chest. Flail chest may also go hand in hand with sternal fracture and cardiac contusion (Box 9.7).

BOX 9.7: Clinical Associations with Flail Chest

Flail chest associations

- Pneumothorax (±tension, especially if ventilated)
- Pulmonary contusion
- Massive haemothorax
- Sternal fracture
- Myocardial contusion
- Respiratory failure

CLINICAL FEATURES

Flail chest will usually be diagnosed on the basis of respiratory distress, abnormal chest wall movements and palpation of fracture crepitus and/or subcutaneous emphysema. There are usually visual clues to the severe chest trauma (Figure 9.5), but this is not always the case and flail chest can present with little in the way of external bruising or abrasions (Box 9.8).

MANAGEMENT

The definitive treatment of severe flail chest (and its associated pulmonary contusion) is positive pressure ventilation. All efforts should be directed to expediting this management.

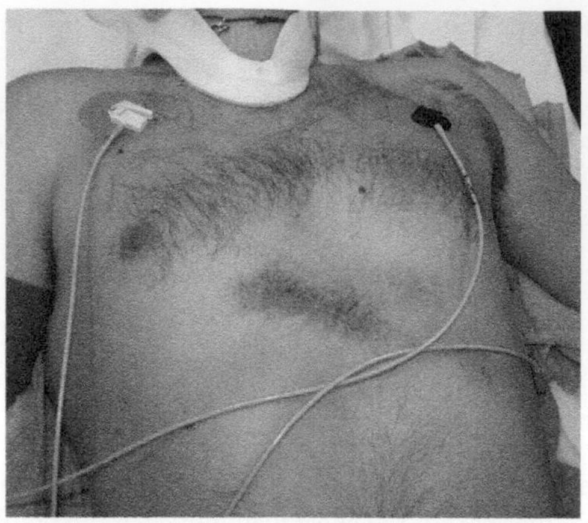

Figure 9.5 External signs of severe blunt trauma (seatbelt marks).

BOX 9.8: Clinical Features of Flail Chest

- Chest pain
- Respiratory distress
- Low SpO_2
- Cyanosis
- Confusion/agitation
- Tachycardia
- Signs of flail (paradoxical movement, asymmetrical movement)
- External signs of blunt chest injury (bruising, swelling and seatbelt marks)
- Crepitus
- Subcutaneous emphysema

Flail chest patients may develop co-existent tension pneumothorax(ces), whilst spontaneously breathing and they are at high risk of rapid tension pneumothorax development when ventilated. If pre-hospital emergency anaesthesia (PHEA) is necessary for other reasons, it should be performed, followed by finger thoracostomy if tension develops.

CARDIAC TAMPONADE

Any breach in the myocardium will allow blood into the pericardial space. When the filling of the pericardial space is rapid, as little as 100 mL is needed within the fixed fibrous pericardium to restrict cardiac filling and cause tamponade (18). If this continues, it leads fairly quickly to either a low output state or cardiac arrest. Pericardial blood invariably clots very rapidly. The vast majority of cardiac tamponades are caused by a penetrating injury inside the cardiac box. However, it can also occur (albeit rarely) from lateral wounds, neck wounds and abdominal wounds. Pericardial effusion is rare following blunt trauma but does occasionally occur.

CLINICAL FEATURES

The predominant features of cardiac tamponade are tachycardia and hypotension, but it is the presence of a penetrating injury which must raise the possibility of the diagnosis. Distended neck veins may occur, but will not be found in the hypovolaemic patient. The presence of muffled heart sounds is exceptionally difficult to establish in the pre-hospital environment and no attempt should be made to elicit pulsus paradoxus. Diagnosis of cardiac tamponade can be effectively made on ultrasound scan if the capability is available.

MANAGEMENT

The definitive treatment for traumatic cardiac tamponade is thoracotomy, pericardial incision and repair of the myocardial defect. Because the blood in the pericardial space is almost invariably clotted, needle pericardiocentesis, although very occasionally providing brief respite, is usually ineffective. For this reason any patient with a wound in the central thoracic area and lateral wounds with associated hypotension should be triaged directly to a major trauma centre.

The pre-hospital trauma team should consider thoracotomy for any patient who has arrested within the previous 10 minutes or who is peri-arrest following a stabbing in the cardiac box (see Appendix B for the management of traumatic cardiac arrest).

Ultrasound scanning (USS) may be used by those skilled in its use to confirm the presence of cardiac tamponade before proceeding to thoracotomy. Pre-hospital thoracotomy is less controversial than it was, and a recent series of 71 pre-hospital thoracotomies by the London *Helicopter Emergency Medical Service* documented 13 survivors (12 with good neurological outcome) when this was undertaken within 10 minutes of arrest (8 of them within 5 minutes of arrest). All of these survivors had cardiac tamponade (19,20). It is of interest that the first successful 'pre-hospital' thoracotomy and cardiac repair was carried out on a kitchen table in Montgomery, Alabama, in 1902.

MEDIASTINAL TRAVERSING INJURY

Mediastinal traversing injuries are high-mortality penetrating wounds, suggested initially by the position of the wounds and confirmed by imaging following arrival in hospital (Figure 9.6). They may have different component injuries including tension pneumothorax, open pneumothorax, massive haemothorax and cardiac tamponade. They require urgent evacuation for surgery.

POTENTIALLY LIFE-THREATENING INJURIES

These injuries are usually not diagnosed until hospital, but the pre-hospital practitioner should be aware of them.

AORTIC (AND OTHER GREAT VESSEL) INJURY

An aortic tear is immediately fatal in about 90% of cases. It is caused by rapid deceleration blunt trauma when the mobile parts of the aorta continue moving leading to tearing at one of the fixed points, usually the ligamentum arteriosum. Survival depends on the development of a contained haematoma, hence the patient may not be shocked. If the scene indicates a sudden deceleration mechanism, this must be communicated to the hospital so that they can seriously consider this diagnosis. Any of the great vessels (aorta, vena cava, subclavian, carotids and

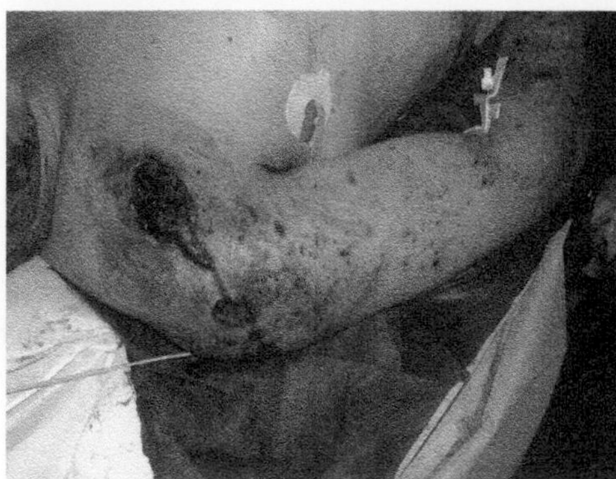

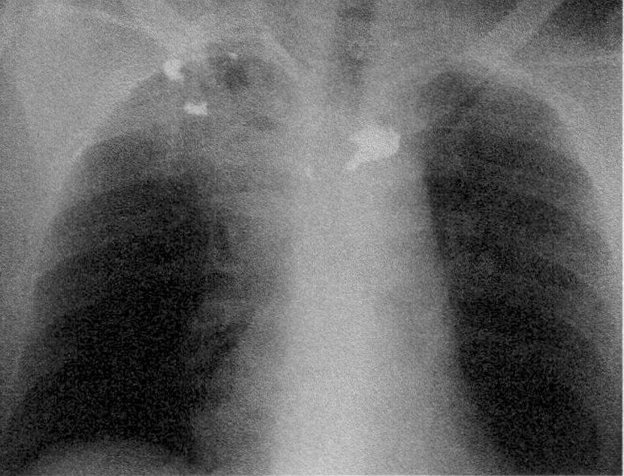

Figure 9.6 Mediastinal traversing wound (entrance wound left shoulder). The diagnosis was confirmed on plain radiograph after arrival in hospital.

hilar vessels) can be damaged in penetrating trauma leading to torrential blood loss. The only chance of survival lies in rapid transport to definitive surgical care.

TRACHEOBRONCHIAL INJURY

Injury to the larynx, trachea and proximal bronchus causes extensive subcutaneous emphysema in the neck, face and/or chest wall. Additional features of tracheobronchial injury are shown in Box 9.9

BOX 9.9: Features of Tracheobronchial Injury

- Laryngeal fractures presenting with hoarseness and crepitus
- Tracheal injuries (often subtle)
- Cough
- Airway obstruction
- Pneumothorax which may tension
- Haemoptysis

MANAGEMENT

Definitive treatment of tracheobronchial injury is to secure the airway, usually in hospital. A very high threshold should be maintained for attempting this pre-hospital and if the decision to proceed is made, the need for a surgical airway must be expected and planned for. If intubation is successful, the tip of the tube must be below the injury and therefore may need to be inserted further than normal.

OESOPHAGEAL INJURY

Oesophageal injury is difficult to diagnose, even in hospital and hence is sometimes known as the 'silent killer'. It will not be diagnosed in pre-hospital care but may be one of the causes of extensive subcutaneous emphysema in the neck or chest.

MYOCARDIAL CONTUSION

Direct blunt trauma to the heart occurs usually as a result of compression against the seatbelt (or steering wheel if unrestrained) during sudden deceleration forces. About 20% of these patients may have a dysrhythmia such as sinus tachycardia, supraventricular tachycardia, ventricular extrasystole, bundle branch block or complete heart block. It can also cause persistent shock despite fluid resuscitation as a result of decreased cardiac contractility and compliance. The diagnosis should be suspected when there are signs of a sternal fracture such as bruising and tenderness.

PULMONARY CONTUSION

Contusion (bruising) of the lung occurs frequently with blunt trauma and plays a major part in the severe respiratory distress found with flail chest.

MANAGEMENT

The definitive treatment of severe pulmonary contusion leading to hypoxaemia is mechanical ventilation, although this may only be required in severe cases or where there are associated injuries.

DIAPHRAGMATIC INJURY

It is difficult to diagnose diaphragmatic injury in the pre-hospital environment, but it must be suspected with any penetrating injury in the lower thoracic or upper abdominal areas.

Diaphragmatic injury also occurs with blunt trauma and may contribute to respiratory distress due to the displacement of abdominal contents into the chest cavity.

PRACTICE POINT

In traumatic cardiac arrest:

The reversible causes are	***Therefore the treatment is***
Hypoxia	Intubation
Hypovolaemia	Ventilation with 100% oxygen
Tension pneumothorax	Bilateral finger thoracostomy
Tamponade	Fluid/blood challenge
	Thoracotomy

MINOR INJURIES

If the patient shows no signs of major chest injury, they may have any one or more of a number of minor problems. These include injury to the chest wall (soft tissue injury to intercostal muscles or rib fractures), sternal fracture, clavicular fracture and simple pneumothorax. The decision to treat these injuries will depend on the presence of other more time-critical injuries and the need for urgent evacuation.

SIMPLE PNEUMOTHORAX

Simple pneumothorax is air in the pleural cavity that is neither under tension nor communicating with the outside. It can be difficult to diagnose clinically but the (ipsilateral) features to look for are poor expansion on the affected side, reduced breath sounds and hyperresonance. Simple pneumothorax may also be diagnosed in the pre-hospital environment by USS. There is no need to treat simple pneumothorax pre-hospital, however, its diagnosis is mainly of importance in monitoring the patient for the development of a tension (particularly if the patient is to be ventilated).

MINOR CHEST WALL INJURY

Minor chest wall injury (without flail segment) requires no action, but these injuries can be disproportionately painful and adequate analgesia should be given. Chest wall injuries present with pain, localised tenderness and hypoventilation and may be particularly debilitating in the elderly or those with chronic respiratory disease.

STERNAL FRACTURE

The main significance of this injury is its association with myocardial contusion. Any patient suspected of sternal fracture must be transferred to hospital. Its features are sternal tenderness with or without bruising and swelling. Occasionally a palpable step in the sternum may be felt and the patient may complain of clicking on inspiration.

PRACTICE POINT

High flow oxygen must be given to all patients with significant thoracic trauma.

GENERAL TREATMENT OF THORACIC TRAUMA

OXYGEN

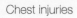

High flow oxygen must be given to all patients with significant thoracic trauma. Care is theoretically needed in the patient with chronic obstructive pulmonary disease (COPD), however, it must be remembered that the majority of patients with significant thoracic trauma are suffering a severe hypoxaemic process. Therefore if any COPD patient is tachypnoeic from significant thoracic trauma high concentration oxygen should still be given. The concentration can always be titrated downwards if the patient's respiratory rate starts to fall as a result of presumed hypercarbia.

INTRAVENOUS ACCESS AND FLUIDS/BLOOD

Unless blood products are available, standard pre-hospital guidelines for pre-hospital fluid administration should be observed with 250 mL fluid bolus (crystalloid or blood if available) given only if the radial pulse is absent (21). Intravenous access may be required before transport to hospital for administration of analgesia, sedation or anaesthesia, or for fluid administration if the patient is trapped.

PENETRATING OBJECTS

In general any penetrating object must be left in situ. It may be possible to gently pack around the protruding part of a penetrating object, but this should not delay evacuation, must not result in movement of the object inside the patient and should not inhibit movement of the object, for example of a knife to the precordium moving with each heartbeat.

ANALGESIA

Reassurance plays an important part in analgesia. It also decreases any anxiety-driven hyperventilation and therefore decreases overall oxygen demand. Local anaesthesia is the standard approach to thoracostomy but does not take away the pain associated with pleural penetration. For this reason judicious use of analgesia in addition to the local anaesthetic can make this slightly less unpleasant for the patient.

PRACTICE POINT

Entonox is absolutely contraindicated due to the risk of increasing the size of a pneumothorax.

TRANSPORT

The importance of critical decision making as an 'intervention' in itself cannot be overstated. For example, this may be the decision to rapidly transfer (with no practical procedures performed) a patient with an anterior stab wound to a major trauma centre. On occasion, critical decisions must also be made with respect to the need to request rendezvous with a pre-hospital trauma team.

A hypoxaemic patient will have better respiratory function if they are sitting at 45 degrees than if lying supine. Patients with penetrating trauma may be transported semi-recumbent unless they are hypotensive in which case lying supine is likely to be preferable. A critical decision is required as to whether the B (breathing) or C (circulating) problem is the greatest risk to the patient and whether there are any procedures that can temporarily improve one or both of these problems.

SUMMARY

The management of thoracic trauma is straightforward as long as the basic principles are followed and the underlying pathological processes are understood. Careful assessment will identify the immediately life-threatening problems. A limited number of interventions will very significantly increase survival rates.

Critical decision-making with regard to evacuation and which interventions should be performed before arrival in hospital are vital components of management.

REFERENCES

1. www.emedicine.medscape.com/article/428723-overview
2. Thoracic trauma, www.trauma.org.
3. Burlew CC, Moore EE, Moore FA, Coimbra R, McIntyre RC Jr, Davis JW, Sperry J, Biffl WL. Western Trauma Association critical decisions in trauma: Resuscitative thoracotomy. *Journal of Trauma and Acute Care Surgery* 2012;73(6):1359–1363.
4. Kaye P, O'Sullivan I. Myocardial contusion: Emergency investigation and diagnosis. *Emergency Medicine Journal* 2002;19(1):8–10.
5. Rutherford RB, Hurt HH, Brickman RD, Tubb JM. The pathophysiology of progressive tension pneumothorax. *Journal of Trauma* 1968;8(2):212–227.
6. Leigh-Smith S, Davies G. Tension pneumothorax: Eyes may be more diagnostic than ears. *Emergency Medicine Journal* 2003;20(5):495–496.
7. Liman ST, Kuzucu A, Tastepe AI, Ulasan GN, Topcu S. Chest injury due to blunt trauma. *European Journal of Cardio-Thoracic Surgery* 2003;23(3):374–378.
8. Leigh-Smith S, Harris T. Tension pneumothorax – Time for a re-think? *Emergency Medicine Journal* 2005;22:8–16.
9. McPherson JJ, Feigin DS, Bellamy RF. Prevalence of tension pneumothorax in fatally wounded combat casualties. *Journal of Trauma* 2006;60:573–578.
10. Leigh-Smith S. Tension pneumothorax prevalence grossly exaggerated. *Emergency Medicine Journal* 2007;24(12):865.
11. Comparative trial of chest seals for battlefield use. Defence Medical Services Report 2012 (unpublished).
12. Britten S, Palmer SH, Snow TM. Needle thoracocentesis in tension pneumothorax: Insufficient cannula length and potential failure. *Injury* 1996;27(5):321–322.
13. Britten S, Palmer SH. Chest wall thickness may limit adequate drainage of tension pneumothorax by needle thoracocentesis. *Journal of Accident and Emergency Medicine* 1996;13(6):426–427.
14. Tintinalli J, Ruiz E, Krome R. *Emergency Medicine: A Comprehensive Study Guide,* 4th ed. New York: McGraw-Hill, 1996.

15. Keel M, Meier C. Chest injuries – What is new? *Current Opinion in Critical Care* 2007;13(6):674–679.
16. Velmahos GC, Vassiliu P, Chan LS, Murray JA, Berne TV, Demetriades D. Influence of flail chest on outcome among patients with severe thoracic cage trauma. *International Surgery* 2002;87(4):240–244.
17. Svennevig JL, Bugge-Asperheim B, Geiran OR. Prognostic factors in blunt chest trauma: Analysis of 652 cases. *Annales Chirurgiae et Gynaecologiae* 1986;75:8–14.
18. Forauer AR, Dasika NL, Gemmete JJ, Theoharis C. Pericardial tamponade complicating central venous interventions. *Journal of Vascular and Interventional Radiology* 2003; 14(2 Pt 1):255–259.
19. Davies, Gareth E. Lockey, David J. Thirteen survivors of prehospital thoracotomy for penetrating trauma: A prehospital physician-performed resuscitation procedure that can yield good results. *Journal of Trauma* 2011;70(5):E75–E78.
20. Thoracotomy, www.trauma.org.
21. Revell M, Porter K, Greaves I. Fluid resuscitation in prehospital trauma care: A consensus view. *Emergency Medicine Journal* 2002;19:494–498.

10 Shock

OBJECTIVES

After completing this chapter the reader will be able to

- Understand the pathophysiology of shock associated with trauma
- Recognise the clinical features of a shock state
- Apply a structured approach to the assessment and management of shock

INTRODUCTION

Physiological shock occurs when there is inadequate organ perfusion and cellular oxygen utilisation (1). In this chapter, the basic pathophysiology and applied therapeutics related to shock following major injury are reviewed. Physiological shock occurs when an imbalance of oxygen supply and demand results in a critical reduction in the oxygen available to the mitochondria. Anaerobic metabolism, lactic acidosis and organ dysfunction follow. The pathophysiologic events in the various shock syndromes are complex and interrelated. In simple terms, physiological shock may result from a change in any combination of intravascular volume, myocardial function, systemic vascular resistance or tissue blood flow. Although there is often an overlap, the clinical classification of shock is usually based on the likely dominant trigger: hypovolaemic, cardiogenic, obstructive or distributive (Figure 10.1). All of these may be present in any single trauma patient (2,3).

PRACTICE POINT

Physiological shock occurs when an imbalance of oxygen supply and demand results in a critical reduction in the oxygen available to the mitochondria.

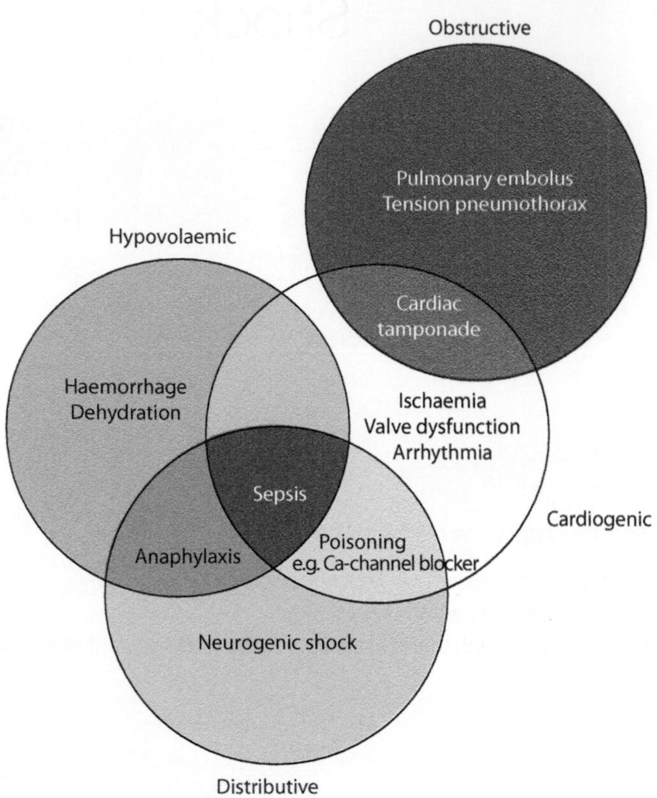

Figure 10.1 The relationship between different types of shock. (Adapted from Shippey B, *Anaesthesia and Intensive Care Medicine* 2010;11:509–511.)

TYPES OF SHOCK

HYPOVOLAEMIC SHOCK

Hypovolaemic shock remains the greatest single contributor to early trauma mortality and, in many respects, reflects the final common pathway for all forms of shock. Cardiac output is dependent on stroke volume and heart rate. Stroke volume, the amount of blood ejected by the left ventricle in one contraction, is influenced by preload, myocardial contractility and afterload. Preload, or diastolic filling, is affected by venous blood pressure, venous tone and the volume of circulating blood. An absolute or relative reduction in the volume of circulating blood can thus reduce cardiac output.

Stroke volume is also dependent on myocardial contractility and afterload. Increased myocardial contractility is a compensatory mechanism in hypovolaemia. However, the hypoxaemia and acidaemia associated with hypoperfusion *depress* myocardial contractility. Similarly, left ventricular afterload, the resistance opposing myocardial ejection of blood, is closely linked to systemic vascular resistance. Increased systemic vascular resistance is also a compensatory mechanism that may, if prolonged, result in both reduced tissue perfusion and increased afterload. Cardiac output is also related to heart rate. Increased heart rate is a compensatory mechanism in hypovolaemia but the potentially adverse consequence is that the increased heart rate is at the expense of the duration of diastole and cardiac filling and, in due course, results in reduced preload. The control of haemorrhage, preservation of intravascular volume and management of the physiological consequences of relative and absolute hypovolaemia are therefore cornerstones of shock management.

CARDIOGENIC SHOCK

Cardiogenic shock occurs when there is decreased cardiac output and evidence of inadequate tissue perfusion in the presence of adequate intravascular volume. It is usually considered in the context of acute myocardial infarction. However, myocardial dysfunction can occur in the context of major trauma both primarily (as a result of direct myocardial injury) and as a secondary phenomenon (in association with, for example, the acute catecholamine excess state seen in traumatic brain injury). Traumatic myocardial dysfunction, as a contributor to physiological shock, is frequently unsuspected and therefore undiagnosed. When it results in, or contributes to, hypoperfusion, the resultant acidaemia further reduces contractility.

PRACTICE POINT

Preservation of intravascular volume and *management of the physiological consequences of hypovolaemia* are the cornerstones of shock management.

OBSTRUCTIVE SHOCK

Obstructive shock occurs when there is a physical obstruction to flow into, or out of, the heart. It is characterised by either impairment of diastolic filling (decreased preload) or excessive afterload or both. Impaired diastolic filling can result from direct venous obstruction, increased intrathoracic pressure or decreased cardiac compliance. In the context of the trauma patient, increased intrathoracic pressure can result from tension pneumothorax and pneumomediastinum. It can also result from mechanical ventilation where there is air trapping, excessive inflation pressures or excessive positive end-expiratory pressure. Cardiac tamponade is the commonest cause of restricted cardiac filling (compliance). Excessive afterload is more often associated with pulmonary embolism or aortic dissection. Obstructive shock, as with cardiogenic shock, may easily be missed in the trauma patient if there is co-existing evidence of hypovolaemia.

DISTRIBUTIVE SHOCK

Hypovolaemic, cardiogenic and obstructive shock are all associated with vasoconstriction and increased systemic vascular resistance. In contrast, *distributive* or *vasodilatory shock* is associated with a failure of vasomotor tone and decreased systemic vascular resistance (4). The systemic release of histamine in anaphylaxis, the loss of sympathetic tone related to disruption of the autonomic pathways in spinal cord injury (neurogenic shock) and the systemic inflammatory response syndrome in sepsis are the commonest precipitants of distributive shock but other causes such as transfusion reactions and poisoning should be considered.

THE BODY'S RESPONSE TO SHOCK

Irrespective of the dominant trigger, the response to diminished tissue perfusion is activation of a wide range of homeostatic mechanisms and an initial phase of compensation.

This compensated phase can be subtle. As tissue perfusion worsens, however, there is a progressive failure of compensatory mechanisms and less subtle signs and symptoms of organ dysfunction will appear. Progressive end-organ dysfunction leads to irreversible organ damage and patient death. In undertaking initial and subsequent assessments of trauma patients, the clinician must therefore be familiar with the different shock syndromes and their subtle symptoms and signs.

THE CLINICAL APPROACH TO THE TRAUMA PATIENT

Haemorrhage is the most common cause of shock in the trauma patient. As highlighted elsewhere, active, rapid identification and control of critical external haemorrhage (<C>) is an essential precursor to shock management. Haemorrhage control, or *haemostatic resuscitation,* involves strategies to both minimise blood loss and optimise coagulation. Blood loss can be controlled by a combination of

- Simple dressings, pressure and elevation
- Haemostatic dressings
- Tourniquets
- Reduction and splintage of fractures
- Careful handling

After arrival at hospital, either interventional radiology or damage control surgery (or both) may be used to definitively stop bleeding.

Coagulopathy associated with trauma may occur for a number of reasons (3,5). Normal coagulation is a balance between haemostatic and fibrinolytic processes. Factors that disrupt this balance include the lethal triad of *acidaemia, hypothermia and hypoperfusion* related to tissue injury as well as haemodilution. A systemic consumptive coagulopathy (a *disseminated intravascular coagulation*) may also occur due to inadequate clotting factors in the face of ongoing consumption. More recently, an acute traumatic coagulopathy has also been characterised (Figure 10.2).

Traumatic coagulopathy is an impairment of haemostasis and activation of fibrinolysis occurring early after injury, and independent of the development of significant acidaemia, hypothermia or haemodilution (6). Some consider this to be an early, partially compensated stage of disseminated intravascular coagulation. The key point is that there are a number of reasons why significant coagulopathy may already be present in the early stages of clinical assessment and why exposure to factors that are known to be associated with coagulopathy should be avoided. This is achieved by controlling blood loss (as mentioned earlier) by minimising any further tissue damage, preventing or correcting acidaemia and hypothermia, and preventing dilutional coagulopathy. In addition factors that are known to exacerbate coagulopathy must be avoided and physiological conditions that actively facilitate clotting created (Box 10.1).

BOX 10.1: Methods of Promoting Effective Haemostasis

- Minimisation of any further tissue damage
- Prevention or correction of acidaemia
- Prevention or correction of hypothermia
- Prevention of dilutional coagulopathy
- Avoidance of any factor known to exacerbate coagulopathy
- Creation of physiological conditions that actively facilitate clotting

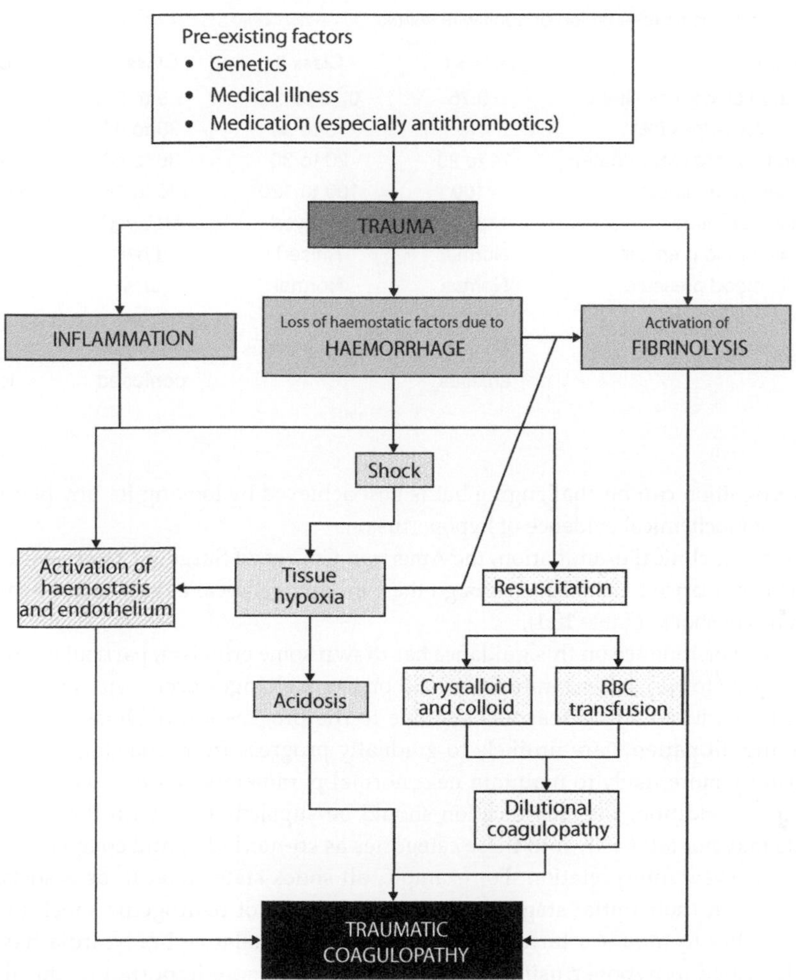

Figure 10.2 Pathophysiology of coagulopathy following injury. (Adapted from Spahn DR et al., *Critical Care* 2013;17(2):R76.)

PRACTICE POINT

Significant coagulopathy may already be present in the early stages of clinical assessment.

The control of haemorrhage and the optimisation of coagulation are key elements of the initial assessment and resuscitation phase. It is equally important to consider and identify any non-haemorrhagic causes of shock (obstructive, cardiogenic or neurogenic) in order to reduce their impact on coagulation and reduce metabolic compromise. Similarly, the full range of wound-protective, lung-protective and neuro-protective strategies should be employed early.

Once primary assessment and immediate threats to life have been addressed, and efforts are under way to minimise any further blood loss and reduce coagulopathy, it is essential to actively look for the features that might reveal an ongoing shock state. These syndromes comprise a combination of the causes of shock and the compensatory physiologic responses.

Table 10.1 Clinical presentation of adult with shock

Parameter	Class I	Class II	Class III	Class IV
Estimated blood loss (litres)	<0.75	0.75 to 1.5	1.5 to 2.0	>2.0
Blood volume loss (%)	<15	15 to 30	30 to 40	>40
Respiratory rate (per minute)	14 to 20	20 to 30	30 to 40	>35 or low
Heart rate (per minute)	<100	100 to 120	120 to 140	>140 or low
Capillary refill time	Normal	Delayed	Delayed	Delayed
Diastolic blood pressure	Normal	Raised	Low	Very low
Systolic blood pressure	Normal	Normal	Low	Very low
Pulse pressure	Normal	Low	Low	Low
Mental state	Slightly anxious	Mildly anxious	Anxious confused	Confused lethargic

Early recognition can be challenging but is best achieved by looking for any physical, physiological or biochemical evidence of hypoperfusion.

In terms of clinical examination, the American College of Surgeons has historically sought to provide guidance to clinicians through the concept of clinical correlates of haemorrhage or the 'grades of shock' (Table 10.1).

Whilst over-reliance on this guidance has drawn some criticism, particularly with respect to the degree to which heart rate and blood pressure changes occur with any given volume of blood loss, it remains a reasonable guide to the progression of shock, bearing in mind that young, fit patients are unlikely to gradually progress from one stage to the next, but significantly more likely to maintain near normal parameters before rapidly decompensating (2,3). In addition, the classification should be supplemented with the knowledge that patients may not fall easily into these categories as co-morbidity and compensatory mechanisms may skew interpretation. For example, all shock states tend to be associated with a tachycardia in their initial stages – with the exception of neurogenic shock (where there is an inability to mount a tachycardia). Paradoxical or relative bradycardia has, however, been described in hypoperfusing trauma patients and, more importantly, the absence of a tachycardia in the presence of other signs of hypoperfusion has been associated with poor outcomes (5). Hypotension itself may, of course, be relative and it is important to interpret vital signs with the patient's baseline in mind. This is particularly important in children, pregnancy, athletes and elderly patients. Pallor, poor capillary refill and cool extremities may represent early peripheral vasoconstriction in the absence of changes in vital signs. So too may be subjectively weak peripheral pulses or an objective but subtle reduction in the pulse pressure. Agitation, confusion or irritability may also be early indicators of relative cerebral hypoperfusion. Sweating may indicate physiologic stress and appear before other abnormalities. Mild tachypnoea may reflect early respiratory compensation for metabolic acidosis. The key is that there should be a low threshold for considering whether these findings might represent a compensated shock state.

Once the patient has arrived in hospital, serum lactate and blood gas analysis (systemic metabolic acidosis and base deficit) can be used to identify hypoperfusion and monitor the progress of the patient's shock state with treatment. It may be that these metabolic changes are evident before the clinician identifies subtle clinical signs (Table 10.2).

Table 10.2 Signs of shock

- Pallor
- Poor capillary refill
- Sweating
- Cool extremities or clamminess
- Weak peripheral pulses
- Reduction in the pulse pressure
- Agitation, confusion or irritability
- Sweating
- Tachypnoea

PRACTICE POINT

The clinician should use all available resources to make a deliberate assessment of whether the trauma patient has any evidence of a shock syndrome. If such a syndrome is obvious, then it should be considered to represent a decompensated state requiring immediate management.

CLINICAL MANAGEMENT

Clinical management of shock needs to be integrated into the wider trauma patient management decision framework. There is limited evidence regarding the best therapeutic approach and judgement will always be required regarding resuscitation priorities and techniques (7–9). In all cases, early access to the circulation is essential, ideally with peripheral intravenous access. If this fails, intraosseous access is recommended (10).

If hypovolaemic shock is identified, management can be considered in terms of whether the bleeding has been controlled and whether the patient is compensating or decompensating. All patients require an approach that reduces further bleeding, optimises coagulation, causes minimal further harm and improves physiology prior to damage control, or definitive surgical repair and/or critical care. This combination has been termed by some as a 'haemostatic resuscitation strategy' (Box 10.2).

BOX 10.2: Compensated Hypovolaemic Shock

The haemostatic resuscitation strategy

- Reduce further bleeding
- Optimise coagulation
- Cause minimal further harm
- Improve physiology
- Consider volume replacement

Blood transfusion is accepted as the basis of treatment for hypovolaemic shock due to trauma. However, for less severe haemorrhage that has been controlled, the clinical literature is limited. In the patient who has sustained haemorrhage (or injuries consistent with haemorrhage), a judgment needs to be made about whether the patient is 'compensating' and the bleeding controlled. This judgement requires assimilation of the physiology in the context of the injury pattern. A patient may have features of controlled haemorrhage and hypovolaemic shock but be maintaining sufficient blood flow to remain alert and conscious. These patients might possibly be safely managed with no intravenous volume expansion or may benefit from moderate restoration of volume with crystalloid solutions.

Current recommendations are that the need for restoration of volume should be carefully considered in the context of the wider fluid and electrolyte requirements of the patient (11). If crystalloids are used for resuscitation at all, they should be warmed and contain sodium in the range 130–154 mmol/L. Colloid solutions based on hydroxyethyl starch should never be used (11). The use of further fluids should be based on the patient's response to initial resuscitation (after a 250–500 mL bolus) and their ongoing fluid requirements. Patients who respond by normalisation of vital signs and other parameters may not require further volume resuscitation, although they may remain at high risk of further bleeding and/or development of coagulopathy.

The patient who is compensating but thought to be actively bleeding should only have crystalloids to replace fluid volume if blood components are not available (packed red cells and pre-thawed fresh frozen plasma pre-hospital with platelets in hospital). Consideration should be given to haemorrhage control and using a more restrictive volume replacement approach until that control is achieved (see later). Patients who are transient responders or show minimal or no response to initial treatment should be considered to have decompensated and have continued uncontrolled bleeding.

DECOMPENSATED HYPOVOLAEMIC SHOCK

For the decompensating patient, there is an immediate risk of death and resuscitation should be directed at controlling bleeding and preservation of life. There is a continuum between shock and cardiac arrest. The risk of imminent cardiac arrest should be recognised and efforts should be made to control any external bleeding; secure the airway; ventilate the patient; minimise the risk of any obstructive causes of shock; gain access to the circulation via intraosseous, peripheral vascular or central venous routes; and prepare for transfusion. The emergency management of the decompensated shock patient is to restore sufficient volume and oxygen-carrying capacity to restore perfusion, with a view to surviving to damage control surgery. Traumatic cardiac arrest protocols are an exemplar of this approach.

For those decompensated shocked patients who are not in cardiac arrest, the concept of permissive hypotension has emerged as a bridge to damage control surgery or interventional radiology. This is the situation where a shocked patient is permitted to remain shocked in order to support haemostatic resuscitation and reduce the risk of further bleeding prior to definitive haemorrhage control. This restrictive approach involves small boluses of 250 mL of blood or crystalloid, depending on availability, to maintain an adequate level of perfusion whilst en route to definitive control.

PRACTICE POINT

Red blood cells and fresh frozen plasma (1:1 ratio) are the fluids of choice for the resuscitation of the shocked trauma patient in volumes sufficient to maintain a palpable radial pulse.

In pre-hospital settings, volume resuscitation should be titrated to maintain a palpable radial pulse. If blood is available, it should be administered in a ratio of 1 unit of pre-thawed fresh frozen plasma or reconstituted plasma to 1 unit of red blood cells. If blood is not available, crystalloid may have to be used. The antifibrinolytic agent tranexamic acid should also be administered as early as possible (and within 3 hours of injury). Once in the hospital setting, there should be no barrier to provision of blood products in a 1:1:1 ratio of red cells, plasma and platelets (10,12,13). This initial fixed ratio protocol should be changed to a protocol guided by laboratory coagulation results as soon as possible. All hospitals should have specific major haemorrhage protocols and access to haematology and transfusion specialists to support this. Physiological parameters such as systolic blood pressure and mean arterial pressure are more likely to be available in hospital, and a permissive hypotensive strategy should be targeted to a systolic blood pressure of approximately 80 to 100 mmHg or a mean arterial pressure of approximately 50 to 65 mmHg. It has been recognised that whilst this permissive hypotensive strategy may buy time, patients may only tolerate it for an hour or so. A hybrid approach has therefore been recommended whereby if definitive control of bleeding has not been achieved within an hour of permissive hypotension, a less restrictive approach is adopted and volume titrated to a systolic blood pressure of approximately 100 to 110 mmHg. In practice, the majority of patients will have reached hospital within an hour of injury.

PRACTICE POINT

Tranexamic acid should be administered within 3 hours of injury.

OVERVIEW

The patient who is obviously in a decompensated shock state with evidence suggesting possible hypovolaemic, cardiogenic and obstructive elements may represent a challenge for the trauma team but the patient's shock state is not concealed. The patient might require immediate transfusion with a range of blood products balanced to replicate whole blood, surgical intervention or a permissive hypotensive strategy as a bridge to surgery or interventional radiology. Whatever the case, the shock syndrome and its component pathophysiology is revealed and targets for resuscitation, no matter how challenging, can be developed.

In contrast, the patient with the same underlying injuries who is compensating represents a much greater challenge. These are the patients who may 'talk and die'. To prevent this, all trauma patients require not only the immediate structured assessment as described in this manual but also a meticulous search for the presence of the shock syndrome. Everyone who is, or might be, bleeding needs to have the possible sources identified and controlled, with minimal further tissue damage, as quickly as possible. This focus on preservation of blood and optimisation of coagulation now takes precedence over the traditional model of immediate fluid challenge. It is the control of haemorrhage, the preservation of intravascular volume and management of the physiological consequences of relative and absolute hypovolaemia that now represent the cornerstones of shock management.

SUMMARY

A haemostatic resuscitation strategy should be used with all trauma patients: control bleeding, optimise coagulation, and make deliberate and informed decisions about volume replacement. In those who are compensating and have bleeding controlled, volume replacement may not be required. If it is, consider blood products and/or crystalloid solutions in the context of wider fluid and electrolyte requirements. In those who are decompensating and where bleeding is not controlled, blood products or crystalloid should be given, depending on availability, to maintain a central pulse. A permissive hypotensive strategy should be followed for one hour. If definitive control cannot be achieved within an hour, a hybrid strategy may be more appropriate, titrating blood or crystalloid to a higher systolic blood pressure for the remaining period until haemostasis is achieved.

REFERENCES

1. Shippey B. Causes and investigation of shock. *Anaesthesia and Intensive Care Medicine* 2010;11:509–511.
2. Vincent J, De Backer D. Circulatory shock. *New England Journal of Medicine* 2013;369: 1726–1734.
3. Spahn DR, Bouillon B, Cerny V, Coats TJ, Duranteau J, Fernandez-Mondejar E, Filipescu D et al. Management of bleeding and coagulopathy following major trauma: An updated European guideline. *Critical Care* 2013;17(2):R76.
4. Demetriades D, Chan LS, Bhasin P, Berne TV, Ramicone E, Huicochea F, Velmahos G et al. Relative bradycardia in patients with traumatic hypotension. *Journal of Trauma* 1998;45:534–539.
5. Landry DW, Oliver JA. The pathogenesis of vasodilatory shock. *New England Journal of Medicine* 2001;345:588–595.
6. Frith D, Brohi K. The pathophysiology of trauma-induced coagulopathy. *Current Opinion in Critical Care* 2012;18:631–636.
7. Curry N, Hopewell S, Doree C, Hyde C, Brohi K, Stanworth S. The acute management of trauma hemorrhage: A systematic review of randomized controlled trials. *Critical Care* 2011;15:R92.
8. Kwan I, Bunn F, Chinnock P, Roberts I. Timing and volume of fluid administration for patients with bleeding. *Cochrane Database of Systematic Reviews* 2014;(3):CD002245.
9. Karam O, Tucci M, Combescure C, Lacroix J, Rimensberger PC. Plasma transfusion strategies for critically ill patients. *Cochrane Database of Systematic Reviews* 2013;(12):CD010654.
10. National Institute for Health and Care Excellence. Major trauma: Assessment and initial management. NICE Guideline NG39, February 2016.
11. National Institute for Health and Care Excellence. Intravenous fluid therapy: Intravenous fluid therapy in adults in hospital. NICE Clinical Guideline CG174, December 2013.
12. Holcomb JB, Tilley BC, Baraniuk S. Fox EE, Wade CE, Podbielski JM, del Junco DJ et al. Transfusion of plasma, platelets, and red blood cells in a 1:1:1 vs a 1:1:2 ratio and mortality in patients with severe trauma: The PROPPR randomized clinical trial. *JAMA* 2015;313:471–482.
13. Holcomb JB, Donathan DP, Cotton BA, del Junco DJ, Brown G, Wenckstern TV, Podbielski JM et al. Prehospital transfusion of plasma and red blood cells in trauma patients. *Prehospital Emergency Care* 2015;19:1–9.

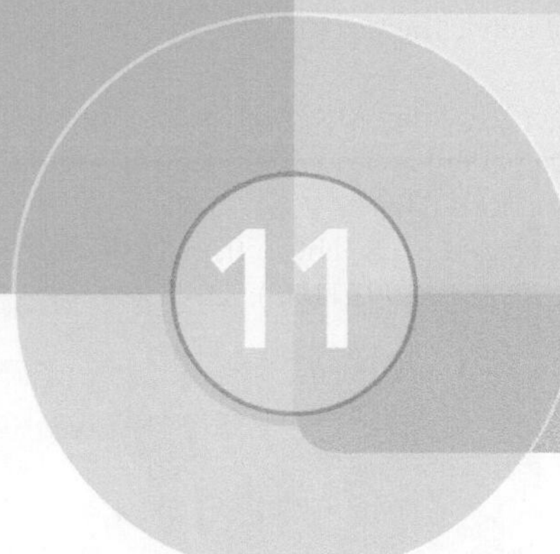

11 Entrapment and extrication

OBJECTIVES

After completing this chapter the reader will

- Be able to determine the need for extrication in the light of a rapid but thorough assessment of the patient and the scene
- Understand the processes used by the emergency services to extricate a patient
- Be able to balance the urgency of the need for extrication with the risks associated with the procedure

INTRODUCTION

The extrication of a trapped patient can be a complex operation. It presents unique hazards and clinical challenges. No two extrications are the same, but the approach of the emergency services follows distinct stages which must be understood by those providing medical assistance at scene. The key role of the clinician is to determine the urgency with which the patient is extracted, bearing in mind that the risks are likely to increase with increasing speed of removal. The clinician must also be able to communicate clearly and effectively with personnel who are used to a hierarchical command structure. Safe extrication is about balancing risks, and the role of the clinician in providing guidance and ensuring responsiveness to clinical priorities is vital.

The patient's condition may demand any of the approaches described later, whether or not they are entrapped. Extrication does not imply entrapment, merely that the patient is in a position where they are unable to safely or comfortably remove themselves from a situation following trauma. Entrapment is conventionally divided into *absolute* or *relative (clinical) entrapment* (Box 11.1).

BOX 11.1: Entrapment–Definitions

Absolute entrapment

Absolute entrapment occurs when a trauma victim is physically trapped by wreckage or other material which renders it impossible for them to move and requires removal.

Relative (clinical) entrapment

Relative entrapment occurs when pain associated with movement is so severe that the casualty cannot be moved until the pain is eliminated by analgesia or anaesthesia.

TYPES OF EXTRICATION

Many patients will be able to remove themselves from a hazardous area at the scene of an accident and will probably already have done so by the time the emergency services arrive. If they have not, they should always be asked if they can 'extricate' themselves and assisted to do so if this is possible. There is no evidence to suggest that patients will put their spines at risk in such circumstances, nor that an assisted self-extrication poses risks to the victim as long as it is carried out carefully and halted in the event of pain. When extrication from a vehicle is needed (Figure 11.1), it is conventionally divided into three types:

- Snatch or immediate rescue
- Controlled release
- Rapid access

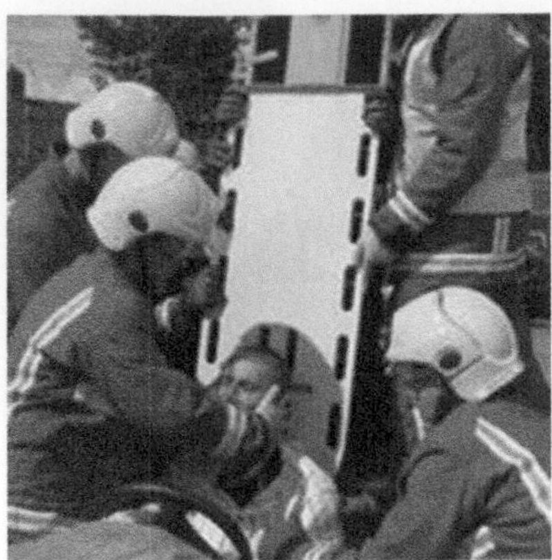

Figure 11.1 Extrication from a road traffic collision.

SNATCH OR IMMEDIATE RESCUE

Snatch rescue is the immediate removal of the patient from the vehicle. Snatch rescue will be needed where there is an immediate risk to the patient or rescuers, for example from fire (or risk of fire), or where the patient's condition necessitates it, for example when they are in cardiac arrest. This rescue may be little more than a controlled pull from the vehicle, with minimal use of tools to create an exit. A snatch rescue will have normally been instituted by the fire service or even members of the public.

CONTROLLED RELEASE

The controlled release is usually plan A in the stable casualty where minimising patient movement is key, whilst maximising their comfort. In this situation the vehicle is dismantled around the patient creating an exit point through which the patient can be carefully removed with full consideration given to potential injuries. Inevitably, this takes a significant amount of time. Before any attempt is made to gain access to a trapped patient or to move them, a clear plan must be in place with which those involved are familiar.

RAPID ACCESS

Rapid access can be seen as plan B, when, in the time-critical casualty, access is necessary to manage the medical condition and extricate the patient. Examples of such situations include when airway manoeuvres in the vehicle are failing, to treat life-threatening ventilation problems or where haemodynamic instability necessitates immediate transfer to definitive care. An extrication path is rapidly created, if necessary by simple removal of a door, possibly with the addition of a B-post rip to allow extrication of the casualty. Extrication is performed as carefully as possible, whilst appreciating the time critical situation and the need for the patient to be out of the vehicle.

The *rapid access* must be planned first in case of deterioration, prior to the full controlled removal being designed and carried out. Rapid access may be the only appropriate option for some seriously injured patients. The fire service will look to the medical team for guidance as to which plan is appropriate. The medical team will need to communicate with the fire commander if the patient deteriorates and resort to plan B is needed.

THE APPROACH OF THE FIRE AND RESCUE SERVICE

The systematic team approach followed by the fire service involves six stages (Box 11.2).

The first three stages should happen simultaneously so as to minimise delay in patient removal.

BOX 11.2: The Fire Service Structured Approach to Extrication

- Scene assessment and scene safety establishment
- Stabilisation and initial access
- Glass management
- Space creation
- Full access
- Extrication

STAGE 1: SCENE ASSESSMENT AND SCENE SAFETY

The fire officer in charge will do a 360° walk around the incident to gather information, noting its extent, hazards, the number and location of casualties, and mechanisms of injury. Based on this information they will begin to formulate tactical rescue plans. At the same time other fire officers will be establishing scene safety, setting up and establishing zones, preparing equipment and initiating early casualty contact. Road traffic collisions present numerous hazards to both casualties and rescuers (also see Box 11.3):

BOX 11.3: Hazards at the Scene of a Road Traffic Collision

- Traffic
- Fire
- Damaged vehicle
- Damaged objects
- Vehicle stability
- Electricity
- Airbags
- Automatic rollover protection devices
- Trip hazards
- Hydraulic equipment hoses
- Hazardous materials

- *Traffic* – The commonest cause of death of rescuers is being struck by another vehicle.
- *Fire* – Fuel leaks coupled with electrical systems, hot exhaust systems and bystanders smoking provide opportunities for ignition. Once alight a number of vehicle components have explosive capabilities.
- *Damaged vehicles* – The wreckage of the vehicle will contain glass, multiple sharp metal edges and hot surfaces.
- *Damaged objects* – Roadside signs and lighting may be unstable.
- *Vehicle stability* – Prior to stabilisation the vehicle may move, potentially causing injuring and trapping rescuers.
- *Electricity* – Short circuiting may lead to sparking and ignition of fuel. There is also the risk of electrocution both from the vehicle's electrical system and from any street furniture that may have been damaged.
- *Airbags* – Un-deployed airbags may provide a significant risk to rescuers who should try to avoid placing themselves in the deployment zone.

- *Automatic rollover protection devices* – Found on convertible cars and normally deployed when a rollover occurs, they can present a hazard if the have failed to deploy
- *Trip hazards* – From equipment and debris.
- Hydraulic equipment hoses may cause high-pressure injection injuries.
- Hazardous materials being transported.

The fire service may well have identified and addressed hazards prior to the arrival of the medical support, however the medical team should perform their own risk assessment on their arrival. The key to minimising risks is to ensure that the team is fully kitted in appropriate personal protective equipment (PPE).

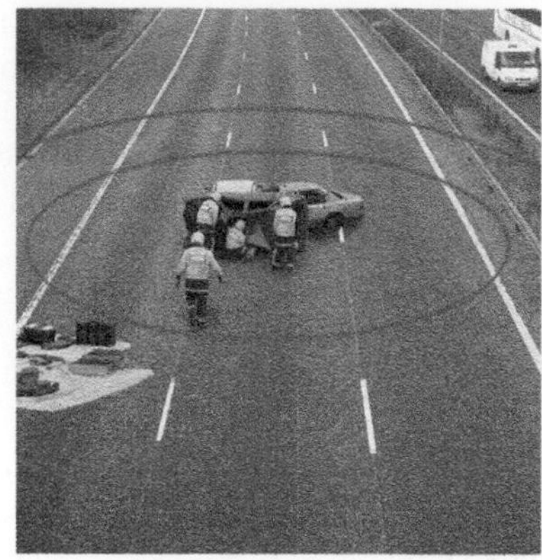

Figure 11.2 The inner (5 m) and outer (10 m) zones.

The fire service will create notional zones around the immediate wreckage (Figure 11.2). The inner zone should only contain personnel directly involved in casualty care and extrication procedures. Eye protection must be worn when inside the inner zone.

The outer zone will include a salvage sheet with a kit dump for equipment needed for the extrication. Personnel without a task are to be found on the edge of the outer zone ready to be allocated tasks as necessary.

STAGE 2: STABILISATION AND INITIAL ACCESS

The fire service will stabilise the vehicle in its current position using blocks, wedges, stepped chocks, pneumatic struts and winches to prevent movement of the vehicle. This may result from the additional load of rescuers or occur following dismantling of the vehicle and whilst moving casualties. Contact with the casualty should occur as soon as possible to allow for triage and life-saving interventions. Access can be through any door that will open or occasionally glass management in the form of removal of window or windscreen may be required.

STAGE 3: GLASS MANAGEMENT

Glass management is the process of making glass safe to allow further access and extrication. This commonly involves shattering the glass using a glass punch, though windows can be simply wound down if they are manual or if the battery has not yet been disconnected. Because of their lamination windscreens normally require sawing. The rear windscreen is often removed intact as part of the tailgate. The casualty, and rescuers, should be protected from inhalation of glass dust.

Once casualty care has been established the patient is then protected from further injury caused by the debris created by the efforts of the rescue team. Protection may be 'hard', such as a teardrop, or 'soft' protection from durable sheeting. The patient should also be given eye protection, ear protection and, if appropriate, reassurance and an explanation of what is happening around them.

STAGE 4: SPACE CREATION

Space creation involves making the largest working space possible around the patient. This may be simply achieved by adjusting the seat position, that is sliding the patient away from the dashboard and reclining the seat. However, electrical seat control systems may no longer be active and seat runners are often structurally disrupted in severe impacts.

Reclining the patient at an early stage may offer a number of advantages including improving perfusion to the brain in patients who are shocked, positioning the patient at an early stage in their clot formation process which will not greatly change prior to arrival at definitive care, moving the patient and rescuer out of the deployment zone of any un-deployed airbags, and making it easier for a single rescuer to maintain cervical spine immobilisation whilst improving eye contact and reassurance. However, fully reclining the patient prior to insertion of an extrication board may make the process more difficult. Also, in circumstances such as when the patient is dependent on postural drainage of facial haemorrhage, any attempt to recline them should be avoided until the very last minute before formal airway control is achieved.

Space creation can be lifesaving, for example in the patient with marked constriction of the chest where asphyxiation is a real possibility without rapid expansion in space to allow them to breathe properly.

Further space creation includes removal of rear parcel shelves and possibly rear seating. Roof removal is often required to give the vertical space required for extrication. Roof removal need not be complete; the roof may be flapped in any direction to give access.

STAGE 5: FULL ACCESS

During this stage, the vehicle is dismantled around the patient in order to maximise access to them so that extrication can occur with minimal manoeuvring along the extrication path.

The fire service will refer to removal of the structural posts of a car as shown in Figure 11.3. Additional techniques may need to be employed when the vehicle shape has been distorted.

A dashboard roll may be needed when the patient's lower limbs are still trapped by the intrusion into the passenger compartment. This involves cuts low down on the A-posts and pushing forward or lifting the dashboard, either with hydraulic rams or spreaders. Alternatively the metalwork of the front wing may need to be pushed forward to gain access to the foot well.

Significant side impacts may rotate the occupant's seat, preventing it from reclining, or altering the extrication path with the result that the patient may have to exit in an oblique direction. Where the vehicle has been wrapped around a tree or piece of street furniture, and no access is available on the side of the impact, a B-post rip (division and folding outwards) on the opposite side will allow removal of a casualty who may well have been rotated with the back of the seat to face the midline of the car.

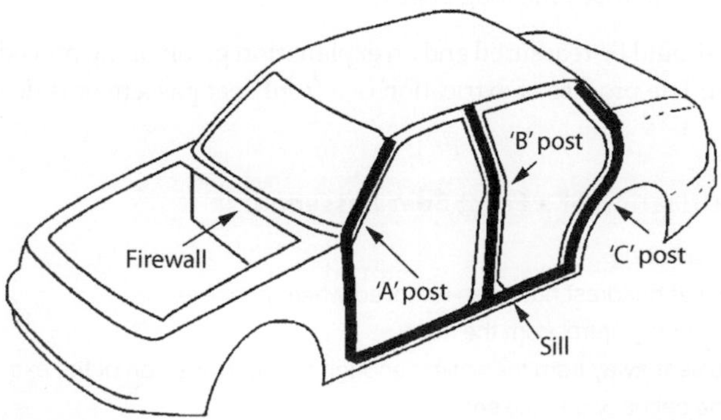

Figure 11.3 The structural components of a car.

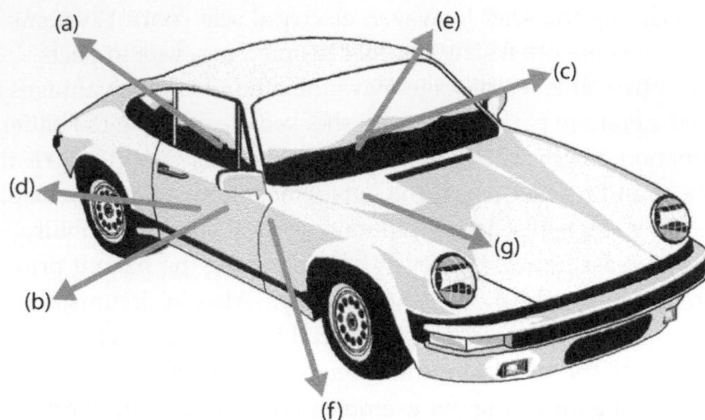

Figure 11.4 Potential vehicle extrication paths: (a) extrication board out to rear; (b) rapid extrication, driver's door; (c) rapid extrication, opposite door; (d) extrication board and rear quarter oblique; (e) extrication board and rear quarter contralateral oblique; (f) extrication board and feet first front quarter oblique; (g) appropriate for minibuses without a front mounted engine.

STAGE 6: EXTRICATION

There are a number of extrication paths that a patient can follow (Figure 11.4). The ideal path in a plan A extrication is on an extrication board out of the rear of the vehicle. However, where the vehicle shape has been distorted, the patient has been unrestrained, or where multiple occupants prevent full access, other directions may need to be used. The alignment of the patient relative to the vehicle structure and any obstructions to extrication will determine the extrication path.

EXTRICATING THE DRIVER

The intended plan must be confirmed with the rescue services and other clinicians, and roles clearly defined and allocated. Ideally at least six people are needed to extricate a patient with minimal movement. The patient's feet must be free and the lower limbs moved away from the steering column. The following personnel are needed:

- Two people on either side lifting at the thighs and pelvis
- Two people lifting either side of the torso
- One to maintain C-spine control
- One to insert and brace the long board

The casualty should be reassured and an explanation given of the procedure. Adequate analgesia is essential. The process of extrication of a front seat passenger is described in Box 11.4.

BOX 11.4: Extrication of a Front Seat Passenger

- Minimise monitoring.
- Check that the headrest has been removed where possible.
- Maintain C-spine control from the front.
- Recline the seat away from the patient enough to allow insertion of the extrication board between the casualty and the seat.
- Recline the patient back onto the extrication board.

- Recline the seat as far as possible to the point at which the extrication path will still clear any of the rear seats or posts.
- Hand over C-spine control to a rescuer at the head end of the board during this time.
- At the command of the rescuer maintaining C-spine control, slide the patient up the extrication board. This rescuer should confirm a distance to be moved with all the other rescuers
- Once the casualty is fully on the extrication board, rest the extrication board in a secure position, often on the top of the rear seats, to enable securing of the patient to the board prior to further movement.
- Carry the patient away from the vehicle to be scooped off the extrication board for transport to definitive care.

EXTRICATING REAR SEAT PASSENGERS

The inability to recline the rear seats increases the difficulty of extrication of casualties from this position. Moving the front seat forward where possible will create space, and door removal and removal of the C-post bodywork will make access easier. Vertical removal of a patient should be avoided as it invariably places too much strain on rescuers as well as being difficult to control. Creating an extrication path through the rear quarter or rotating the patient out through the rear door are two feasible options.

OVERTURNED CARS

An overturned car with a patient still restrained in their seat provides an interesting challenge. Where the casualty has slid out of their seat or where the A-posts have been flattened by the force of the rollover, their head may come to rest against the roof, possibly forcing their neck into flexion. Severe flexion can cause an ischaemic cord injury and, when present, this is a time-critical situation.

There are two possible methods of extrication.

METHOD 1

The patient is lowered face first onto a extrication board. Access is gained via the rear of the car and space created for the extrication path through the rear.

With the patient still retrained by their seat belt the seat is reclined so that the patient ends up suspended facing the ground or roof. Two straps or fire hoses are passed across the front of the patient, one at the level of the pelvis, the other at the level of the chest, and held under tension to suspend the patient against their seat. The seat belt can then be cut and by gradual release of tension on the fire hoses, the casualty is lowered face first down onto a padded extrication board. Once the patient has been slid out of the vehicle on the extrication board, the patient can then be log rolled (if there is no concern regarding pelvic injuries) off the extrication board directly onto a scoop stretcher, or sandwiched between an extrication board and scoop stretcher and rotated supine.

METHOD 2

The *front roll manoeuvre*. If the patient has slipped out of their seat and come to rest with the crown of their head facing towards the front of the car, then it is likely that they have rotated out of their seat to the point that their upper spine and neck are close to perpendicular with the ground.

This rotation from the seat can be then continued so that the patient exits through the front window void. Space can be created in the overturned car through a *rear oyster* in which the B- and C-posts are cut and hydraulic rams lift the floor of the car vertically away from the roof.

HGVS/VANS

Vehicles other than cars provide specific challenges. The patterns of intrusion will differ given the different forces involved in the impact. It is often not possible or advantageous to recline seating as the extrication pathway is likely to be obstructed by trailers or loads. The cab of a heavy goods vehicle (HGV) is well above ground level so extrication must take place 10 feet up in the air. However, the principles are the same. A platform will normally be created around the cab to enable safe working at height. The fire service will follow the same management stages, but the possible extrication pathways will be limited.

EXTRICATION DEVICES

A number of *commercial extrication jackets* are available (Figure 11.5). These devices are designed to be applied securely to the casualty whilst in the vehicle, and are structured to maintain the head, neck and torso in alignment during the extrication process. They aim to minimise movement and provide handles for lifting and manoeuvring the patient.

ALTERNATIVE EXTRICATION TECHNIQUES

Mainstream UK practice involves stabilising the vehicle in the position in which it came to rest, which fortunately in the majority of cases is on all four wheels. In cases where the vehicle comes to rest on its side or roof, extrication can be performed once the vehicle has been stabilised in that position. Alternatively, as is practised in other countries, the vehicle is repositioned on all four wheels in a controlled manner, prior to extrication continuing. Proponents of this technique argue the extra time taken to right the vehicle is outweighed by the time saved carrying out the conventional extrication that follows. More commonly when there is significant intrusion into the passenger compartment from an immovable object, such as a tree or other vehicle, it is necessary to winch the vehicle away from the immovable object in order to allow access and release of entrapment.

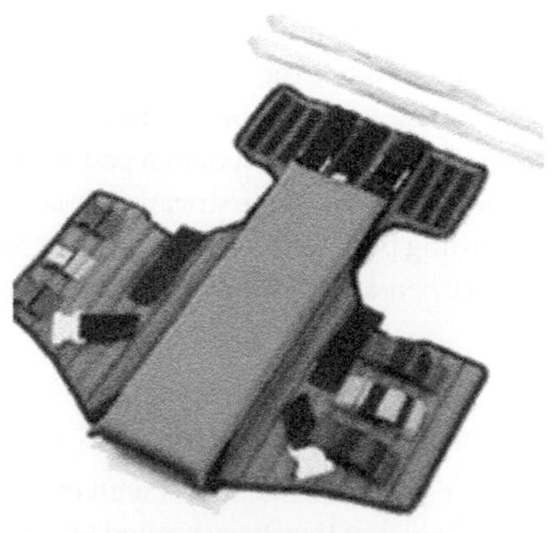

Figure 11.5 A commercial extrication device.

The ever developing technology seen in vehicles poses increasing challenges to the fire service: for example structural composites that cannot be cut through and crash protection systems with multiple airbags. Most fire services have specialised teams with extended training and experience in managing difficult extrications. In situations where extrication is expected to be challenging, ensuring the attendance of such a team with additional skills and equipment is valuable.

THE NEED FOR EXTRICATION

Decision-making regarding the mode of extrication is challenging for the medical team. Traditional decision-making balances the need for controlled extrication aiming to avoid movement and further injury, especially spinal injury, against the time taken to achieve it and the consequent delay to definitive care.

Pre-hospital management of spinal injuries is an evolving field. There is a body of expert opinion that, given the magnitude of difference between the energy involved causing the primary traumatic insult and that transferred during patient handling, there is little chance of causing or worsening an existing spinal injury during medical handling of the patient. This position challenges current practice which places significant emphasis on minimising movement of the spinal column whenever possible.

For the co-operative patient, there is evidence suggesting that the most effective method of getting a patient out of a car with the least amount of movement of their head and neck is for the patient to simply step out of the vehicle, assuming they are physically capable of doing so and are not trapped.

With the unconscious or seriously injured patient, the need to provide definitive care is pressing. Adding on-scene time with extensive and prolonged extrication techniques and precautions aimed at minimising movement of the spinal column for a *potential* spinal injury may not be in the patient's best interests given the higher likelihood of injury elsewhere. Recognising that hypoxia and poor perfusion are detrimental to spinal cord injuries should drive the medical team to treat these and expedite transfer to hospital. Given the current balance of evidence, spinal immobilisation measures should not hamper care or delay transfer. As such, complex evacuation plans might not be appropriate for the unconscious or critically injured patient.

IMMOBILISATION AND PACKAGING

Preparing the patient for transfer to definitive care is an important stage in the patient's journey. Ensuring the patient is safe, secure, as comfortable as possible and protected from further deterioration helps to deliver the patient to hospital in the best possible condition.

IMMOBILISATION

Patients in the United Kingdom are fortunate in that transfer times to definitive care are usually relatively short compared to other regions of the world. Most patients will be at hospital well under an hour from leaving the scene. The pre-hospital clinician has to judge whether immobilisation of the spine is warranted and then package the patient so that they arrive at definitive care in the best condition possible.

PRACTICE POINT

The majority of conscious patients without distracting injuries will 'manage' their own cervical spines.

Spinal cord injuries carry significant morbidity and mortality, though fortunately the incidence is relatively rare. Injury to the bony spinal column occurs in about 10% of *major* trauma patients; injury to the spinal cord in under 2%. The vast majority of patients immobilised in the pre-hospital arena have no injury. However, in most cases, pre-hospital management centres on recognising the potential for injury to the spinal cord, as opposed to identifying an actual injury. The potential for injury is based on the mechanism of injury and the clinical findings, whilst management relies on attempting to avoid further injury by minimising movement through immobilisation.

Current practice, aimed at minimising further movement of the spinal column in the belief that it will avoid further deterioration of a neurological injury, is not one fully supported by evidence. The evidence is weak both for and against current practice. There is evidence supporting the view that immobilisation might be harmful and worsen outcome. It has been argued that, given the significant force required to cause the primary fracture and injury, further movement is unlikely to cause further damage to the cord. The lack of evidence to determine best practice makes it difficult to move away from the widespread practice of immobilisation, especially given the fear that further deterioration could carry devastating consequences. Treating hypoxia and hypoperfusion as part of the patient's overall care may also help to reduce secondary spinal injury and should not be impaired by immobilisation.

The gold standard for immobilisation is considered to be the correct application of an appropriately sized cervical collar secured in neutral alignment to a firm surface with blocks and tape or straps. Manual in-line immobilisation (or stabilisation) – *MILS* – is the term given to the practice of holding the patients head in a neutral position before instigation of triple immobilisation. Immobilisation is nearly always performed once the patient has returned to neutral alignment. In rare cases where the nature of the injury prevents this happening, and gentle attempts to bring the head into the midline have failed, the patient should be immobilised in a pain- and paraesthesia-free position. Pre-existing disease, such as ankylosing spondylitis, may prevent neutral alignment as may immediate pain or neurological symptoms on movement. In such cases immobilisation should be in the position in which the patient is found.

Manual in-line stabilisation without a cervical collar in place is pragmatic whilst assessment and treatment is ongoing. Application of a collar need only occur, if indicated, when the patient is due to be moved and packaged for transfer to hospital. Wearing a correctly applied collar is uncomfortable and not without the risk of harm: minimising duration of application is in the patient's interests and likely to be appreciated by the alert patient.

The emphasis in spinal cord management is invariably on the cervical spine. However, injuries can occur along the length of the spinal cord. Clinical vigilance and the current practice of minimising movement through immobilisation relates to the whole length of the spinal column and should not be missed.

PRACTICE POINT

Mobile patients who are not complaining of neck pain do not need to be compelled into triple immobilisation!

RULES FOR CLEARING C-SPINE

Recognising that the majority of patients are immobilised unnecessarily has driven the development of algorithms that enable the pre-hospital clinician to reliably identify those patients who do not warrant immobilisation. These decision tools are extensions of the guidelines developed for in-hospital clearance of the cervical spine in the emergency department.

UK practice continues to use the NEXUS criteria as a tool for identifying patients who do not need immobilisation. If the patient satisfies all criteria then injury to the cervical spine can be reliably excluded (Box 11.5).

PRAGMATIC COLLARING

Some practitioners utilise the Canadian C-Spine Rule in addition to, or instead of the, NEXUS criteria. Again the rule asks a series of questions to identify who not to immobilise (Box 11.6).

The importance of experience and judgment should not be ignored in avoiding unnecessary immobilisation, which is not a risk-free procedure. If an ambulatory patient is deemed to be in need of immobilisation the technique of a vertical takedown is no longer appropriate and should not be used. In the majority of cases the co-operative patient should be asked to lie themselves down on the ambulance stretcher with the least degree of movement of their cervical spine.

BOX 11.5: The NEXUS Criteria

If the patient

- Is alert
- Is not intoxicated
- Has no vertebral tenderness or deformity
- Has no focal neurological deficit
- Has no painful distracting injury

then spinal immobilisation is not necessary.

BOX 11.6: The Canadian C-Spine Rule

1. Is any high-risk factor present that mandates radiography?
   Age 65 years or more
   Dangerous mechanism of injury
   - A fall from greater than one metre or five stairs
   - An axial load to the head, e.g. diving
   - A high-speed motor vehicle collision (combined speed >100 km/hr)
   - A rollover motor vehicle accident
   - Ejection from a motor vehicle
   - An accident involving motorised recreational vehicles
   - A bicycle collision

   Paraesthesia in the extremities
2. If none of the above is present, is any low-risk factor present that allows safe assessment of range of motion?
   - Simple rear-end motor vehicle collision
   - Sitting position in ED
   - Ambulatory at any time since injury
   - Delayed onset of neck pain
   - Absence of midline C-spine tenderness
3. If no high-risk factors are present, and the patient does not have any of the low risk factors rotation can be assessed: can the patient actively rotate their neck 45 degrees to the left and right?

Patients capable of neck rotation do not need to be immobilised.

PACKAGING

Preparing the patient for transfer to definitive care is an important stage in the patient's journey. Ensuring the patient is safe, secure, as comfortable as possible and protected from further deterioration helps to deliver the patient to hospital in the best possible condition.

Current best practice focuses on minimal patient handling. The principle of minimising movement is part of this approach. Planning ahead is essential, aiming to minimise and streamline the patient's movements, reducing overall scene time as well as overall movement, both on scene and at definitive care. The long spinal board is no longer considered appropriate for transport to definitive care – it should be used for extrication only. Not only are spinal boards uncomfortable with an increased risk of tissue pressure damage, but log-rolling to place the patient on the board may not be appropriate.

The scoop stretcher is the recommended platform for the majority of transfers to hospital within the UK. The ability to insert the blades of the scoop under the patient with little more than a 10° tilt to each side helps to minimise movement. Their removal is just as quick and simple, although in many cases the patient will remain on a scoop stretcher throughout resuscitation and CT scanning, following which it will be removed, as this facilitates easy and rapid handling.

For lengthy journeys to definitive care there is an increased risk of tissue pressure injuries caused by immobility and unchanged pressure contact points with the scoop stretcher. In these situations a vacuum mattress will conform to the patient's body distributing contact pressure more evenly. In addition patients report a greater degree of comfort.

Avoiding hypothermia is very important for trauma patients as it directly impacts on outcome. Proprietary waterproof, windproof and insulating blankets help to mitigate temperature loss. Active warming blankets are also available.

Once suitably packaged, a pragmatic approach to transport to hospital can be used. The compliant patient will appreciate the reasoning behind the use of immobilisation and keep their head still. Loosening the cervical collar, coupled with reassurance and reminding of the need to remain still, may well make their journey more bearable. Similarly in anaesthetised patients, who are unable to move, loosening the collar may aid cerebral perfusion.

SUMMARY

Effective extrication and packaging requires effective and coordinated team working, as well as some basic technical knowledge. The expertise of the rescue services and clinicians are absolutely complementary. Recent changes in guidelines have promulgated a more pragmatic and thoughtful approach to possible spinal injury, recognising that full immobilisation is not a procedure without risks. In this area, as in all other aspects of pre-hospital care, there is no substitute for practice in realistically simulated scenarios.

FURTHER READING

Benger J, Blackham J. Why do we put cervical collars on conscious trauma patients? *Scandinavian Journal of Trauma, Resuscitation and Emergency Medicine* 2009;17:44.

Calland V. Extrication of the seriously injured road crash victim. *Emergency Medicine Journal* 2005;22:817–821.

Connor D, Greaves I, Porter K, Bloch M, on behalf of the Consensus Group Faculty of Pre-Hospital Care. Pre-hospital spinal immobilisation: An initial consensus statement. *Emergency Medicine Journal* 2013;30:1067–1069.

Engsberg JR, Standeven JW, Shurtleff TL, Eggars JL, Shafer JS, Naunheim RS. Cervical spine motion during extrication. *Journal of Emergency Medicine* 2013;44:122–127.

Hauswald M. A re-conceptualisation of acute spinal care. *Emergency Medicine Journal* 2013; 30:720–723.

Hauswald M, Ong G, Tandberg D, Omar Z. Out-of-hospital spinal immobilization: Its effect on neurologic injury. *Academic Emergency Medicine* 1998;5:214–219.

Kwan I, Bunn F, Roberts I, on behalf of the WHO Pre-Hospital Trauma Care Steering Committee. Spinal immobilisation for trauma patients. *Cochrane Database Systematic Review* 2001;(2):CD002803.

Moss R, Porter K, Greaves I. Minimal patient handling: A faculty of pre-hospital care consensus statement. *Emergency Medicine Journal* 2014;30:1065–1066.

Stuke LE, Pons PT, Guy JS, Chapleau WP, Butler FK, McSwain NE. Prehospital spine immobilization for penetrating trauma—Review and recommendations from the Prehospital Trauma Life Support Executive Committee. *Journal of Trauma* 2011;71:763–769.

Valliencourt C, Stiell IG, Beaudoin T, Maloney J, Anton AR, Bradford P, Cain E et al. The out-of-hospital validation of the Canadian C-Spine Rule by paramedics. *Annals of Emergency Medicine* 2009;54:663–671.

12 Head injury

OBJECTIVES

After completing this chapter the reader will

- Have an understanding of the pathophysiology of head injuries
- Have a systematic approach to the assessment of the head injured patient in the pre-hospital environment
- Be able to formulate a strategic management plan for the treatment of head-injured patients in the pre-hospital environment

INTRODUCTION

'Head injury' is a term that encompasses injury to the scalp, skull and brain. *Traumatic brain injury* (TBI) is often used as it captures the importance of the neurological insult to the brain tissue. TBI is an insult to the brain tissue from an external force, leading to temporary or permanent impairment of cognitive, physical and psychosocial functions, with an associated diminished or altered state of consciousness (1).

Traumatic brain injury remains a leading cause of death and disability in young individuals. However, its epidemiology is changing and improvements in road safety are now being offset by increases in fall-related injuries in an ageing population. In all age groups there is a male predominance (2). Other populations at high risk of sustaining TBI include low-income individuals, the unmarried, members of ethnic minority groups, residents of inner cities, individuals with a history of substance abuse and those who have suffered a previous TBI (1).

In the United Kingdom 1.4 million people attend emergency departments with a head injury each year. A meta-analysis of 23 European countries revealed a combined hospitalisation and fatal TBI incidence of 235 per 100,000 people, although there was large variability between centres (3,4). In the UK 10.9% of these injuries are classified as either moderate or severe (5). Survivors commonly have neurocognitive defects (such as impaired attention, inability to form visuospatial associations or poor executive function), psychological health issues (30%–70% develop depression), or increased impulsivity, and many display lack of self-regulatory behaviours which can affect relationships and integration in society (3). As a consequence, TBI of all levels of severity is a major cause of death, disability and economic cost to society.

The leading causes of TBI are road traffic collisions (RTCs), falls, assaults and violence, sports and recreation activities. Alcohol use is implicated in 25%–65% of cases (6). There is no effective treatment which will reverse the effects of primary TBI, but measures can be taken to prevent it through changes in socio-economic, behavioural and environmental factors (for example legislation and enforcement of seat belts, helmets and airbags).

The medical management of brain-injured patients is complex and includes specialised pre-hospital care, transport to an appropriate treatment centre, in-hospital acute care and, for some, long-term rehabilitation (5). Ischaemia has a key role in all forms of brain injury and preventing ischaemia (or *secondary*) injury is at the core of all neuroprotective strategies. Prompt medical care in the pre-hospital setting has the potential to influence outcomes by preventing, or at least reducing, secondary brain injury.

PATHOPHYSIOLOGY OF TRAUMATIC BRAIN INJURY (TBI)

Primary brain injury occurs at the moment of trauma. It results from the physical mechanism of injury, for example blunt or penetrating trauma, acceleration/deceleration forces or even blast waves from an explosion. These physical mechanisms can be classified as impact loading, impulsive loading and static loading (1,7).

IMPACT LOADING

Impact loading may be caused by a direct blow to the head. Such a collision of the head with a solid object causes traumatic brain injury through mechanical force resulting in deformation of brain tissue as a result of compression, stretching or shearing.

IMPULSIVE LOADING

In impulsive loading, for example due to a motor vehicle accident, the head is set in motion and then the moving head is stopped abruptly without being directly struck or impacted by a mechanical force. This usually results in diffuse axonal injury.

STATIC LOADING

In static loading, the effect of speed of occurrence may not be significant. Static loading results from a slowly moving object trapping the head against a fixed rigid structure and gradually squeezing the skull. This causes comminuted fractures that may be enough to deform the brain.

Primary injuries may manifest as focal lesions such as skull fractures, intracranial haematomas, cranial nerve lesions, lacerations, contusions and penetrating wounds, or more widespread damage including diffuse axonal injury (7,8). *Coup and contre-coup cerebral contusions* result from a combination of vascular and tissue damage. There is injury at both the site of impact to the skull (*coup*) and on the opposite side of the head (*contre-coup*). The impact accelerates first the skull and then its contents away from it. As the skull stops, the brain then impacts on the internal surface of the skull resulting in damage. *Diffuse axonal injury* is characterised by extensive, generalised damage to the white matter tracts of the brain as a result of shearing forces (Box 12.1).

Neurological damage due to trauma evolves over the ensuing hours and days: this is termed *secondary brain injury*. Improved outcomes result when these delayed insults, which have the

BOX 12.1: A Classification of Brain Injury

Localised injury

- Skull fracture
- Cerebral lacerations
- Cerebral contusions
- Penetrating wounds
- Cranial nerve injuries

Generalised injuries

- Diffuse axonal injury
- Hypoxic brain injury

effect of reducing cerebral blood flow, are prevented or appropriately treated (9). Reduced cerebral blood flow and associated reduction in the delivery of oxygenated blood to cerebral tissues leads to ischaemia and neuronal cell death. Causative factors include hypoxia, hypotension, raised intracranial pressure (ICP) and anaemia (for example through haemorrhage). Hyperthermia and epileptic seizures cause an increased cerebral metabolic rate and oxygen consumption which can be catastrophic in the face of reduced oxygen delivery. The brain is dependent on a continual supply of glucose for cellular function and hypoglycaemia risks neuronal cell death. Hyperglycaemia on the other hand increases cerebral metabolism and therefore oxygen demand, which in the context of impaired perfusion and the resultant restrictions to oxygen delivery can also contribute to poor outcomes.

At a cellular level a complex cascade of processes occurs that results in secondary brain injury. Damaged neurons bring about the release of inflammatory neurochemical mediators. These mediators are responsible for altered vessel permeability, oedema, neuronal ischaemia, necrosis and cell death. Heightened metabolism in the injured brain is stimulated by a further increase in the circulating levels of catecholamines contributing to a vicious cycle of ischaemia, cell death and tissue oedema (1,10).

INJURY TYPES

INTRACRANIAL HAEMORRHAGE

EPIDURAL/EXTRADURAL HAEMATOMA (EDH)

Epidural/extradural haematoma (EDH) is common following head trauma. A collection of blood forms between the inner surface of the skull and outer layer of dura. In 80% of cases EDH is associated with a skull fracture. The bleeding source is usually a torn middle meningeal artery. Occasionally it can result from venous blood from a torn sinus. Commonly patients have a period of lucidity followed by decreasing consciousness, although this is not invariable and cannot be relied upon in diagnosis.

SUBDURAL HAEMATOMA (SDH)

In *subdural haematoma (SDH)* a collection of blood accumulates in the potential space between the dura and subarachnoid mater of the meninges. It results from stretching and tearing of bridging cortical veins as they cross the subdural space to drain into an adjacent dural sinus.

SUBARACHNOID HAEMORRHAGE (SAH)

Subarachnoid haemorrhage (SAH) is a collection of blood within the subarachnoid space and is caused by lacerations of the superficial microvessels in the subarachnoid space.

INTRACEREBRAL HAEMORRHAGE (ICH)

The term *intracerebral haemorrhage (ICH)* encompasses a number of entities that share the finding of an acute accumulation of blood in the parenchyma of the brain. ICH occurs secondary to lacerations or contusion of the brain following trauma.

NEUROPHYSIOLOGICAL EFFECTS OF TRAUMATIC BRAIN INJURY

The Monroe–Kellie doctrine states that the skull is essentially a 'rigid box' with three components:

- *Brain tissue* (85%)
- *Cerebrospinal fluid* (10%)
- *Blood* (5%).

None of these components are appreciably compressible. If one component increases in volume the other components must accommodate this additional volume. When the body can no longer compensate for these changes the intracranial pressure (ICP) rises. Raised ICP can be caused by any space-occupying lesion including haematoma, obstructed flow of cerebral spinal fluid (hydrocephalous), brain oedema or through vasodilatation (as a result of hypoxia and hypercarbia).

Once the compensatory mechanisms are exhausted, the ICP rises exponentially. Areas of focal ischaemia may occur as perfusion of the brain (and hence supply of oxygen and glucose) becomes increasingly compromised. This is a crucial period where interventions can influence longer-term morbidity or even mortality. If the ICP reaches a critical threshold, then global ischaemia, brain herniation and death are the likely outcomes. Signs of cerebral herniation include abnormal pupils (asymmetric, dilated or unreactive), progressive neurological deterioration, extensor posturing and compromised brainstem function (bradycardia, hypertension and irregular respiration).

To prevent the consequences of raised ICP it is important to have an understanding of the neurophysiology behind it. Normal cerebral blood flow is approximately 50 mLs/100g/min. In the first few hours after severe head injury, cerebral blood flow can fall to 25 mLs/100g/min. Irreversible neuronal damage occurs once cerebral blood flow drops below 18 mLs/100g/min. Therefore following traumatic injury the brain is susceptible to further ischaemic insult. As cerebral blood flow is difficult to measure, cerebral perfusion pressure is used as a surrogate marker for cerebral perfusion. Cerebral perfusion pressure is determined by the following calculation:

$$\text{Cerebral perfusion pressure (CPP)} = \text{Mean arterial pressure (MAP)} - \text{Intracranial pressure (ICP)}$$

CPP represents the pressure gradient driving cerebral blood flow (CBF) and hence oxygen delivery. In head trauma the ICP is assumed to be raised above 20 mmHg (as the ICP cannot be directly measured in the pre-hospital setting).

Under normal circumstances autoregulation ensures that cerebral blood flow is constant over a range of cerebral perfusion pressures. Autoregulation occurs by involuntary alteration of the resistance of cerebral blood vessels. As the blood-brain barrier becomes damaged, these homeostatic mechanisms are lost and cerebral blood flow becomes proportional to cerebral perfusion pressure. Those areas of the brain that are ischaemic, or at risk of ischaemia become critically dependent on an adequate cerebral blood flow, and therefore cerebral perfusion pressure (11).

To prevent further neuronal death (secondary brain injury), this flow of well-oxygenated blood must be maintained. Maintaining an adequate CPP is the cornerstone of modern brain injury therapy. Pre-hospital hypotension (defined as a single observation of systolic blood pressure <90 mmHg) has a significant negative impact on outcome from brain injury (12).

The partial pressures of carbon dioxide ($PaCO_2$) and oxygen (PaO_2) influence ICP through changes in cerebral blood flow and blood volume. $PaCO_2$ exerts the greater influence, with a 15%–30% increase in cerebral blood flow per kilopascal (kPa) increase in $PaCO_2$. Increases in blood volume in this compromised 'rigid box' contribute further to increases in ICP, thus reducing cerebral blood flow. Hyperventilation can have the opposite effect of reducing the blood volume, however the vasoconstriction can be so profound that this itself compromises blood flow. Normocapnia should be maintained. Hypoxaemia is a strong predictor of poor outcome in the TBI patient (12). Low oxygen tensions (PaO_2<8 kPa; SpO_2<90%) cause cerebral vasodilatation, and cerebral blood flow rises rapidly in an attempt to maintain oxygen delivery.

PRACTICE POINT

Hypoxia and hypotension should be avoided!

SYSTEMIC EFFECTS OF TRAUMATIC BRAIN INJURY

A number of systemic complications may be seen after a head injury. These can present within hours or days following the primary insult. Of particular importance in the pre-hospital phase are the cardiovascular effects. These are common and are associated with increased morbidity and mortality. An initial catecholamine surge is driven by the central neuroendocrine axis due to direct damage or as a protective effect to maintain cerebral perfusion. Disruption of brainstem function brings about neurogenic hypotension and the systemic response to neuroinflammatory mediators can contribute to a systemic inflammatory response and myocardial dysfunction. The clinician may encounter hypertension or hypotension (more than expected for the associated injury pattern), ECG morphological changes (ST-segment changes, flat/inverted T waves and prolongation of the QTc interval), arrhythmias and myocardial dysfunction. In severe cases this can lead to cardiogenic shock and pulmonary oedema (13).

APPROACHES TO THE CLASSIFICATION OF TBI

Being able to determine the type of traumatic brain injury is less important in the pre-hospital environment than an accurate overall assessment of the clinical state of the patient. In most cases, an accurate diagnosis will only be possible on CT scanning after arrival in hospital. It is the seriousness of the brain injury in terms of conscious level that will influence the pre-alert and handover to the hospital as well the most appropriate transfer destination. The most useful tool for assessing conscious level is the *Glasgow Coma Scale (GCS)* score (Box 12.2) (14). An alternative is AVPU:

- A – Alert
- V – Responds to voice
- P – Responds to painful stimuli
- U – Unresponsive

AVPU is rapid, reproducible and suitable for rapidly changing pre-hospital conditions.

In addition, there is no absolute agreement on some of the definitions used in the classification systems. This is especially true of the clinical severity classifications. Literature review has shown there to be numerous definitions for what encompasses a mild, moderate or severe traumatic brain injury. In the pre-hospital setting the mechanism, the distinction between isolated head injury and head injury as part of multi-trauma and the Glasgow Coma Scale based classifications are used most commonly. The GCS score may be invalidated by medical sedation or anaesthesia, paralysis or intoxication.

BOX 12.2: Classification of TBI, Clinical Severity

Glasgow Coma Scale

The GCS score comprises the values from three component tests (eye, motor and verbal scales).

Eyes

1 = No response
2 = Open in response to pain
3 = Open in response to speech
4 = Spontaneous

- Motor

1 = No response
2 = Extension to painful stimuli
3 = Abnormal flexion to painful stimuli
4 = Flexion/withdrawal to painful stimuli
5 = Localises painful stimuli
6 = Obeys commands

- Verbal

1 = No response
2 = Incomprehensible sounds
3 = Inappropriate utterances
4 = Disoriented, confused
5 = Oriented, converses normally

Other features which must be identified in determining the magnitude of a traumatic brain injury include whether the injury is blunt or penetrating and whether it is isolated or associated with extracranial injuries (50% of cases are associated with extracranial injuries including cervical spine injuries) (15). Other factors include the length of loss of consciousness or amnesia and the presence of neurological deficit on history taking or examination. Using the Glasgow Coma Scale score injuries are classified as

- Severe (GCS 3–8)
- Moderate (GCS 9–13)
- Mild (GCS 14–15)

INITIAL ASSESSMENT AND MANAGEMENT OF TBI

Emergency medical service personnel are often the first healthcare providers for patients with TBI. Pre-hospital assessment and treatment are critical links in providing appropriate care (12). The primary survey (as described in Chapter 6) ensures systematic assessment and management of patients. The main aim of pre-hospital treatment is to deliver adequate oxygen to the (already damaged) brain by optimising oxygenation of the blood and maintenance of cerebral perfusion. There is a window of opportunity in which to manage hypoxia and hypotension and prevent progression of secondary TBI before changes become irreversible. When pre-hospital data is reviewed, oxygen saturation below 90% is found in 44%–55% of cases and hypotension in 20%–30%. Trauma renders the brain more vulnerable to these insults, and hypoxia and hypotension are strongly associated with poor outcomes (12,14,15).

The cause of the initial traumatic head injury must always be established and any possible medical cause such as epileptic seizure or diabetes resulting in hypoglycaemic coma must be identified. The involvement of alcohol and recreational or other drugs should be considered. However, a depressed conscious level should only be ascribed to intoxication after a significant brain injury has been excluded, and this is unlikely to be possible until after arrival in hospital and appropriate investigation (8,16). It is essential to be aware of the potential for non-accidental injuries in both children and adults, especially the elderly, and there may be safety issues for medical personnel. As much scene information as possible about the mechanism of injury and potential confounding factors should be gathered. Such information provides a global overview of the situation for the receiving medical team in hospital.

CATASTROPHIC BLEEDING

Sources of obvious massive haemorrhage must be identified and controlled. Maintenance of the circulation has relevance for maintaining cerebral perfusion, and early external haemorrhage control to maintain the blood pressure is important (12). Bleeding from scalp wounds may occasionally be catastrophic.

AIRWAY

There may be evidence of airway obstruction with blood, vomit, foreign bodies or soft tissue swelling. Associated facial or cranial trauma must be identified. Signs include bruising, lacerations, fractures, boggy swellings, CSF leak from the ears or nose, and Battle's sign suggestive of a base of skull fracture. Airway management needs to be prompt, as patients with a depressed level of consciousness are less capable of protecting their own airway. The airway should be cleared and initially maintained with simple airway manoeuvres or airway adjuncts as required. Simple measures include jaw thrust and chin lift (to allow for cervical spine control); head tilt should be a last resort. Adjuncts, including supraglottic airway devices and suction, should be used where necessary, although all can raise ICP. There is a theoretical risk that nasopharyngeal airway devices may enter the cranium via a basal skull fracture. However, if the airway is in jeopardy and no other airway devices are appropriate, their use should still be considered. In practice, penetration of the cranium is unlikely with careful insertion and would require a very large basal skull defect indeed. If the skill set is available, intubation is the definitive airway procedure, allowing the airway to be secured and optimal ventilation and oxygenation to be achieved. Mobile medical teams with the appropriate skill set can provide drug-assisted intubation (see later). However, there is always a need to balance the delay on scene resulting from achieving a secure airway with rapid transfer to the receiving hospital following simple manoeuvres.

CERVICAL SPINE IMMOBILISATION

Cervical spine injury is common in this patient group. The risk increases with the severity of TBI (15). Spinal immobilisation should therefore be established and maintained in patients with reduced consciousness. Where possible ability to move the limbs should be documented in addition to any notable signs or symptoms of spinal cord injury (for example diaphragmatic breathing, hypotension without obvious cause, bradycardia, priapism and loss of pain below a dermatomal level) (16,17).

BREATHING

The catastrophic consequences of hypoxia mandate a thorough assessment of breathing and ventilation. Hypoxia, hyperventilation and hypoventilation all require treatment. Oxygen saturations and respiratory rate will guide the assessment. Even a single episode of hypoxia (SpO_2 <90%) should be avoided. High concentration oxygen should be administered via a non-rebreathing mask aiming for an oxygen saturation greater than 95% (even in those with COPD), as this provides a safety margin should the partial pressure of oxygen deteriorate rapidly. Ventilation may need to be assisted if saturations are below 90% on high concentration oxygen, the respiratory rate is less than 10 or greater than 30, or chest expansion appears inadequate (8).

The decision to intubate and ventilate a head-injured patient is a balance of benefit versus risk: whether to stay on scene to secure a definitive airway and institute controlled ventilation, or scoop and run to the nearest neurosurgical centre for rapid definitive treatment using simple effective airway adjuncts meanwhile? Intubation requires a skill set that not all pre-hospital medical personnel have. However, knowledge of the reasons *for* and the process *of* intubation will allow individuals who do to prepare for intubation and potentially reduce vital time on scene.

Box 12.3 provides guidance regarding which patients should be considered for intubation and ventilation (16).

BOX 12.3: Indications for Intubation and Ventilation Following Head Injury

- Coma – Not obeying commands, not speaking, not eye opening (GCS ≤ 8)
- Loss of protective laryngeal reflexes
- Spontaneous hyperventilation
- Irregular respirations
- Significantly deteriorating conscious level (1 or more points on the motor score) even if not coma
- Unstable fractures of the facial skeleton
- Copious bleeding into the mouth (e.g. from skull base fracture)
- Seizures
- Combative patients who benefit from induction of anaesthesia for their own safety

Intubation in traumatic brain injury can be challenging and the decision to do so should not be taken lightly. Patients can be combative and there may be associated facial trauma with soiling and deformity of the airway. Manual in-line immobilisation of the cervical spine must be maintained throughout the intubation process with due regard to potential injury during airway manoeuvres thus making siting an endotracheal tube more difficult.

Anaesthetic and paralysing agents facilitate rapid control of the airway by a competent laryngoscopist. Ketamine is preferred for trauma anaesthesia. Evidence suggests that previous concerns raised regarding changes in the intracranial pressure following ketamine administration are limited (15). A high-dose opiate (for example fentanyl) may be used in conjunction with ketamine to reduce the response to laryngoscopy. Once intubated, the patient should continue to be ventilated with appropriate sedation, muscle relaxation and analgesia en route to hospital. When using sedatives and analgesics, attention must be paid to potential undesirable side effects which might contribute to secondary injury (for example haemodynamic instability) (9). Deep sedation and muscle paralysis reduce the cerebral metabolic demands and allow optimisation of ventilation to prevent hypoxia and preserve normocapnia. Prophylactic hyperventilation causes cerebral vasoconstriction, may worsen ischaemia and secondary brain injury, and is contraindicated. Recommendations suggest a $PaCO_2$ of 4.5–5.0 kPa (18). There is a gradient between the arterial and end-tidal concentrations of carbon dioxide ($EtCO_2$) of 0.5–1.0 kPa. Routine use of capnography in these patients guides the adjustment of ventilation to target an $EtCO_2$ of 4.0–4.5 kPa.

CIRCULATION

Systemic hypotension increases the morbidity and mortality from traumatic brain injury. Hypotension in the early phases is unlikely to be caused by the head injury, and other sources of blood loss should be sought and addressed. In many polytrauma patients, anti-fibrinolytic agents (tranexamic acid) will be given as per local protocols (19). Trials are ongoing to determine the efficacy of tranexamic acid in isolated head injury (20). The blood pressure should be supported with fluid and vasopressors to maintain adequate cerebral perfusion. Hypotonic solutions such as dextrose should not be used for resuscitation. Scalp lacerations can cause significant blood loss and should be attended to during the primary survey. If associated cardiovascular side effects (arrhythmias, ventricular dysfunction, changes in ECG morphology) are encountered, treatment should be supportive and management focused on the underlying head injury (13).

DISABILITY

Conscious level is easily assessed using the AVPU system. There is limited evidence for using the GCS in the pre-hospital environment as a reliable indicator of the severity of TBI (15), but its use together with pupillary function may guide subsequent decision-making with regard to the management of the injury. An accurate assessment of GCS, neurological signs (sensory or motor deficit) and pupillary size and reactivity should be recorded at presentation and subsequently to establish a trend. The presence of drugs or alcohol and the addition of sedative agents can influence the GCS, making interpretation of trends difficult. The presence of such agents should be clearly documented and communicated to the receiving hospital team.

Seizures may occur acutely following traumatic head injury and should be managed as for any convulsion (by protection from harm, protection of the airway, oxygenation, and medication such as a benzodiazepine). These seizures may precipitate further adverse events in the injured brain because of a dramatic increase in the cerebral oxygen requirement. Opinions vary greatly about routine anti-seizure prophylaxis. Prophylactic anticonvulsants are indicated to decrease the incidence of early (within 7 days of injury) post-traumatic seizures, *but are not indicated in the pre-hospital context* (9). Patients who are suffering seizures post head injury should be considered for induction of anaesthesia and subsequent intubation and ventilation.

EXPOSURE AND ENVIRONMENT

There is as yet no confirmation from a high-quality randomised controlled trial that prophylactic hypothermia improves outcome or reduces mortality following traumatic brain injury. Previous research has suggested that using therapeutic hypothermia to reduce ICP might be beneficial in TBI. However this was studied as part of the Eurotherm3235 trial and no improvement in clinical outcomes was found compared to standard of care (10).

ADDITIONAL INTERVENTIONS

Pain should be managed effectively, as it can lead to a rise in ICP. Hypoglycaemia and hyperglycaemia are associated with poor outcome from traumatic brain injury. Hypoglycaemia should be treated promptly to avoid a cerebral metabolic crisis. Conversely, administration of hypoglycaemic agents is not indicated in the pre-hospital environment. Tight glycaemic control (blood glucose <6.7 mmol/L) has been shown to increase the incidence of hypoglycaemic events and a more tolerant approach (mild hyperglycaemia) should be accepted aiming to keep the blood glucose <10 mmol/L (21).

The use of steroids to reduce cerebral oedema and ICP following TBI is not recommended. The majority of available evidence indicates that steroids do not improve outcome or lower ICP in severe TBI. There is also strong evidence that steroids are deleterious. The MRC CRASH Trial 2005 (corticosteroid randomisation after significant head injury) was a large international double-blind randomised placebo-controlled trial of the effect of early administration of a 48-hour infusion of methylprednisolone on the risk of death and disability after head injury. The risk of death was higher in the corticosteroid group than in the placebo group (22). Similarly the results of two randomised, controlled trials of the neurosteroid progesterone showed no benefit with respect to a functional outcome at 6 months (23).

Obstructing cerebral venous drainage can further compound the problem of maintaining adequate cerebral perfusion. If possible the trolley should be slightly head-up, with the head in a neutral position, and ties and collars loosened sufficiently so as to not cause venous congestion. The administration of mannitol has been common practice in the management of TBI with suspected or actual raised ICP. There are two described mechanisms of action of mannitol: an immediate plasma-expanding effect, which reduces the haematocrit, increases the deformability of erythrocytes (and thereby reduces blood viscosity), increases CBF, and increases cerebral oxygen delivery, as well as a delayed osmotic gradient effect (15–30 min), which mobilises water across an intact blood-brain barrier into plasma (9,14). The risks of mannitol therapy include a rebound phenomenon with reversal of the osmotic gradients allowing water to pass back into the extracellular space of the brain and reduced cerebral perfusion due to hypovolaemia, as a result of the diuretic effect. Despite widespread current use there is insufficient reliable evidence to make recommendations on the use of mannitol in the management of patients with traumatic head injury and insufficient data on the effectiveness of pre-hospital administration (24). Mannitol crystallises at low temperatures, which reduces its suitability for pre-hospital use.

Hypertonic saline (HS) can also be used for osmotherapy. The principle effect on ICP is thought to be due to osmotic mobilisation of water across the intact blood-brain barrier, which reduces cerebral water content. Effects on the microcirculation may also have a role. HS dehydrates endothelial cells and erythrocytes, which increases the diameter of the vessels and deformability of erythrocytes and leads to plasma volume expansion with improved blood flow. It was thought that HS would benefit patients with TBI, as it has the potential to preserve or even improve haemodynamic parameters. However, current evidence is not strong enough to make recommendations on the use, concentration and method of administration of HS. Consequently, in adults there is insufficient evidence to support the use of HS over mannitol for osmotherapy at present (9,14).

TRANSFER

Pre-hospital recognition of traumatic brain injury and an effective management strategy are essential to the patient's recovery. Vital actions in the pre-hospital setting include (12,14):

- Information gathering by emergency medical call-takers and dispatchers to determine if the patient potentially has a significant brain injury.
- Dispatching the optimal personnel and equipment to the scene and allocating the correct response.
- Carrying out a rapid and accurate assessment of the overall neurological situation through evaluation of the mechanism of injury, the scene, and the patient examination.
- Initiating the appropriate clinical interventions and management strategy to prevent or correct hypotension or hypoxaemia and to address other potential threats to life or limb. At this step the decision regarding the level of responder dispatched to the scene impacts on patient care.
- Selecting the most appropriate transport mode.
- Selecting the most appropriate destination facility to allow for rapid detection and treatment of operable lesions.

Standby calls to the chosen destination should be made for all patients with a GCS less than or equal to 8 to ensure appropriately experienced professionals are available for their treatment and to prepare for imaging. The current primary investigation of choice for the detection of acute clinically important brain injuries is CT imaging of the head (16).

The patient needs to be transferred to the most appropriate facility for management of the injury. Ideally this should be a major trauma centre (MTC) with a neurosurgical capability. This limited resource may not always be directly accessible and will depend on the regional configurations of the trauma network. The receiving emergency department may be required to continue the supportive pre-hospital management and identify the extent of head and associated injuries before promptly referring on to the neurosurgical centre. A provisional *written* radiology report should be made available within 1 hour of the scan being performed (16).

Patients requiring an onward emergency transfer to a neuroscience unit should be accompanied by a doctor with appropriate training and experience in the transfer of patients with acute brain injury. The doctor should be familiar with the pathophysiology of head injury, the drugs and equipment they will use, and with working in the confines of an ambulance (or helicopter if appropriate). They should also have a dedicated and adequately trained assistant and adhere to the minimum monitoring standards (18).

HEAD INJURY IN CHILDREN

Of the 1.4 million attending emergency departments annually with a head injury, between 33% and 50% are children under 15 years of age (16). During the treatment process, families should have as much access to their child as is practical. In children, as in adults, global or regional ischaemia remains an important secondary insult to the acutely injured brain. Paediatric values for blood pressure, cerebral blood flow and cerebral metabolic rate differ from that of an adult. A CPP threshold of 40–50 mmHg may be considered with age-specific thresholds for infants at the lower end and adolescents at the upper end of this range (25). The blood pressure should be maintained at a level appropriate for their age. The paediatric version of the Glasgow Coma Scale should include a 'grimace' alternative to the verbal score to facilitate scoring in pre-verbal children (16).

SUMMARY

Traumatic head injury is common. Avoidance of hypoxia and hypotension is key to preventing secondary injury. Effective management techniques and appropriate decision-making regarding patient destination are essential.

REFERENCES

1. Dawodu ST. Traumatic Brain Injury (TBI) – Definition, epidemiology, pathophysiology. March 6, 2013. http://emedicine.medscape.com/article/326510-overview.
2. Murray G, Teasdale GM, Braakman R, Cohadon F, Dearden M, Iannotti F, Karimi A et al. The European Brain Injury Consortium survey of head injuries. *Acta Neurochirurgica* (Wien) 1999;141(3):223–236.
3. Roozenbeek B, Maas AIR, Menon DK. Changing patterns in the epidemiology of traumatic brain injury. *Nature Reviews Neurology* 2013;9:231–236.
4. Tagliaferri E, Compagnone C, Korsic M, Servadei F, Kraus J. A systematic review of brain injury epidemiology in Europe. *Acta Neurochirurgica* (Wien) 2006;148:255–268.
5. Yates PJ, Williams WH, Harris A, Round A, Jenkins R. An epidemiological study of head injuries in a UK population attending an emergency department. *Journal of Neurology, Neurosurgery, and Psychiatry* 2006;77:699–701.
6. Critchley G, Memon A. Epidemiology of head injury. In *Head Injury*, PC Whitfield, EO Thomas, F Summers, M Whyte, PJ Hutchinson (eds.). Cambridge University Press, 2009, 1–11.
7. Ganacher RP. *Traumatic Brain Injury: Methods for Clinical and Forensic Neuropsychiatric Assessment*. 2nd ed. CRC Press, 2008, 2–17.
8. Fisher JD, Brown SN, Cooke MW (eds.). *UK Ambulance Service Clinical Practice Guidelines*. 2006.
9. Brain Trauma Foundation. Guidelines for the management of severe traumatic brain injury. *Journal of Neurotrauma* 2007;24(sup 1):S7–S13.
10. Andrews PA, Sinclair HL, Battison CG, Polderman KH, Citerio G, Mascia L, Harris BA et al. Hypothermia for Intracranial hypertension after traumatic brain injury (the Eurotherm 3235 trial). *N Engl Med J* 2015;373:2403–2412.
11. Cerebral perfusion pressure. Trauma.org 2000;5:1. http://www.trauma.org/archive/neuro/cpp.html.
12. Brain Trauma Foundation. Guidelines for prehospital management of traumatic brain injury 2nd edition. *Prehospital Emergency Care* 2007;12(Supp 1):S1–S52.

13. Gregory T, Smith M. Cardiovascular complications of brain injury. *Continuing Education in Anaesthesia, Critical Care & Pain* 2012;12(2):67–71.
14. Maas A, Stocchetti N, Bullock R. Moderate and severe traumatic brain injury in adults. *Lancet Neurology* 2008;7:728–741.
15. Dinsmore J. Traumatic brain injury: An evidence-based review of management. *Continuing Education in Anaesthesia, Critical Care & Pain* 2013;13(6):189–195.
16. National Institute for Health and Care Excellence (NICE). Head injury. Clinical guideline CG176. 2014. www.guidance.nice.org.uk/cg176.
17. Bonner S, Smith C. Initial management of acute spinal cord injury. *Continuing Education in Anaesthesia, Critical Care & Pain* 2013;13(6):224–231.
18. Association of Anaesthetists of Great Britain and Ireland. *Recommendations for the Safe Transfer of Patients with Brain Injury.* London: Association of Anaesthetists of Great Britain and Ireland, 2006.
19. CRASH-2 Collaborators. The importance of early treatment with tranexamic acid in bleeding trauma patients: An exploratory analysis of the CRASH-2 randomised controlled trial. *Lancet* 2011;377(9771):1096–1101.
20. Dewan Y, Komolafe EO, Mejia-Mantilaa JH, Perel P, Roberts I, Shakur H. CRASH-3 – Tranexamic acid for the treatment of significant traumatic brain injury. *Trials* 2012;13:87.
21. Vespa P, McArthur DL, Stein N, Huang SC, Shao W, Filippou M, Etchepare M, Glenn T, Hovda DA. Tight glycaemic control increases distress in traumatic brain injury: A randomized controlled within-subjects trial. *Critical Care Medicine* 2012;40(6):1923–1929.
22. Edwards P, Arango M, Balica L, Cottingham R, El-Sayed H, Farrell B, Fernandes J et al. Final results of MRC CRASH, a randomized placebo-controlled trial of intravenous corticosteroid in adults with head injury-outcomes at 6 months. *Lancet* 2005;365:1957–1959.
23. Schwamm LH. Progesterone for traumatic brain injury – Resisting the sirens' song (Editorial). *New England Journal of Medicine* 2014:371(26):2522–2523.
24. Wakai A, McCabe A, Roberts I, Schierhout G. Mannitol for acute traumatic brain injury. *Cochrane Database of Systematic Reviews* 2013;(8):CD001049.
25. Kochanek PM, Carney N, Adelson PD, Ashwal S, Bell MJ, Bratton S, Carson S et al. Guidelines for the acute medical management of severe traumatic brain injury in infants, children, and adolescents – second edition. *Pediatric Critical Care Medicine* 2012;13 (Suppl 1):S1–S82.

13

Spinal injuries

OBJECTIVES

After completing this chapter the reader will

- Understand the importance of secondary injury prevention
- Be able to perform an accurate neurological assessment
- Be competent to manage the treatment and handling of a patient with an established or suspected spinal injury

INTRODUCTION

Spinal injury can be one of the most devastating outcomes following major trauma. It causes significant morbidity and mortality, and spinal injury patients very often need long-term, complex and costly care. Fortunately, the incidence of spinal injury is reasonably low: in the range of 19 to 88 cases per 100,000 population for spinal fractures and 14 to 53 per million population for a spinal cord injury (1–6). Spinal fractures or dislocations without cord injury were found to occur in 9.6% of patients presenting with major trauma in one cohort study; in the same study 1.8% of patients had a cord injury (7). Spinal injuries typically affect young adults with the incidence decreasing with age before increasing again in patients over 75. There is a 2:1 male to female ratio. Spinal injuries following apparently minor trauma are an important component of the increasingly common phenomenon of *'silver trauma'*.

MECHANISMS OF INJURY

Certain mechanisms of injury offer some predictive value for the presence of a spinal injury. Falls from greater than 2 m, then sports injuries (to include leisure activities such as horse riding) followed by road traffic collisions (RTCs) have the highest odds ratios for spinal fractures and dislocations. For actual spinal cord injuries, sports injuries show the highest association followed by falls greater than 2 m and then RTCs. However, the relative rarity of sports-related incidents means that they account for just 1.8% of all injuries. This is in comparison to RTCs which account for the majority (37%), then falls of greater than 2 m (30%), and falls of less than 2 m (23%).

PRACTICE POINT

Where no neurological examination is possible, a high index of suspicion should be maintained in the unconscious patient, especially in patients with concomitant chest injuries and those presenting after a high-risk mechanism: RTCs, sports injuries and falls of over 2 m.

ASSOCIATED INJURIES

As might be expected, there is an association between chest, abdominal and pelvic injuries and the presence of a spinal cord injury, simply reflecting the increased forces undergone by the patient during the trauma. Concurrent chest injuries demonstrate the strongest association. Spinal injuries are also associated with a reduced Glasgow Coma Scale (GCS) score, with the likelihood increasing as the GCS score decreases. However, although the likelihood of spinal injury increases with reducing GCS score it is important to remember that the majority (69%) of all injuries are seen in patients with a GCS score of 15.

DISTRIBUTION OF INJURIES

The traditional teaching regarding the pre-hospital management of spinal injuries has emphasised, almost to the exclusion of other areas, injuries to the cervical spine. However, injuries at all levels of the spinal column can have profound consequences (8). The majority of *cord injuries* are seen in the cervical region (45%), but the incidences of injury elsewhere are thoracic spine (28%), lumbar (23%) and multiple spinal levels (1%). Only 25% of all *spinal fractures and dislocations* involved the cervical spine, with 28% the thoracic, 37% the lumbar, and injuries at multiple levels accounting for a tenth (7) (Figure 13.1).

PRACTICE POINT

Spinal injuries are seen in about 1 in 10 patients with major trauma.

ANATOMY

The vertebral column is made up of 33 vertebrae: 7 cervical, 12 thoracic, 5 lumbar, 5 sacral and 4 coccygeal. The sacral and coccygeal vertebrae are fused forming the sacrum and coccyx, respectively. The spinal column is most vulnerable to injury at the junctions between articulating regions – the cervicothoracic junction, the thoracolumbar junction, and to a lesser extent at the lumbosacral junction (Figure 13.2).

The spinal cord runs from the foramen magnum down the spinal canal ending between T12 and L3, but usually at about L1. The cauda equina, made up of the lumbar, sacral and coccygeal spinal nerves, continues below this. The spinal cord is divided into 31 segments with each segment having a motor and sensory nerve root. Each motor nerve root supplies a distinct group of muscles and each sensory root receives innervation from a specific area of skin. Testing sensation and motor function allows the mapping of neurological injury to a specific level. An injury is classified according to the lowest level that still has full neurological function. (The sensory

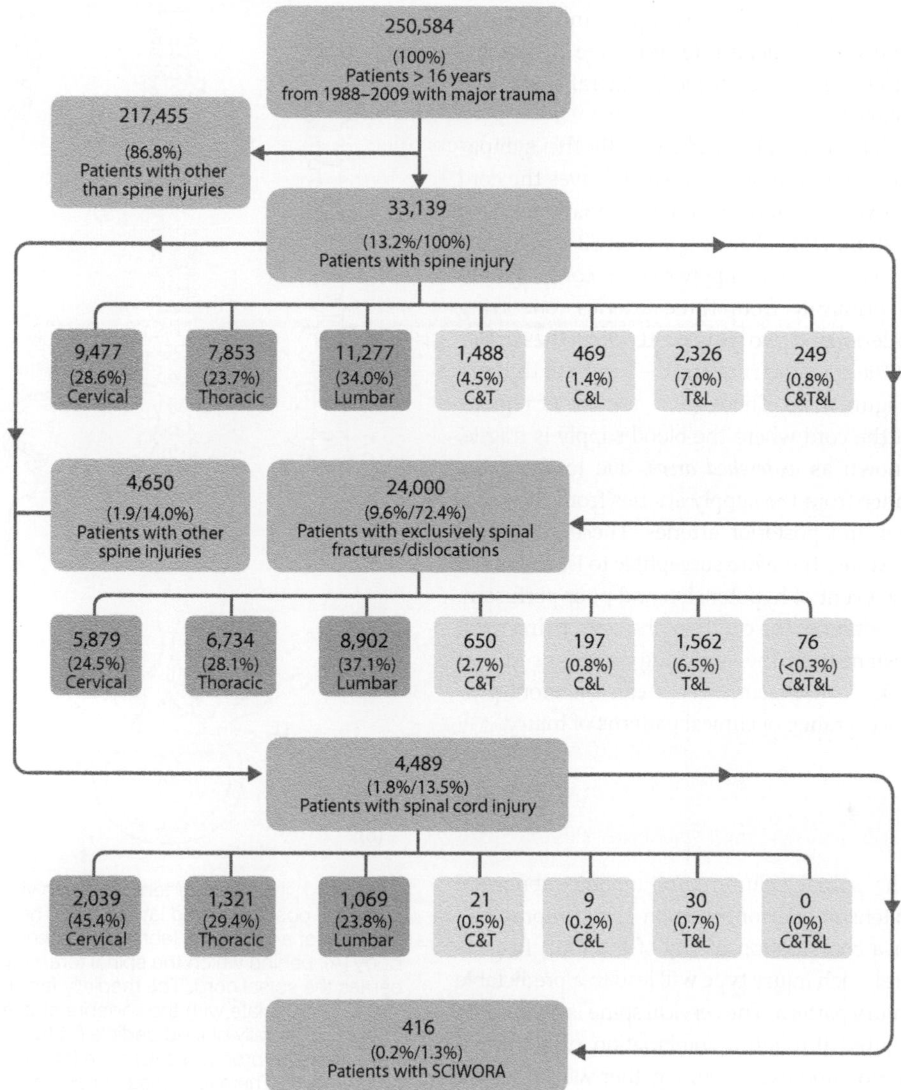

Figure 13.1 The incidence of spinal fractures and cord injuries from TARN. (Reproduced by permission of TARN and redrawn by Andrew Dakin, Department of Clinical Illustration QEHB.)

levels are illustrated in Figure 13.3 and Table 13.1; a limited list of myotomes is also included in Table 13.1.)

Not only can the level of injury be quantified on examination, but the nature and location of the injury within the cord may also be determined. Specific areas of the cord contain specific nerve components, for example the motor fibres lie within the lateral and anterior regions of the cord, whilst the posterior region contains sensory functions such as proprioception and vibration. Using this information it is possible to identify areas of damage (Figure 13.4). The motor fibres also decussate (cross the midline) before descending in the spinal cord. Therefore injuries produce signs on the opposite side (*contralateral*). The same applies to the sensory modalities of light touch, proprioception and vibration sense the fibres which carry them also decussating. The fibres for the modalities of pain and temperature do not decussate, therefore symptoms can be identified on the ipsilateral side to the injury.

The cord also carries both the sympathetic nervous system, which leaves the cord between C7 and L1, and the parasympathetic system, which leaves between S2 and S4.

The vascular supply to each cord segment is primarily from three arteries: one lying anterior and two lying posterior on the surface of the cord and running the length of the cord (Figure 13.5). There are a number of regions of the cord where the blood supply is fragile, known as *watershed areas,* due to their distance from the supply arteries from the anterior and posterior arteries. These watershed areas are therefore susceptible to ischaemia in the event of hypotension and poor perfusion. In addition, the centre of the cord, being most distant from the supplying arteries is also at risk. An ischaemic insult can therefore produce a range of clinical patterns of injury.

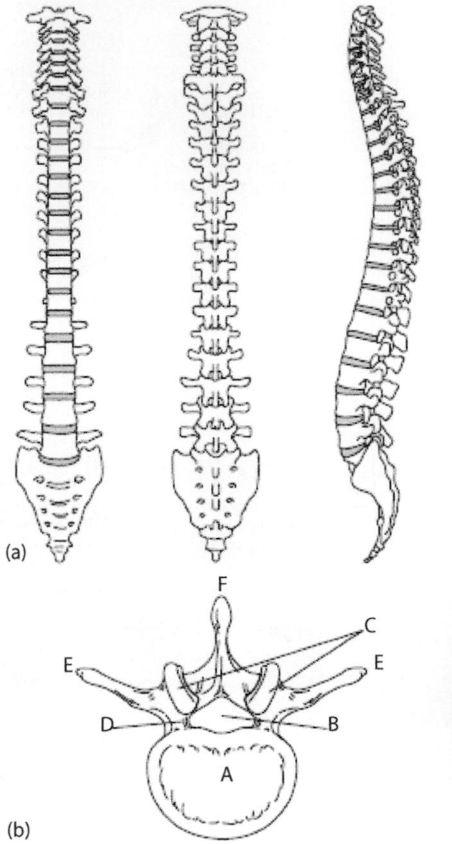

(a)

F
C
E
E
D
B
A

(b)

Figure 13.2 (a) The vertebral column viewed anteriorly posteriorly and laterally. (b) The anatomy of a typical vertebra with a dense bony body (A), behind which the spinal foramen (B) carries the spinal cord. The medially facing facet joints (C) articulate with the vertebra above. There is a laterally placed pedicle (D) from which the transverse processes (E) arise for muscular attachments. There is a posterior spinous process (F).

MECHANISMS OF INJURY

The spinal column can undergo abnormal extension, flexion, rotation and compression, or a combination of any of the four. In general, each injury type will lead to a predictable injury pattern. The cervical spine is commonly injured through a combination of abnormal flexion and extension, together with rotation. Hyperflexion is commonly seen in RTC injuries and from activities such as diving. If there is the addition of rotation, as seen in significant RTCs and major impact trauma, the extent of the injury will be correspondingly more severe. Hyperextension injuries tend only to be found in the cervical and lumbar regions of the spinal column.

Compression injuries are normally associated with falls from height. Wedge fractures, when the vertebral body is compressed at its anterior border, are caused by compression and forward flexion. These are the most common fractures seen in the lumbar and thoracic regions. The C1 vertebra can also be compressed following transmission of force applied directly to the crown of the head.

PRIMARY AND SECONDARY INJURY

The injury to the spinal cord can be separated into primary and secondary neurological damage. *Primary neurological injury* is damage to neural tissue resulting directly, from the

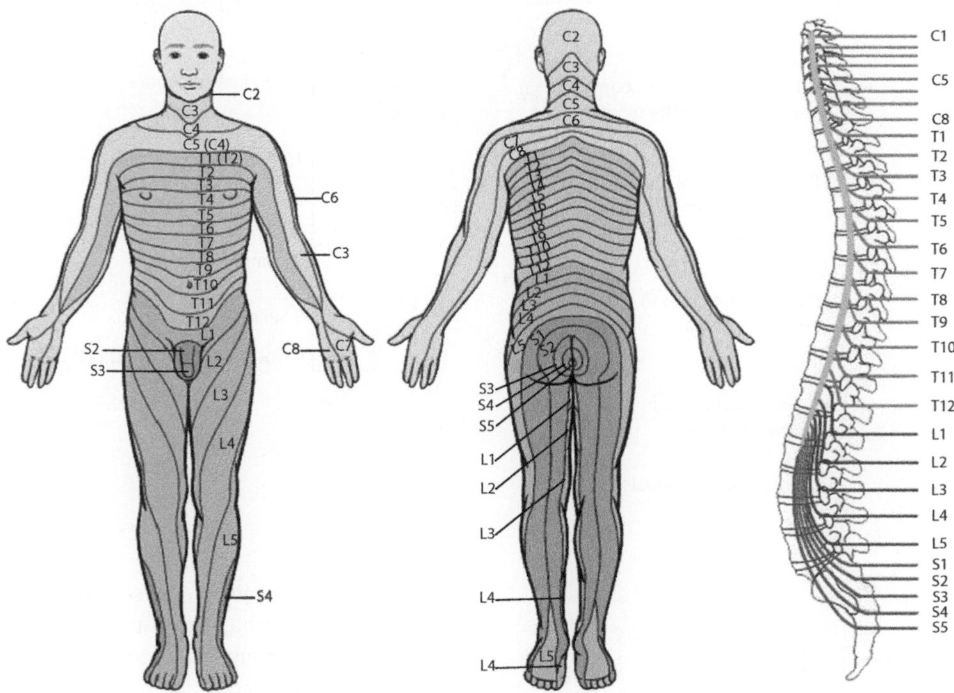

Figure 13.3 Dermatones.

Table 13.1 Segmental values for dermatomes and myotomes

Segment	Representative dermatomes	Representative myotomes
C5	Sensation over deltoid	Deltoid muscle
C6	Sensation over thumb	Wrist extensors
C7	Sensation over middle finger	Elbow extensors
C8	Sensation over little finger	Middle finger flexors
T1	Sensation over inner aspect of elbow	Little finger abduction
T4	Sensation around nipple	–
T8	Sensation over xiphisternum	–
T10	Sensation around umbilicus	–
T12	Sensation around symphysis	–
L1	Sensation in inguinal region	–
L2	Sensation on anterior upper thigh	Hip flexors
L3	Sensation on anterior mid-thigh	Knee extensors
L4	Sensation on medial aspect of leg	Ankle dorsiflexors
L5	Sensation between first and second toes	Long toe extensors
S1	Sensation on lateral border of foot	Ankle plantar flexors
S3	Sensation over ischial tuberosity	–
S4/5	Sensation around perineum	–

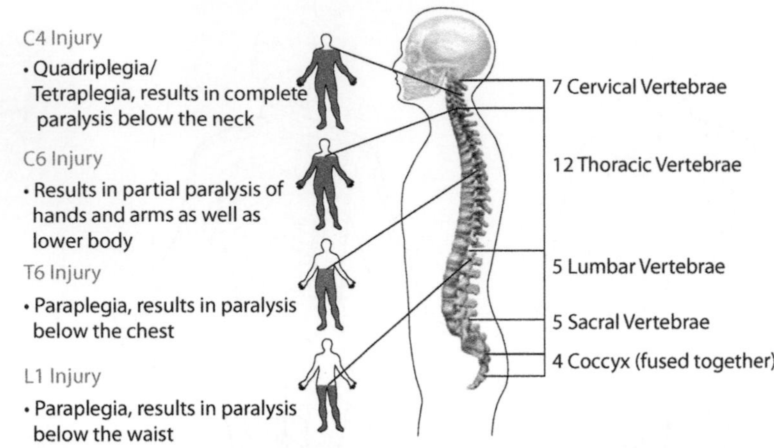

Figure 13.4 Cord damage levels.

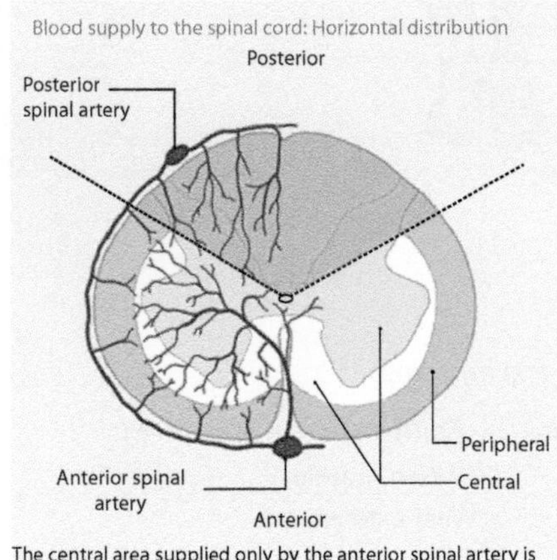

Figure 13.5 Cross section of the spinal cord.

mechanism of injury. Causes of primary injury include damage to the cord from the abnormal movement undergone by the spinal column and cord, damage from bony fragments or fractures, or compression from haematomas and soft tissues. These mechanisms frequently reduce the volume of the canal. The primary injury directly disrupts the nerves and causes haemorrhage within the white, and particularly, grey matter.

Secondary neurological injury is the ongoing injury to tissue following the initial traumatic insult. This can continue for a number of hours as oedema develops, further compressing neurones and compromising perfusion to tissues. Secondary injury often extends above the area of initial primary injury by up to two spinal levels. It is at about 8 hours post injury that ischaemia develops into infraction and necrosis and becomes irreversible. The common causes of secondary neurological damage are

- Hypoxia
- Hypoperfusion
- Further mechanical disruption

Trauma patients are frequently globally hypoxic and hypoperfused due to the extent of their concomitant injuries. Recognising and addressing these issues is key to survival, let alone to minimising spinal cord injury. There is debate regarding the importance of minimising further mechanical disruption by limiting further movement of the spinal column, which has for so long been a central tenet of pre-hospital spinal management (9). Efforts to improve oxygenation and perfusion should not be hampered by spinal immobilisation.

NEUROGENIC SHOCK AND SPINAL SHOCK

Neurogenic shock is the term given to hypotension associated with the loss of sympathetic autonomic outflow following a high (above T6) cord injury. The loss of sympathetic outflow leads to uninhibited vasodilatation and a redistributive shock, along with uninhibited vagal responses, namely profound bradycardia. Classically, patients present with a triad of hypotension, bradycardia and peripheral vasodilatation.

The term *spinal shock* is unhelpful, but its use persists. Spinal shock is defined as the *complete loss of all neurological function below the level of cord injury.* This period of flaccid paralysis and areflexia lasts for 24 to 72 hours, and therefore prevents full assessment of the true extent of injury and neurological deficit. Full recovery can be seen after periods of profound paralysis. The term spinal shock therefore is effectively spinal *concussion;* it certainly has nothing to do with inadequate perfusion.

PRE-HOSPITAL ASSESSMENT AND MANAGEMENT

The pre-hospital management of spinal injuries is centred on the recognition of an injury or, far more frequently, the recognition of the *possibility* of an injury or potential injury. The patient is therefore managed with the aim of minimising further cord damage by minimising further movement of the spinal column (9,10).

The belief that minimising further movement of the spinal column will avoid further deterioration of a neurological injury is not one fully supported by evidence (11). The evidence is weak both for and against current practice. Indeed, there is evidence supporting the view that immobilisation might be harmful and worsen outcome (12). The principle has been put forward that given the considerable force required to bring about the primary fracture and injury, subsequent movement is unlikely to cause further damage to the cord (13). The lack of evidence to determine best practice makes it difficult to move away radically from the practice of widespread immobilisation, given that an injury can cause devastating consequences, although current practice is more pragmatic than previously.

INITIAL MANAGEMENT

Current pre-hospital management follows the <C>ABCDE method. Consideration is given to minimising further movement in the cervical, and also the wider spinal column, only once catastrophic haemorrhage and life-threatening airway compromise have been managed. Examination for any spinal injury, and its extent, is undertaken once other more pressing issues have been addressed, and is usually delayed until after arrival in hospital. Treating hypoxia and hypoperfusion as part of the patient's overall care will also help to reduce secondary spinal cord injury.

IMMOBILISATION

The 'gold standard' of triple immobilisation is seen as the correct application of an appropriately sized cervical collar, and securing the head, in neutral alignment, to a firm surface with blocks and tape or straps (Figure 13.6) (14). Manual in-line immobilisation (or stabilisation) is the term given to the practice of holding the patients head in a neutral position before instigation of triple immobilisation. Immobilisation is nearly always performed once the patient has returned to neutral alignment. In rare cases the injury may make this impossible: should the patient report

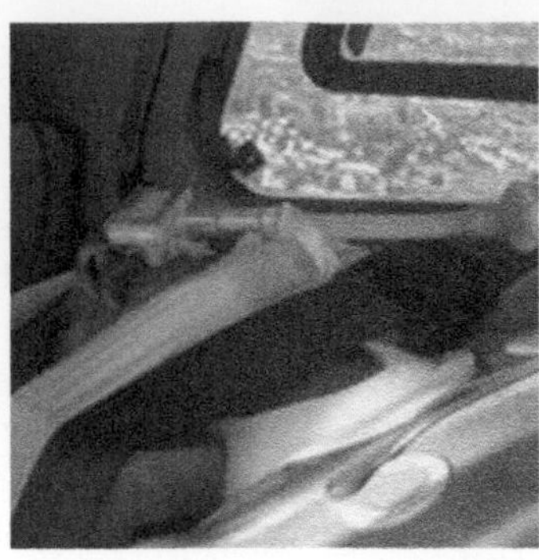

Figure 13.6 Triple immobilisation.

pain or paraesthesia on gentle movement of the head towards the neutral position, then no further movement should occur with the patient being immobilised in the pain- or paraesthesia-free position.

More commonly pre-existing disease, such as ankylosing spondylitis, will prevent neutral alignment. In such cases immobilisation should be in the normal alignment for that patient (15).

The previous practice of ensuring manual in-line immobilisation as soon as possible has been de-emphasised with the adoption of a more pragmatic approach. Requiring one clinician to be solely responsible for 'immobilising the neck' is often not an efficient use of resources. This can sometimes be delegated to a bystander or other emergency services responder, as it is a relatively unskilled task. Alternatively, and most simply, the conscious patient can be advised not to move their neck until further assessment has been made. The unconscious patient is unlikely to move their neck independently and so the head can be moved, and secured, in a neutral position, without manual support where possible.

THE AGITATED PATIENT

The uncooperative, combative patient presents the greatest challenge. Their risk of spinal injury is higher given that the mechanism of injury is likely to have been severe enough to cause serious head injury (a common cause of agitation), yet they are not in a position to cooperate. Manual immobilisation is of value in this situation, as it can rapidly react to the movements of the patient, and the constant attention and reassurance of a clinician can have a calming effect. However, the movements the patient is making should not be forcibly restricted by the immobilising clinician, as there is the potential for further harm if restraint requires noticeable strength. Sedation and pre-hospital anaesthesia are increasingly commonly used, not just to facilitate immobilisation but also as part of the overall care for the patient. If this is not possible or appropriate, some patients may tolerate a collar alone. Otherwise, no immobilisation should be applied and in no circumstances should forcible restraint, either manually or with straps or tape, occur.

A similarly pragmatic approach is taken to the timing of the application of a cervical collar. Manual in-line stabilisation without a cervical collar in place is acceptable whilst assessment and treatment is ongoing. Application need only occur, if indicated, when the patient is due to be moved and packaged for transport. Wearing a correctly applied collar is not comfortable and not without the risk of harm; therefore minimising duration of application is in the patient's interests.

Again it is important to stress the possibility of injuries in the spinal column other than the cervical region. Devastating injuries can occur along the length of the spinal cord. Clinical vigilance and the current practice of minimising movement through immobilisation, when indicated, applies to the whole length of the spinal column.

ONGOING MANAGEMENT

Further management commonly involves an assessment as to whether spinal immobilisation precautions are indicated or necessary. Although over 13% of patients suffering *major trauma* have a spinal injury, the incidence in patients presenting to the emergency department following blunt trauma is approximately 2% (16,17). It is well recognised that a vast number of patients, approaching 98% of all immobilised patients, are immobilised without any spinal injury being subsequently found.

Spinal immobilisation is not without negative consequences. Apart from being uncomfortable and distressing for some patients (18), it can restrict ventilation (19,20), increase intracranial pressure (21–23), hamper the drainage of vomit and blood with an increased risk of aspiration (24), obstruct efforts at airway management (25), and cause tissue pressure damage (26). In addition the financial costs of transport, examination and investigation of unnecessary injuries which are clinically unlikely is also significant. The time taken to immobilise patients on scene can be up to 5 minutes (27). This can be a significant delay in time-critical patients.

PRACTICE POINT

If there is associated head injury, the cervical collar should be loosened or removed, and the patient immobilised with head blocks and tape.

Therefore appropriate efforts should be made to use spinal immobilisation only in patients who require it. No pre-hospital algorithm has been validated; current guidelines on cervical spine immobilisation (28,29) are based on an extrapolation of in-hospital practice which itself is based on the NEXUS and Canadian C-spine rules which aim to identify patients in need of further cervical spine imaging. The ability of pre-hospital providers to correctly apply the rules has been demonstrated (30–36).

The National Emergency X-Radiography Utilization Study (NEXUS) was an observational study of cervical spine radiography in blunt trauma patients (16). This study of 34,069 patients stated that significant injury to the cervical spine could be excluded without the need for imaging if five criteria each indicative of low risk could be met:

1. No midline cervical tenderness
2. No focal neurological deficit
3. Normal alertness
4. No intoxication
5. No painful distracting injury

Midline tenderness was reported in up to 58% of patients without a neck injury (17) and no definition regarding what comprises a distracting injury was initially given. Attempts at a definition suggest that more proximal injuries (upper limb, ribs, in other words closer to the neck) are more distracting, together with those reported to give a pain score of more than 7 out of 10 (37).

The Canadian C-Spine Rule is based on high- and low-risk factors, generating a series of three questions (Table 13.2) (17). It is based on a prospective cohort study of 8924 blunt trauma patients who were not walking after an incident with a dangerous mechanism of injury but alert, stable, had neck pain, or had no neck pain but had a visible injury above the clavicle.

The NICE guidance is based primarily on the Canadian C-Spine Rule but combined with the 'absence of midline tenderness' from the NEXUS rules in an attempt to increase sensitivity (29).

MANAGEMENT OF PENETRATING TRAUMA

Spinal immobilisation is very rarely warranted for penetrating head and neck injuries (38). Immobilisation is associated with doubling of the mortality rate, possibly due to increased on-scene time for application of immobilisation and therefore delayed transport to definitive care (39).

Table 13.2 The Canadian C-Spine Rule

1. Is any high-risk factor present that mandates radiography?
   Age 65 years or more
   Dangerous mechanism of injury
   - A fall from greater than one metre or five stairs
   - An axial load to the head, e.g. diving
   - A high-speed motor vehicle collision (combined speed >100 km/hr)
   - A rollover motor vehicle accident
   - Ejection from a motor vehicle
   - An accident involving motorised recreational vehicles
   - A bicycle collision

   Paraesthesia in the extremities
2. If none of the above is present, is any low-risk factor present that allows safe assessment of range of motion?
   - Simple rear-end motor vehicle collision
   - Sitting position in ED
   - Ambulatory at any time since injury
   - Delayed onset of neck pain
   - Absence of midline C-spine tenderness
3. If no high-risk factors are present, and the patient does not have any of the low risk factors rotation can be assessed: can the patient actively rotate their neck 45 degrees to the left and right?

Patients capable of neck rotation do not need to be immobilised.

Patients who need immobilisation in these circumstances will usually have clear indications of a spinal injury (40).

EXAMINATION

As highlighted earlier, consideration should be given to the whole spinal cord, as well as examination for cervical tenderness. Where possible, the length of the column should be examined for tenderness and alignment. In the majority of cases a detailed examination will occur after arrival in hospital. Should the patient be found in a position that enables examination, then the opportunity to examine the back should be considered. Delaying evacuation from the scene to logroll the patient for examination is not appropriate.

Consideration should be given to the presence of neurogenic shock, classically presenting with hypotension, bradycardia and peripheral vasodilatation below the level of the injury. This is rare. The diagnosis is one of exclusion and other more common reasons for hypotension should be considered first. In addition a spinal injury may mask the classical signs of hypotension when the two co-exist. A spinal injury causing neurogenic shock is unlikely if there is no neurological deficit or if the level of injury is below T6.

PACKAGING AND TRANSPORT

Current best practice focuses on minimal patient handling (41). The principle of minimising movement is fundamental to this approach. Planning ahead is essential: If it is thought that immobilisation is warranted, then the process of packaging for immobilisation and transport should be considered early in the patient's management. This will streamline the patient's movements, reducing time as well as overall movement, both on scene and at definitive care. The principles of minimal handling are

- Use a long spinal board, if necessary, for extrication only
- Transfer the patient using a scoop stretcher combined with a minimal tilt to allow insertion of the scoop blades

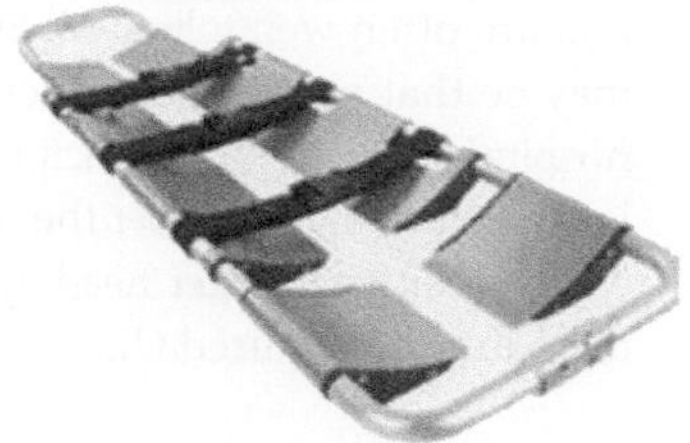

Figure 13.7 A scoop stretcher.

Immobilisation for transport to definitive care should take the form of

- A scoop stretcher if the total scoop time will be less than 45 minutes
- A vacuum mattress if a prolonged transport time is likely

Immobilisation for transport should no longer be performed on a rigid long spinal board due to the increased discomfort and risk of tissue pressure damage. Immobilisation for short transfers to definitive care should be carried out using a modern scoop stretcher (Figure 13.7). In addition to being more comfortable, and potentially having a lower risk of tissue pressure damage, use of a scoop stretcher should shorten timelines and transfers at definitive care.

Logrolling a patient is no longer considered the optimum method when positioning a patient for immobilisation. A minimal tilt of 10° to 15° is sufficient to insert the blades of the scoop stretcher. Minimising movement will help to reduce movement of the spinal column as well as adhering to the principles of careful patient handling.

Once the patient is packaged for transfer to definitive care, a pragmatic approach to immobilisation can be employed. In the compliant or the anaesthetised patient, the collar can be loosened to improve comfort and limit potential increases in intracranial pressure.

PAEDIATRIC SPINAL INJURY

Fortunately, devastating spinal injuries are rare amongst the paediatric population. Nevertheless they present a challenge in the pre-hospital setting.

One specific type of injury seen in children under the age of 8 is *spinal cord injury without radiological abnormality (SCIWORA)*. This occurs as a result of the increased hypermobility and laxity of the paediatric spinal column, which can withstand trauma without fracturing. The underlying cord however is still damaged from the abnormal flexion, extension, compression, distraction or rotation. Although no bony abnormality will be seen on plain X-ray or CT, the injury will be identified using MRI scanning.

The management of paediatric spinal injuries or potential injuries is a challenge. Immobilising an injured, frightened child will often be an additional traumatic experience for them. Again a pragmatic approach should be taken. The NEXUS criteria included patients under the age of 16, but there is inevitably an age limit below which young children will be unable to give meaningful information. Distress will be just as great a distraction as a 'distracting injury'. Some reassurance can be taken from the rarity of significant spinal injuries in the paediatric population.

At its simplest, and least upsetting, manual in-line stabilisation without any collar is appropriate and tolerated by many. If a child is already restrained in a car seat, then transfer to definitive care in that car seat may solve many issues. Vacuum mattresses and splints can be useful and are often well tolerated. Simple makeshift head roll supports have their advocates. But it may be that no immobilisation is tolerated, in which case the child should be transported to hospital following the principles of minimal handling with as little movement as is possible. It is important to remember the normal anatomical position for the age of the child. In the infant, with a relatively larger head, lying flat will lead to abnormal flexion and so support under the torso may be required (42).

SUMMARY

The pre-hospital management of spinal injuries is currently being scrutinised. Whilst recognising the devastating consequences of these reasonably rare injuries, the practice of routine immobilisation is being challenged. A more pragmatic approach, in the absence of robust evidence and reflecting concerns that immobilisation may harm patients, is being adopted. Decision tools may help to identify patients who need immobilisation and, importantly, those who do not.

Pre-hospital spinal management should not distract from, or delay, the management of life-threatening injuries. The whole length of the spine, not just the cervical spine, should be considered when managing patients, who should be managed expediently following the principles of minimal handling.

REFERENCES

1. Pirouzmand F. Epidemiological trends of spine and spinal cord injuries in the largest Canadian adult trauma center from 1986 to 2006. *Journal of Neurosurgery Spine* 2010;12(2):131–140.
2. Lenehan B, Boran S, Street J, Higgins T, McCormack D, Poynton AR. Demographics of acute admissions to a National Spinal Injuries Unit. *European Spine Journal* 2009; 18(7):938–942.
3. Hu R, Mustard C, Burns C. Epidemiology of incident spinal fracture in a complete population. *Spine* 1996;21(4):492–499.
4. Dryden DM, Saunders LD, Rowe BH, May LA, Yiannakoulias N, Svenson LW, Schopflocher DP, Voaklander DC. The epidemiology of traumatic spinal cord injury in Alberta, Canada. *Canadian Journal of Neurolological Sciences* 2003;30(2):113–121.
5. Jackson AB, Dijkers M, Devivo MJ, Poczatek RB. A demographic profile of new traumatic spinal cord injuries: Change and stability over 30 years. *Archives of Physical Medicine and Rehabilitaion* 2004;85(11):1740–1748.
6. Pickett W, Simpson K, Walker J, Brison RJ. Traumatic spinal cord injury in Ontario, Canada. *Journal of Trauma* 2003;55(6):1070–1076.
7. Hasler RM, Exadaktylos AK, Bouamra O, Benneker LM, Clancy M, Sieber R, Zimmermann H, Lecky F. Epidemiology and predictors of cervical spine injury in adult major trauma patients: A multicenter cohort study. *Journal of Trauma and Acute Care Surgery* 2012;72(4):975–981.
8. Goldberg W, Mueller C, Panacek E, Tigges S, Hoffman JR, Mower WR. Distribution and patterns of blunt traumatic cervical spine injury. *Annals of Emergency Medicine* 2001;38:17–21.
9. American College of Surgeons. *Advanced Trauma Life Support for Doctors*. 8th ed. Chicago: American College of Surgeons, 2009.

10. Theodore N, Hadley MN, Aarabi B, Dhall SS, Gelb DE, Hurlbert RJ, Rozzelle CJ, Ryken TC, Walters BC. Prehospital cervical spinal immobilization after trauma. *Neurosurgery* 2013;72(Suppl 2):22–34.
11. Kwan I, Bunn F, Roberts IG. Spinal immobilisation for trauma patients (review). *The Cochrane Library* 2009;(1).
12. Hauswald M, Ong G, Tandberg D, Omar Z. Out-of-hospital spinal immobilization: Its effect on neurologic injury. *Academic Emergency Medicine* 1998;5(3):214–219.
13. Hauswald M. A re-conceptualisation of acute spinal care. *Emergency Medicine Journal* 2013;30:720–723.
14. Podolsky S, Baraff LJ, Simon RR, Hoffman JR, Larmon B, Ablon W. Efficacy of cervical spine immobilization methods. *Journal of Trauma* 1983;23(6):461–465.
15. Thumbikat P, Hariharan RP, Ravichandran G, McClelland MR, Mathew KM. Spinal cord injury in patients with ankylosing spondylitis: A 10-year review. *Spine* 2007;32(26):2989–2995.
16. Hoffman JR, Mower WR, Wolfson AB, Todd KH, Zucker MI. Validity of a set of clinical criteria to rule out injury to the cervical spine in patients with blunt trauma. National Emergency X-Radiography Utilization Study Group. *New England Journal of Medicine* 2000;343(2):94–99.
17. Stiell IG, Wells GA, Vandemheen KL, Clement CM, Lesiuk H, De Maio VJ, Laupacis A et al. The Canadian C-spine rule for radiography in alert and stable trauma patients. *JAMA* 2001;286(15):1841–1848.
18. Chan D, Goldberg R, Tascone A, Harmon S, Chan L. The effect of spinal immobilization on healthy volunteers. *Annals of Emergency Medicine* 1994;23(1):48–51.
19. Bauer D, Kowalski R. Effect of spinal immobilization devices on pulmonary function in the healthy, nonsmoking man. *Annals of Emergency Medicine* 1988;17(9):915–918.
20. Totten VY, Sugarman DB. Respiratory effects of spinal immobilization. *Prehospital Emergency Care* 1999;3(4):347–352.
21. Kolb JC, Summers RL, Galli RL. Cervical collar-induced changes in intracranial pressure. *American Journal of Emergency Medicine* 1999;17(2):135–137.
22. Davies G, Deakin C, Wilson A. The effect of a rigid collar on intracranial pressure. *Injury* 1996;27(9):647–649.
23. Mobbs RJ, Stoodley MA, Fuller J. Effect of cervical hard collar on intracranial pressure after head injury. *ANZ Journal of Surgery* 2002;72(6):389–391.
24. Lockey DJ, Coats T, Parr MJA. Aspiration in severe trauma: A prospective study. *Anaesthesia* 1999;54:1097–1098.
25. Goutcher CM, Lochhead V. Reduction in mouth opening with semi-rigid cervical collars. *British Journal of Anaesthesia* 2005;95(3):344–348.
26. Hewitt S. Skin necrosis caused by a semi-rigid cervical collar in a ventilated patient with multiple injuries. *Injury* 1994;25(5);323–324.
27. Arishita GI, Vayer JS, Bellamy RF. Cervical spine immobilization of penetrating neck wounds in a hostile environment. *Journal of Trauma* 1989;29(3):332–337.
28. Joint Royal Colleges Ambulance Liaison Committee. Neck and back trauma. 2006.
29. National Institute for Health and Care Excellence. Triage, assessment, investigation and early management of head injury in infants, children and adults. Clinical guideline [CG56]. 2007.
30. Vaillancourt C, Stiell IG, Beaudoin T, Maloney J, Anton AR, Bradford P, Cain E et al. The out-of-hospital validation of the Canadian C-Spine Rule by paramedics. *Annals of Emergency Medicine* 2009;54(5):663–671.

31. Armstrong BP, Simpson HK, Crouch R, Deakin CD. Prehospital clearance of the cervical spine: Does it need to be a pain in the neck? *Emergency Medicine Journal* 2007;24:501–503.
32. Brown LH, Gough JE, Simonds WB. Can EMS providers adequately assess trauma patients for cervical spinal injury? *Prehospital Emergency Care* 1998;2:33–36.
33. Domeier RM, Frederiksen SM, Welch K. Prospective performance assessment of an out-of-hospital protocol for selective spine immobilization using clinical spine clearance criteria. *Annals of Emergency Medicine* 2005;46:123–131.
34. Domeier RM, Swor RA, Evans RW, Hancock JB, Fales W, Krohmer J, Frederiksen SM, Rivera-Rivera EJ, Schork MA. Multicenter prospective validation of prehospital clinical spinal clearance criteria. *Journal of Trauma* 2002;53:744–750.
35. Stroh G, Braude D. Can an out-of-hospital cervical spine clearance protocol identify all patients with injuries? An argument for selective immobilization. *Annals of Emergency Medicine* 2001;37:609–615.
36. Domelier RM, Fredericksen SM, Welch K. Prospective performance assessment of an out-of-hospital protocol for selective spine immobilization using clinical spine clearance criteria. *Annals of Emergency Medicine* 2005;46:123–131.
37. Heffernan DS, Schermer CR, Lu SW. What defines a distracting injury in cervical spine assessment? *Journal of Trauma* 2005;59:1396–1399.
38. Barkana Y, Stein M, Scope A, Maor R, Abramovich Y, Friedman Z, Knoller N. Prehospital stabilization of the cervical spine for penetrating injuries to the neck—Is it necessary? *Injury* 2000;31:305–309.
39. Haut ER, Kalish BT, Efron DT, Haider AH, Stevens KA, Kieninger AN, Cornwell EE 3rd, Chang DC. Spine immobilization in penetrating trauma: More harm than good? *Journal of Trauma* 2010;68:115–120.
40. Connell RA, Graham CA, Munro PT. Is spinal immobilization necessary for all patients sustaining isolated penetrating trauma? *Injury* 2003;34:912–914.
41. Moss R, Porter K, Greaves I et al. Minimal patient handling: a faculty of prehospital care consensus statement. *Emergency Medicine Journal* 2013;30:1065–1066.
42. Nypaver M, Treloar D. Neutral cervical spine positioning in children. *Annals Emergency Medicine* 1994;23:208–211.

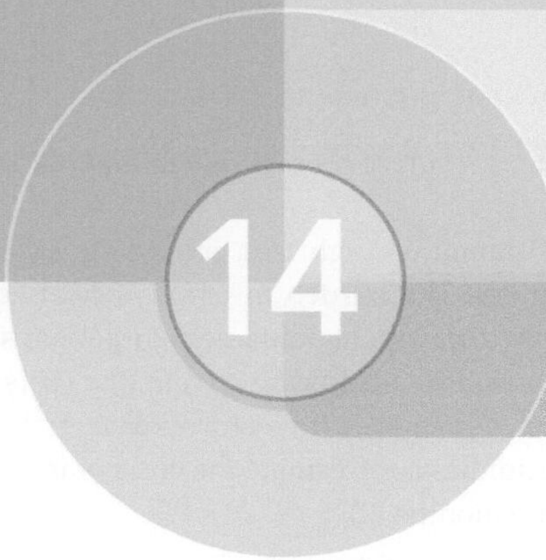

14 Musculoskeletal trauma

OBJECTIVES

After completing this chapter the reader will

- Be aware of the common presentations of musculoskeletal trauma
- Understand the significance of musculoskeletal trauma in the multiply injured patient
- Understand the basic techniques required for the management of musculoskeletal trauma in the pre-hospital environment

INTRODUCTION

Musculoskeletal trauma encompasses a broad range of injury and injury patterns. It is the most common type of trauma encountered by the pre-hospital practitioner ranging from simple strains and sprains through to complex polytrauma associated with high-energy transfer to the limbs and axial skeleton. Minor injury is one of the most common reasons for presenting to emergency departments and calling for the help of the statutory ambulance services. Many of these injuries can be dealt with using simple measures including analgesia, advice and arranging appropriate follow-up. For more complicated injuries, referral to hospital specialists, in-patient treatment and operative intervention will be necessary. This chapter outlines the epidemiology of musculoskeletal injury, before describing the general principles of management. Specific regional injuries are then considered in turn.

EPIDEMIOLOGY

Approximately 10,000 people per year are killed as a result of trauma in the United Kingdom (1). Head injuries make up the largest group, accounting for approximately one-third of deaths. Limb injuries appear within the 20% of people killed by 'multiple injuries', but also on their own, with lower limb injuries accounting for 25% of all trauma mortality. The bulk of this group occurs in the ageing population as a result of fragility fractures, but femoral shaft fractures also appear high on the list. Musculoskeletal injuries kill people by contributing to blood loss (for example open fractures of the femoral shaft) or as a result of septicaemia or embolic phenomena as secondary sequelae of the injury itself.

Whilst the mortality burden of musculoskeletal trauma is high as a proportion of total injury, the vast majority of patients survive their injury. The burden in terms of healthcare cost is considerable, with pre-hospital care, emergency department admission, in-patient stay, and associated operative costs and hospital follow-up. For the healthcare system, the costs are measurable, however, for the patient, the costs are even greater, with lost workdays, travel to and from clinics and the psychosocial burden. Some studies approximate the costs of multiple fractures as being as high as £35,000 per patient over 6 months (2).

ASSESSMENT

Assessment of patients with musculoskeletal trauma must follow the paradigm laid out in Chapter 6. Many musculoskeletal injuries present with obvious pain and deformity: this can distract the clinician towards treating the musculoskeletal injury and away from life-threatening injuries in other body systems. Only those musculoskeletal injuries associated with life-threatening external haemorrhage (<C>) present a requirement for immediate intervention including elevation, pressure, haemostatic dressing and tourniquets.

PRACTICE POINT

Do not focus on the musculoskeletal injury unless it is causing massive haemorrhage: search aggressively for other life-threatening injuries before returning to the obvious injury.

Other musculoskeletal injuries which should be detected and managed during the primary survey include those with associated vascular injury, lesser degrees of external blood loss and pelvic fractures. These require prompt and effective treatment. A pelvic binding device should be placed in every case where pelvic injury is suspected.

The majority of musculoskeletal injuries will be formally identified during the E (exposure) component of the primary survey, although less obvious injuries may not be found until the secondary survey if there is time to perform one before the patient arrives in hospital.

The most common presenting complaint is pain in the affected bone or joint, with a history of trauma to that area. For those who are conscious, the patient will often make the diagnosis, although the patient's assessment of the seriousness of the injury is unreliable. Catecholamines and cytokines may mask initial pain, allowing the patient to continue to use the affected limb, although this is unusual in significant long bone fractures. This is also true for those who are under the influence of drugs or alcohol. Focused questioning relating to numbness or altered sensation will elicit clues to underlying neurological involvement or injury and is important when completing documentation.

The mechanism of injury will often give a clue as to the likely injuries or injury patterns. For example, patients falling from height and landing on their feet may well have calcaneal or ankle fractures, but transmitted force may fracture the tibial plateaux, the hip, the spinal column or base of skull. Knowing the mechanism allows these injuries to be suspected and the affected areas examined. Although an exact history of the mechanism of injury can be difficult to obtain, every attempt should be made to achieve this. Triangulating a history from the patient, the first person to find the patient and the first person on scene is often helpful in this regard.

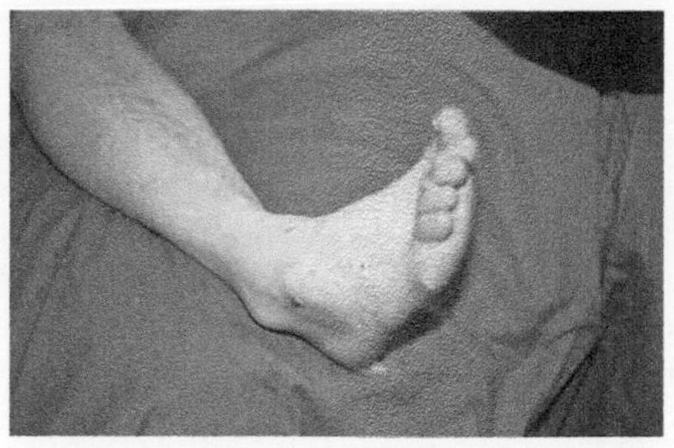

Figure 14.1 Deformity and tenting of the skin in a fracture dislocation of the ankle.

Any history elicited from the patient may focus the clinician towards certain injuries, but this should not prevent a systematic examination. Missed injuries are a common source of morbidity, complaint and litigation (3). The pre-hospital clinician often sets the tone for the in-hospital care. It is therefore imperative that the patient is examined as much as the situation safely allows, and any abnormal findings or suspected injuries conveyed verbally and in writing to the in-hospital or primary care teams.

The most common findings on physical examination include tenderness over the fracture, dislocation and deformity. For certain joints and bones the extent of deformity can be subtle. Comparison with the non-affected side is useful. To be meaningful, the patient should be fully exposed, with clothing removed by cutting where necessary, within the limits of dignity and environmental exposure. Clothing removal also facilitates application of splints and binders.

PRACTICE POINT

The patient should be appropriately exposed to permit examination of the affected limb. Once examined, the patient should be covered for dignity and environmental control.

Where fracture or dislocation is suspected, the affected area should be gently palpated, noting any tenderness and its exact location. The neurovascular status of the limb should be checked (distal pulses, capillary refill in digits and the sensation in the dermatomes supplied by distal radicular nerves). The skin should be examined for any redness, bruising, tenting or breaches (Figure 14.1). Any disruption to the skin should lead to a high index of suspicion of an open fracture and the patient treated accordingly. Finally, in the absence of obvious fractures, it is important to ask the patient to move or use the limb. Pain or inability to use the limb properly should lead to the suspicion of injury.

DIGITAL PHOTOGRAPHY

Photographs offer the advantage of highlighting the initial deformity of the limb, in particular when there is an open fracture, whilst (hopefully) preventing repeated and unnecessary examination. Digital cameras offer a rapid means of taking photographs at the scene of the accident, helping with identification of mechanism of injury and deformity of limbs prior to reduction. The information must remain confidential and, ideally, patient consent should be obtained. In any case, the patient must be informed that the image has been taken (4). Printed copies of the image should be added to the patient's notes and the digital copy immediately deleted to prevent accidental distribution.

PRACTICE POINT

Whilst useful in passing on information to the hospital teams, great care should be taken to make sure images are stored securely or deleted. Where possible, the patient should be informed images have been taken.

ANALGESIA/SEDATION

Many injuries will cause such severe pain that general patient management is difficult. In these circumstances, it is necessary to administer analgesia prior to other activities, such as extrication, clothing removal or movement of the patient. Small aliquots of intravenous opiates are usually effective. Inhaled nitrous oxide/oxygen (Entonox®) is useful if the patient is conscious and able to self-administer the gas. Other agents such as methoxyfluorane (Penthrox®), fentanyl lozenges and intravenous paracetamol offer alternatives. Occasionally, it is necessary to sedate the patient to achieve rapid control of the situation and the patient's pain. Small intravenous doses of midazolam (for example 0.5–1 mg) or ketamine (30–60 mg) usually suffice. It can be dangerous to administer sedation where other life-threatening injuries are present or when access to the patient's airway is restricted.

PRACTICE POINT

Having excluded life-threatening injuries in the primary survey, attention should focus on pain control.

IMMEDIATELY LIFE-THREATENING MUSCULOSKELETAL INJURIES

Musculoskeletal injuries may be life threatening per se or be an indicator of other associated internal injuries. Certain pelvic fractures (see later) are associated with exsanguination and should be immobilised as part of the second C in the primary survey (<C>ABCDE). Equally, open fractures or soft tissue injuries with arterial or major venous bleeding should already have been treated as part of haemorrhage control (<C>). Failure to address these injuries promptly can lead to exsanguination, propagation of acute traumatic coagulopathy, cardiac arrest and death. Simple, rapid measures are usually sufficient. Pelvic binders should be applied at the level of the greater trochanters and tightened according to manufacturers' instructions (Figure 14.2).

Tourniquet use was previously considered controversial. However, recent experience in military conflicts has seen development of tourniquet technology and a surge in its use (5). Where direct pressure and elevation are ineffective, a commercially available tourniquet must be applied. Partial or complete amputation of the limbs may require such measures, as may penetrating vascular injury. In the lower limbs, a second proximal tourniquet is occasionally required in circumstances where haemorrhage has not been arrested by the distal one (6). Failure to tighten the tourniquet enough is common. Appropriate tightness is painful and supplemental analgesia necessary. If the tourniquet is under-tightened it will fail to prevent arterial flow and will encourage distal venous engorgement, worsening haemorrhage and reducing the viability of the distal limb.

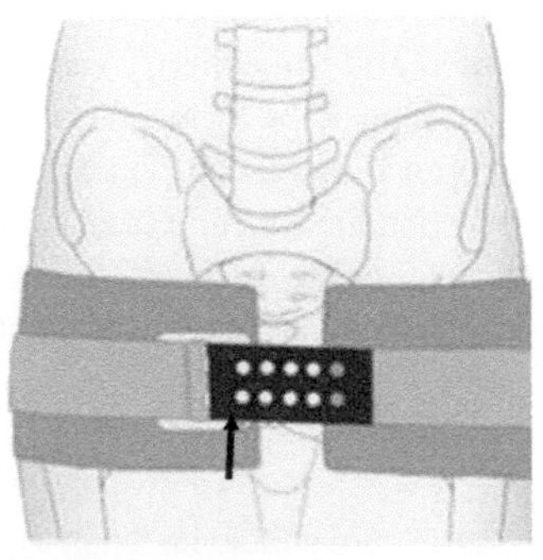

Figure 14.2 A pelvic binder applied at the correct level of the greater trochanters.

OPEN FRACTURES

Open fractures, where the periosteum of the bone has been exposed to external contamination, are at high risk of complications arising from infection. Systemic sepsis is a serious condition with an associated mortality, prolonged in-hospital stay, and delay in recovery and rehabilitation. Localised osteomyelitis of the bone is associated with a substantial morbidity. Patients often need frequent visits to the operating theatre for repeated wash out and debridement, sometimes followed by complex reconstructive orthoplastic procedures and may require lengthy courses of antibiotics. As a result, every effort must be made to prevent infection. Antibiotics are recommended as early as possible where open fractures are present, ideally administered within an hour of injury (7,8). A single dose of a broad-spectrum antibiotic is sufficient, such as co-amoxiclav (1.2 g for an adult; 30 mg per kg for a child). For penicillin-allergic patients, a third-generation cephalosporin or clindamycin may be appropriate. In most cases, antibiotic therapy can be administered after arrival in hospital.

There is no evidence for the routine administration of antibiotics in wounds other than those associated with open fractures. Formal pre-hospital irrigation of wounds is not recommended, although gross contamination should be removed. Where the patient is unlikely to get to help in a reasonable timeframe, gentle irrigation with sterile 0.9% sodium chloride to remove gross contamination is a sensible approach. Iodine-based dressings should not be used.

SPLINTS

Splinting limbs has a number of benefits:

- Anatomical or near anatomical reduction is usually the most comfortable position for the limb.
- Ongoing blood loss from fracture sites (including open fractures) is reduced.
- Relocation of the periosteum prevents the release of ongoing inflammatory mediators, which contribute to ongoing pain, neurological damage and help to drive coagulopathy.
- The risk of fat embolism is reduced.
- Packaging of the patient for transport is facilitated.

A variety of commercially manufactured splints are available to maintain anatomical alignment once reduction has been performed. They all work on similar principles (Box 14.1).

BOX 14.1: Technique for Applying a Kendrick® Splint and Sager® Splint

Kendrick® splint

- Apply the ankle hitch and tighten the stirrup.
- Apply the upper thigh strap at the top of the thigh and tightly into the crotch.
- Snap out the traction pole and ensure it is correctly seated
- Place the pole against leg, ensuring the pole extends 8 inches past the foot. Place the pole into receptacle in the thigh strap.
- Secure elastic strap around knee.
- Place yellow tab over dart end. Apply traction by pulling red tab.
- Finally, apply the thigh and ankle straps.

Sager® splint
- Apply the ankle hitch.
- Place the crutch in the groin against the pubic symphysis.*
- Extend the splint to 8 inches past the foot.
- Attach the ankle hitch to the splint.
- Applying gentle upwards pressure on the splint, slowly pull the handle downwards to apply traction.
- Apply the thigh and groin slings.

*In the male patient the external genitalia should be gently moved from between the crutch and the pelvis to avoid painful trapping of soft tissue.

For femoral fractures, traction splints apply traction against the pelvis. A further strap is placed around the ankle. All available splints then apply a force between these two points along the limb to maintain it in reduction and reduce post-fracture shortening. The *Kendrick®* and *Sager®* splints are the most commonly used in the pre-hospital environment (Figure 14.3). The Kendrick® traction splint has the advantage that it is lightweight and can be used in patients with suspected concomitant pelvic injury, however using a Sager® splint allows splintage of two legs with a single device.

For distal long bone injuries, traction is usually not required. The limbs can be held in anatomical alignment by simple box splints, vacuum splints or disposable casts. The malleable SAM® splint is useful for smaller patients and children, and is lightweight. It consists of an aluminium wire mesh within a soft foam outer covering. The splint can be moulded to provide maximum support to a joint or limb.

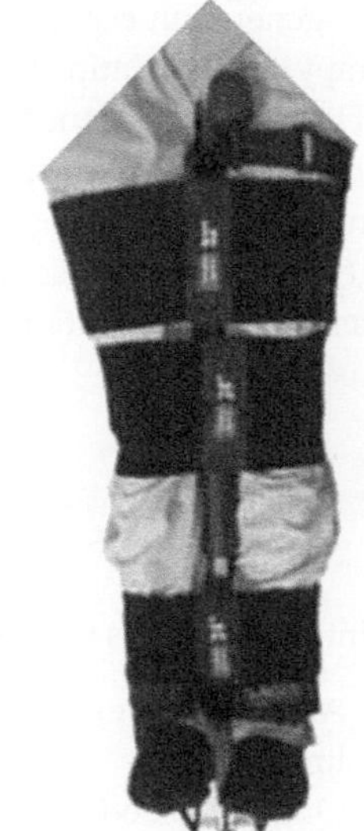

Figure 14.3 The Sager splint in use.

The application of splints can usually wait until the secondary survey/packaging phase, with the exception of pelvic slings, which should be applied during the primary survey (see earlier). Splinting a limb can be achieved by instructing other members of the team to hold the limbs in anatomical reduction, whilst other tasks are performed and the splints made ready. It should be remembered that the splints themselves only *maintain* traction that has been applied by the practitioner. Analgesia, anaesthesia or procedural sedation are usually required before the limb is reduced and the splint applied. All of this should be undertaken with the patient appropriately monitored.

CRUSH INJURIES

Where tissue is crushed, for example by falling masonry or machinery, it may become devitalised. External compression of the tissues prevents perfusion and the cells become ischaemic and die. As they die, they spill their acidic, potassium-rich internal fluid into surrounding structures and blood vessels. If the limb is trapped for an extended period of time, these metabolites may be released into the systemic circulation causing dangerous arrhythmias, which may in turn precipitate cardiac arrest. Secondary rhabdomyolysis can cause renal failure which may require in-patient renal dialysis.

Consensus guidelines (9) recommend loading the patient with intravenous fluids in the rescue phase, prior to release of the affected limb. This desire may need to be balanced with the need to limit haemorrhage by over-infusion. There is no evidence supporting the use of tourniquet application or amputation to prevent the systemic sequelae of crush injury on release of the affected limb. Renal impairment often ensues as a result of release of myoglobin and other toxic metabolites. Sodium bicarbonate administration may help ameliorate such effects and can be considered in the pre-hospital environment where necessary.

AMPUTATION

Amputation is a rarity in pre-hospital practice (10). It may be *traumatic* or *therapeutic* (11). Traumatic amputation occurs when such force is applied to the limb that it is severed by cutting (*guillotine* amputation) or tearing. Military practitioners will be more familiar with traumatic amputation than those in the civilian world, as it is a feature of blast injury. Depending on the mechanism, the nature of the forces involved may mandate a search for other life-threatening visceral injuries, although amputation due to isolated entrapment of a limb in machinery is relatively common. Blood loss from the amputation may be, but is not invariably, severe. Exsanguinating haemorrhage from the proximal stump should therefore be controlled using pressure, haemostatic dressings or a tourniquet tightened until the bleeding stops (<C>). This will usually be painful, therefore cannulation and analgesia will be required. The distal fragment should be wrapped in saline-soaked gauze and transported with the patient where practicable.

Therapeutic amputation may be required when the patient's life is at threat. This is a rarity and there is usually time to re-evaluate the extrication and call for a second opinion. Occasions when this is not possible include the following:

- The patient's life is at threat from other scene hazards.
- The patient's physiology is rapidly deteriorating and they are at imminent risk of cardiac arrest but remain trapped.
- The patient is deceased and they are preventing access to live casualties.
- The limb is unsalvageable as evidenced by experienced assessment of severe tissue disruption or near-complete amputation (10).

To perform an amputation, a proximal tourniquet should be applied. The patient should be cannulated, monitored and procedural sedation given by a trained practitioner. Ketamine is the agent of choice as it provides relative haemodynamic stability. The limb should be prepared with iodine or a chlorhexidine-based antiseptic. A distal circumferential incision should be made through the skin, muscle and ligaments. A Gigli saw can then be used to cut through the bone. The bone edges are likely to bleed and a dressing should be applied. The patient should then be transported to hospital. Cadaveric studies indicate that a simple hacksaw may be as easy to use as a Gigli saw, particularly for the inexperienced (12).

IN-HOSPITAL MANAGEMENT

The in-hospital teams follow the same principles as pre-hospital teams. The patient receives a further primary and secondary survey, and a full history is obtained. This helps plan necessary investigations and defines ongoing treatment. It is common UK practice to perform a *trauma CT scan* (head, neck, chest abdomen and pelvis) on patients who have been exposed to high mechanisms, have altered physiology or anatomically significant injuries. This should happen rapidly and allows full radiological diagnosis of internal injuries as well as musculoskeletal injuries, such as rib fractures, clavicular fractures, scapular fractures and pelvic fractures. The CT scout film will also often reveal limb injuries which can then be formally x-rayed. Treatment priorities will be determined by critical injuries identified during the primary survey or revealed on radiological investigation.

REGIONAL INJURIES

The remainder of this chapter will consider the pre-hospital management of injuries by region.

SCAPULA

The scapula articulates with the ribs, the clavicle (via the acromioclavicular joint) and the humerus, via the glenoid cavity. Numerous muscular attachments keep the scapula in position and its position on the posterior thoracic wall offers it a fair degree of protection. Consequently, scapular fractures are relatively rare. When they do occur, it is usually a result of direct and severe force applied to the back. Confident pre-hospital diagnosis of scapular fracture is difficult and its main significance is as a marker of significant force applied to the thorax which is likely to produce other injuries. Patients usually present with lateral back pain, made worse on movement of the arm, particularly anterior movement at the shoulder. Analgesia is the mainstay of pre-hospital management.

CLAVICULAR FRACTURE

The clavicle forms the attachment of the upper limb onto the axial skeleton. Both the sternoclavicular joint and the acromioclavicular joint are held together by tough ligamentous attachments.

Sternoclavicular dislocation is a very rare injury, but can cause life-threatening airway compromise as posterior displacement may put pressure on the trachea. It these circumstances it may be necessary to pull the clavicle forward manually if signs and symptoms of airway compromise are present.

Falling directly onto the point of the shoulder can break the strong ligamentous attachments and result in acromioclavicular joint dislocation. The diagnosis may be suspected when the patient gives a history of landing on their shoulder with a prominent distal end of the clavicle with tenderness. The pre-hospital treatment is a broad arm sling and analgesia (Figure 14.4).

The clavicle itself can fracture at any point along its length. The most common mechanism is by falling onto an outstretched hand (or putting the hand up prior to impact). Pain, point tenderness and a sagging of the arm on the affected side are hallmarks of a clavicular fracture. The conscious patient will want to support the arm to take the weight of the humerus off the clavicle and a broad arm sling is the treatment of choice.

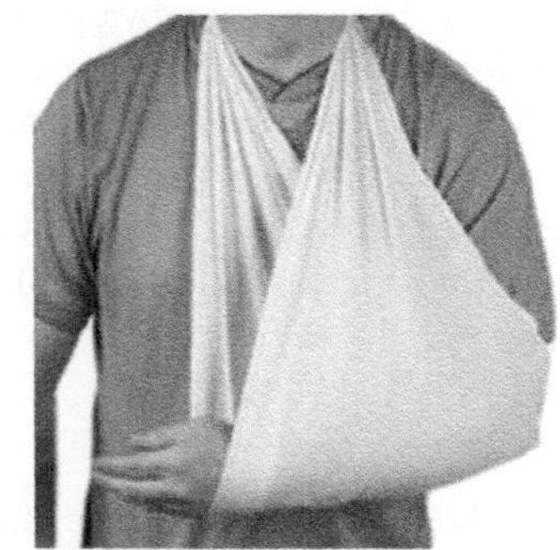

Figure 14.4 Application of a broad arm sling.

GLENOHUMERAL DISLOCATION ('DISLOCATED SHOULDER')

The most common shoulder dislocation is anterior dislocation; the other forms are rare. Dislocation occurs as a result of forced external rotation when the arm is abducted. This may occur during a fall onto an outstretched hand. Inevitably, there is some damage to the ligamentous structures of the shoulder, which puts the patient at risk of recurrent dislocation. The patient will present with severe pain and inability to move the arm. It is usually self-splinted in the position of dislocation and there is characteristic squaring of the shoulder. Pre-hospital treatment should normally be restricted to analgesia. Pre-hospital reduction of a dislocated shoulder is not usually appropriate. Depending on the mechanism of injury and the age of the patient, there may be associated fractures; in the obese the diagnosis may be made in error and the precise nature of the dislocation is not always clear. In addition, significant analgesia and/or sedation is generally required, especially in first dislocations. There may be specific circumstances when reduction is appropriate, but this should only be undertaken by those with considerable experience.

The precise method of reduction, if it is to be attempted, must be the one with which the operator is most comfortable and experienced. Kocher's method involves external rotation followed by adduction and internal rotation, but many practitioners do not favour this method owing to the risk of damage to the shoulder joint during its execution (13). Other techniques involve gentle external rotation of the humerus and external rotation with abduction. The axillary nerve runs around the neck of the humerus and is at risk during dislocation and relocation. The patient should be examined for altered sensation in the regimental badge area on the lateral aspect of the shoulder.

HUMERAL FRACTURES

The humerus usually fractures as a result of the application of direct force to the bone itself, such as being struck with a baseball bat or other object. In those with weakened bones, for example as a result of osteoporosis or metastatic spread of tumours, the bone can break as a result of relatively little indirect force, such as falling onto the elbow or an outstretched hand.

Pain is located to the upper arm, deformity may be present, although it is less likely with proximal fractures in the elderly where significant and early proximal bruising may be seen. The radial nerve winds around the midshaft of the humerus as it runs towards the elbow. Signs of radial nerve involvement include wrist drop and altered sensation to the back of the hand. Pre-hospital management includes analgesia and the application of a splint. For patients with an isolated humeral fracture, a 'collar and cuff' may suffice. This has the effect of utilising the lower arm and elbow as a weight to pull the humerus out to length and maintain anatomical reduction. If the patient has multisystem injuries and is lying flat, the arm should be allowed to rest in a position of comfort. Malleable splints may be useful for midshaft fractures.

DISLOCATED ELBOW

The elbow is vulnerable to injury from direct trauma, for example when a patient lands directly on the elbow itself. Dislocation is possible if force is applied along the length of the forearm whilst the arm is flexed at the elbow. Elbow injuries are extremely painful. The arm should be examined fully to assess for neuromuscular injury as the radicular nerves run through the elbow and are therefore vulnerable to damage.

Treatment is reduction to anatomical alignment, which is usually achieved by flexing the forearm at the elbow and palpating for anatomical reduction of the coracoid process of the ulna. This should not be attempted pre-hospital.

FOREARM AND WRIST FRACTURES

The radius and ulnar may be broken either as a result of direct force or indirect force transmitted when landing awkwardly on the wrist. Sudden deceleration in a road traffic collision where the patient grabs the steering wheel results in force being transmitted and can result in bilateral fractures. The most common cause is a fall onto an outstretched hand in the elderly. Management of the fracture includes the covering of any wounds, provision of analgesia and placement in a splint. Vacuum splints, box splints or SAM splints provide useful options in the field. Patients with open fractures should be given antibiotics.

The proximal row of carpal bones articulates with the distal aspect of the radius and ulna, whilst the distal row articulates with the metacarpals. The scaphoid bone, located in the well of the 'anatomical snuffbox', is vulnerable if the patient falls onto an outstretched hand. Diagnosis is not possible without imaging, and the patient with a painful wrist following a fall is likely to require hospital assessment. Management consists of analgesia and the application of a splint or sling. Malleable splints are useful.

METACARPAL FRACTURES

Metacarpal fractures, most commonly of the fifth metacarpal, usually arise form punching another person or more commonly a hard surface. There is swelling and tenderness over the affected metacarpals, and sometimes angulation of the metacarpal or 'loss' of the knuckle may be seen. Neighbour strapping prior to review in hospital for imaging is appropriate.

PHALANGEAL FRACTURES

The bones of the fingers may break if struck directly, or if the patient lands awkwardly on them. Adjacent fingers offer a useful splint to which the affected finger can be immobilised. Where open, wounds should be covered with saline-soaked gauze. Any amputated distal fragments should be wrapped in a saline-soaked gauze and transported with the patient to hospital.

THE HIP

Injury to the hip usually results in the patient complaining of pain in the joint itself, the proximal femur or the groin. Elderly patients and those with osteoporosis are particularly prone to fragility fractures of the neck of the femur. The exact location of the fracture within the femoral neck determines the surgical treatment, but cannot be determined by the pre-hospital clinician. This is an injury with significant long-term morbidity, particularly in older patients. Patients usually complain of pain associated with a fall, often onto the hip itself. The affected leg may be externally rotated and shortened when the patient is in the supine position. A history of minimal or no trauma and signs suggestive of proximal femur fracture should raise the possibility of a pathological fracture. Analgesia will be required for extrication and transfer. Intravenous opiates are appropriate. Where skill and expertise are available, a femoral nerve block offers good analgesia of the hip, which usually lasts for several hours. In the elderly, femoral neck fractures may appear to be associated with surprisingly little discomfort until the patient is moved.

The head of the femur may dislocate from the acetabulum in high-energy injuries, although significantly less energy is required to dislocate a hip prosthesis. This usually occurs as a result of transmitted force along a flexed leg. In the most common type of dislocation (posterior dislocation) the patient presents with the leg in flexion at the knee, the hip internally rotated and the leg abducted. In all cases the neurovascular status should be assessed, including in the case of clinically posterior dislocations the function of the sciatic nerve. The powerful upper leg muscles work against spontaneous reduction and a general anaesthetic is usually required for relocation. Attempts at re-location in the pre-hospital phase are not generally practical or appropriate.

THE PELVIS

The pelvis is formed by the illium, ischium and the pubic bones and their articulations with the sacrum. It houses the pelvic viscera, including the bowel, bladder and reproductive organs, and conducts the nerves which supply the lower limb. The bones are held together by tough ligaments (sacrospinous, sacrotuberous and sacrocoxygeal). Several arterial and venous plexuses travel through the pelvis and are particularly susceptible to injury. Pelvic fractures have been associated with up to 50% mortality at the scene of accidents and so should be treated with respect (14). Pelvic fractures should be suspected during high-mechanism injuries and a systematic search for other associated injures must be made. These are present in up to 40% of patients.

The pelvis fractures in three principle ways, relating to the direction of energy transferred through it (15). *Anterior-posterior fractures* occur when force is applied to the anterior superior iliac spines. The force causes the pelvis to open out, so-called *open book* fractures. The pubic ramus widen at the front and, if severe enough, the force will cause tearing of the sacroiliac joint. This leads to rupture of pelvic blood vessels and the risk of exsanguination. Motorcyclists are particularly at risk of pelvic fractures, as the petrol tank and handlebars catch the pelvis as the rider leaves the bike during a collision.

Lateral compression (LC) pelvic fractures occur when force is applied across one hemipelvis, such as when being run over by a car. The iliac wing, sacroiliac joint and pubic rami are all at risk of fracture. Haemorrhage is also likely. As the bone rotates inwards, it can damage the pelvic viscera, making bowel, bladder and reproductive organ injury more likely. Lateral compression injuries are associated with significant morbidity when the viscera are involved (16). They should be suspected when the transmission of force is lateral to the pelvis, such as lateral impact road traffic collisions or 'run over'–type mechanisms.

Vertical shear injuries can occur when the patient falls from height, landing on one foot. Force is transmitted along the leg, through the acetabulum. A moment is created and the contralateral hemipelvis rotates around the fixed point as it continues to 'fall'. This causes sacroiliac joint disruption, which can be severe. There is a high risk of neurovascular damage, with exsanguination from torn vessels and long-term injury to sciatic and possibly femoral nerves.

In the primary survey, suspected pelvic fractures should be managed by the application of a pelvic sling. Commercial slings, such as the TPOD® and SAM® sling, are particularly useful. If such a splint is not available, the feet can be tied together with a narrow-folded triangular bandage and a sheet applied tightly and circumferentially around the greater trochanters. Motorcycle leathers are quite tight and often maintain a broken pelvis in a reasonable degree of alignment. If no other slings are available, the leathers should be left uncut. When applying a pelvic binder, the binder should be placed against the skin; all overlying clothing should be removed.

PRACTICE POINT

Do not 'spring' the pelvis: splint it effectively and move on.

FEMORAL SHAFT FRACTURES

Femoral fractures result from direct or indirect force applied to the bone. Given the strength of this bone, the forces involved are usually large and a search for other associated injuries should be made. The patient will usually complain of severe thigh pain, and swelling and deformity are usually obvious. The patient will not be able to bear weight. Femoral fractures are associated with significant blood loss into the leg itself, which may not be visible. Open femoral fractures should be treated aggressively to prevent circulatory shock.

The powerful muscles of the thigh act to prevent manual reduction of the fracture. Opiate intravenous analgesia is essential and the affected limb should be placed in a traction splint after manual correction of the deformity during which the leg should be pulled out to near its normal length. Once the splint is in place, the patient's analgesic requirements normally drop dramatically.

PATELLAR DISLOCATION

Patellar dislocation usually occurs as a result of sudden twisting of the knee or occasionally a result of a direct blow. Some patients will be able to reduce the patella themselves, particularly if dislocation has occurred before. The patient experiences pain and an inability to weight-bear and the leg is held flexed. The trick to reduction is to gradually extend the knee with gentle pressure on the patella in a lateral to medial direction, whilst offering reassurance. Entonox® is useful for analgesia and as a distraction. The patient should be advised to attend hospital, as these injuries may be associated with bony fractures and may require specific imaging. All will require physiotherapy to reduce the risk of recurrent dislocation.

KNEE DISLOCATION

Knee dislocation occurs as a result of a high-energy injury and is a rare injury. It is usually part of a multisystem trauma. (Patellar dislocation is often referred to by lay people as knee dislocation.) This is a serious injury which is often limb-threatening. It is inevitably associated with rupture of several of the knee ligaments, and the popliteal artery is particularly vulnerable to compression over the distal aspect of the femur. This compromises the blood supply to the distal limb and risks ischaemia and myonecrosis.

The diagnosis is usually obvious if the dislocation persists, however, it may spontaneously relocate prior to the arrival of the pre-hospital practitioner. Residual pain may be confused with patellar, meniscal or tibial plateau injury. The leg should be splinted with the dislocation reduced under analgesia and the patient transferred to hospital for expert assessment (16,17).

LOWER LEG FRACTURES

The tibia and fibula are commonly fractured and may break separately or together, depending on the mechanism of injury. Since the tibia lies immediately subcutaneously, open fractures are relatively common. Because these injuries are often obvious, they may distract rescuers. The diagnosis is usually straightforward, as there is pain, swelling and obvious deformity, although this is not always the case. Conscious patients are usually unable to bear weight on the affected limb.

The limb should be thoroughly examined for any sign of an open injury which should be covered if found, after removal of any gross contamination. The patient can usually be managed with intravenous or inhalation analgesia, and the limb straightened and placed in a splint. Box splints, malleable casts and vacuum splints are all sensible options, although the latter are favoured by the National Institute for Health and Care Excellence (NICE) (7).

PRACTICE POINT

Open fractures are managed by removal of gross contamination (particulate dirt, debris, etc.) and coverage with a wet sterile dressing. Wound lavage is not required.

ANKLE FRACTURES

The ankle is a complex joint involving articulation of the tibia, fibula, calcaneum and talus. A number of ligaments hold the bones in position and contribute to ankle stability. If force is applied across the ankle or in inversion/eversion, a fracture can result. This often results from falling or landing awkwardly. Various classification systems exist for ankle fractures, but they are of little use to the pre-hospital practitioner.

Diagnosis is made on the basis of pain and deformity. If the ankle is not grossly deformed but swollen, ligamentous injury may have occurred. Simple sprains can be diagnosed by the application of the Ottawa ankle rules (18). If there is deformity, the patient is unable to weight-bear or there is tenderness over either malleolus or over the fifth metatarsal, hospital assessment is appropriate.

SUMMARY

Individual musculoskeletal injuries are rarely life-threatening, but such injuries must be immediately recognised and managed. These injuries, which include pelvic and femoral fractures may not always be obvious. Some fractures may not be of significance in themselves but may be important as markers of the severity of the trauma or the likelihood of other potentially critical injuries elsewhere. In most cases, even dramatic-looking fractures or soft tissue injuries require only the simplest pre-hospital management and must not be allowed to distract from the identification and treatment of other less obvious but more immediately critical injuries. The key to the management of these injuries once they have been identified is analgesia and splintage followed by transfer to hospital for assessment: precise anatomical diagnosis of an injury is rarely possible and will not affect the treatment required at scene.

REFERENCES

1. Office for National Statistics. Deaths Registered in England and Wales 2011.
2. Bonafede M, Espindle D, Bower A. The direct and indirect costs of long bone fractures in a working US population. *Journal of Medical Economics* 2013;16(1):169–178.
3. Pfeifer R, Pape HC. Missed injuries in trauma patients: A literature review. *Patient Safety in Surgery* 2008;2:20.

4. General Medical Council. Making and using visual and audio recordings of patients. 2011.
5. Lee C, Porter K, Hodgetts T. Tourniquet use in the civilian setting. *Emergency Medicine Journal* 2007;24:584–587.
6. Faculty of Pre-Hospital Care, Royal College of Surgeons of Edinburgh. Interim position statement on the site of application of tourniquets. 2013.
7. National Institute of Health and Care Excellence (NICE). Fractures (complex) assessment and management. NICE guideline [NG37]. February 2016. Accessed July 1, 2016. https://www.nice.org.uk/guidance/ng37/chapter/Recommendations#hospital-settings.
8. British Orthopaedic Association Standard for Trauma. The management of severe open lower limb fractures (BOAST 4). 2009.
9. Greaves I, Porter K, Smith J. Consensus statement on the early management of crush injury and the prevention of crush syndrome. *Journal of the Royal Army Medical Corps* 2003;149:255–259.
10. Porter K. Prehospital amputation. *Emergency Medicine Journal* 2010;27(12):940–942.
11. O'Meara M, Porter K. Extremity trauma. In *ABC of Pre-Hospital Emergency Medicine*, T Nutbeam, M Boylan (ed.). Oxford: Wiley, 2013.
12. Leech C, Porter K. Man or machine? An experimental study of pre-hospital amputation. *Emergency Medicine Journal* 2016. 2016;33:641–644.
13. Limb D, Rankine J, Sloan J, Aldous S. Soft tissue injuries: 7 shoulder and elbow. *Emergency Medicine Journal* 2009;26:426–433.
14. Scott I, Porter K, Laird C, Greaves I, Bloch M. The pre-hospital management of pelvic fractures: An initial consensus statement. *Emergency Medicine Journal* 2013;30:1070–1072.
15. Burgess AR, Eastridge BJ, Young JW, Ellison TS, Ellison PS Jr, Poka A, Bathon GH, Brumback RJ. Pelvic ring disruptions: Effective classification system and treatment protocols. *Journal of Trauma* 1990;30(7):848–856.
16. Brenneman FD, Deepak K, Boulanger BM, Tile M, Redelmeier DA. Long-term outcomes in open pelvic fractures. *Journal of Trauma* 1997;42(5):773–777.
17. Piper D, Howells N. Acute knee dislocation. *Trauma* 16(2):70–78.
18. Stiell I, McKnight RD, Greenberg GH, McDowell I, Nair RC, Wells GA, Johns C, Worthington JR. Implementation of the Ottawa ankle rules. *JAMA* 1994;271(11):827–832.

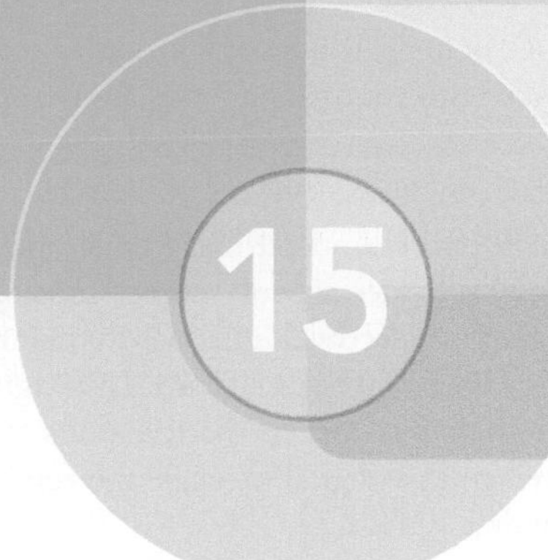

Analgesia, sedation and emergency anaesthesia

OBJECTIVES

After completing this chapter the reader will

- Understand the different options available for the management of pain
- Understand the potential hazards of sedation and anaesthesia
- Be aware of the importance of teamwork and drills in successful sedation and anaesthesia

INTRODUCTION

The effective and safe management of pain is an essential element of pre-hospital care. Pain must be managed because it is unpleasant and distressing, but also in order that necessary procedures can be carried out. In some cases it will be the procedure itself which mandates anaesthesia or analgesia, and in this situation a judgement must be made regarding the necessity of the intervention before the patient arrives in hospital. Whilst anaesthesia in particular offers immense benefit to the trauma victim, it is perhaps the most potentially hazardous component of pre-hospital care and not one to be undertaken lightly.

ANALGESIA

Pain is defined as *an unpleasant sensory and emotional experience associated with actual or potential tissue damage or described in terms of such tissue damage* (1). It is exhibited in a variety of ways: psychosocial factors play a major part in both perception of pain and the individual's ability to cope with it. There is significant interpatient variability in the pain experienced with similar injuries. *Analgesia* is *the inability to feel pain while still conscious* (2) and is often inadequately achieved following injury (3).

Effective analgesia is kind, improves patient compliance, allows better assessment and facilitates emergency procedures demonstrating logistic, physiological and long-term psychological benefits (4).

PHYSIOLOGY OF PAIN

The pain pathway is complex and some elements remain poorly understood. In a simplistic model, a painful stimulus in a particular area of the body activates sensory nerves (nociceptors) in that area. Axons from these nociceptors relay signals as electrical impulses to their cell bodies in the dorsal root ganglion and then onto the dorsal horn of the spinal cord. This 'signal' then ascends the spinal cord mainly through the spinothalamic tract to the thalamus from where it is relayed to areas of the cerebral cortex. It is when this 'signal' reaches the cerebral cortex that it is converted into a conscious sensation of pain.

Concurrent sympathetic stimulation causes tachycardia and vasoconstriction together with hyperventilation, decreased urinary tract tone and gastric emptying, and the cortical functions of fear and anxiety. Cumulatively, these may cause harm by increasing myocardial workload and reducing peripheral perfusion.

ASSESSMENT OF PAIN

Numerous pain-scoring systems are in use. The commonest are the *visual analogue scale (VAS)*, *verbal numerical rating scale (NRS)* and the *verbal categorical rating scale (VRS)*. The VAS and NRS are both equally sensitive in detecting changes in pain score and more sensitive than the VRS (5). In children, the Wong-Baker FACES pain scale is commonly used as a validated measure of pain (6). Whichever scale is used, it is important to realise that as a general rule the patient's pain is what they report it to be, not what the clinician thinks it is or thinks it should be. In pre-hospital care only the *verbal numerical rating system* is likely to be of value (where 0 is no pain and 10 the worst pain the patient has ever suffered).

Analgesia should be titrated to the pain that the patient reports, although in order to avoid giving too much analgesia, some awareness of the likely pain levels associated with particular injuries should be maintained. Whatever the initial pain score, it is vital to measure pain severity using the same system after analgesia has been provided. Pain measurement scores work best for the assessment of the effectiveness of analgesia and a decreasing pain score is the initial goal.

MANAGING PAIN

The ideal analgesic is one that is simple to use, has no adverse effects or drug interactions, and completely controls the patient's pain: such an agent does not exist. Often multiple analgesic modalities are needed for optimal results. Analgesia can be broadly classified into non-pharmacological and pharmacological.

NON-PHARMACOLOGICAL

Non-pharmacological methods of managing pain include

- Reassurance
- Positioning
- Physical methods
- Immobilisation and splinting
- Reduction of dislocations and fractures

Reassurance, particularly, is important but often forgotten. The patient who feels that they are in safe hands will be more confident in the outcome, calmer and cooperative and their pain perception will be reduced. Some patients may be reluctant to move from a position of comfort they have adopted and should not be compelled to do so unless there is a pressing reason, in which case alternative analgesia may be required to allow transport or further investigations.

Pain from burns is amenable to physical methods such as cooling or covering the burn wound to limit exposure to air. Ideally, fractures and dislocations should be reduced into their anatomical position to decrease ongoing pain. However, this may not be immediately possible due to the constraints of the environment, lack of expertise or other treatment priorities. Immobilisation and splinting provide some pain relief in these situations by reducing limb movement.

PHARMACOLOGICAL

There are numerous agents available for the relief of pain. Most can be administered through more than one route. Each route and drug has its own advantages and disadvantages. The clinician needs to tailor the analgesia to the patient's needs, taking into consideration injury, physiological status and skill available. The various routes for analgesia with their pros and cons are given in Table 15.1.

Table 15.1 Routes of analgesia

Route	Pro	Con
Oral	Easy to use No specific training required Ideal for mild pain scores	Slower onset of action Supine positioning of patient limits its use Not easily titrated Variable absorption
Inhalational	Patient controlled analgesia Rapid onset	Needs specific equipment Nausea and vomiting Not all patients can co-ordinate
Rectal	Simple to use Quicker onset than oral	Patient preference may limit acceptance
Nasal	Very useful in small children Non-invasive	Complex drug calculations needed Variable absorption depending on nasal secretions/blood
Buccal	Rapid onset Potent drugs available in this route	Limited availability
Intravenous/ intraosseous	Quick onset Can titrate to effect Widely used, most clinicians will be familiar with use	Needs training in cannulation/ intraosseous access
Intramuscular	Useful for situations where cannulation cannot be achieved	Cannot titrate Potential for 'build up' of potent drugs
Transdermal	Painless	Slow and variable onset
Subcutaneous (local anaesthetic only)	Very effective pain relief Variety of agents available depending on speed and duration of analgesia needed	Need training in nerve blocks to be effective Potential to damage nerves

Table 15.2 Pharmacodynamic properties of commonly used opioids

Drug	Speed of onset	Duration of action	Relative potency	Other routes in common use
Morphine	10 minutes	2–4 hours	1	Oral or intramuscular
Diamorphine	5 minutes	2–4 hours	1.5	Intranasal
Fentanyl	2–5 minutes	15–30 minutes	75–125	Intranasal or buccal
Alfentanil	1 minute	5–10 minutes	10–25	

OPIOIDS

Opioids are a commonly used class of analgesic in acute trauma. Morphine is the most commonly used, but other opioids in common use include fentanyl, alfentanil and diamorphine. There are varying rates of onset, peak effect and duration. Table 15.2 details the pharmacodynamic properties of the commonly used opiates when given intravenously.

Opioids act on three types of receptors in the central nervous system (CNS) to produce their effect: mu, kappa and delta (μ, κ and δ). The varying affinity of each drug to the different receptors is responsible for their differing pharmocodynamic actions. The main immediate adverse effects of opioids are nausea, vomiting, drowsiness and respiratory depression. These can be minimised by giving titrated doses in small aliquots, by administering an antiemetic and by combining them with other analgesic strategies in order to reduce the opioid dose and duration of action.

NON-STEROIDAL ANTI-INFLAMMATORY DRUGS (NSAIDs)

Non-steroidal anti-inflammatory drugs (NSAIDs) reduce prostaglandin synthesis through inhibition of cyclooxygenase 1 and 2 (COX 1, COX 2) to produce analgesic, antipyretic and anti-inflammatory effects. COX 1 inhibition reduces gastro-protection and may cause gastrointestinal side effects. Eighty percent of asthmatics can safely take NSAIDs without respiratory effects. It is advisable not to give an NSAID to an asthmatic if they have not taken one before, but they can safely be prescribed if the asthmatic patient has taken them in the past. Renal dysfunction may occur and NSAIDs should be avoided in those with known renal disease and in the elderly, although single doses are extremely unlikely to cause significant problems.

Common NSAIDs include ibuprofen, diclofenac, naproxen and ketoprofen. Ibuprofen has the lowest side effect profile, while naproxen and diclofenac have higher efficacy but more side effects. Newer NSAIDs (for example ketorolac) are selective COX 2 inhibitors and have a better safety profile than older NSAIDs.

PARACETAMOL

Paracetamol has long been the first choice of analgesia at the bottom of the pain ladder. It has almost no side effects and very few people are allergic to it. The exact mechanism of action is not understood but it is thought to be via selective COX 2 inhibition. Paracetamol in combination with ibuprofen is a highly effective combination analgesic (7).

Intravenous (IV) paracetamol is a popular and effective analgesic. There is some evidence that IV paracetamol is as effective as IV morphine and with a low side effect profile. It can be used in most trauma patients (8).

KETAMINE

Ketamine is a phencyclidine derivative. It provides profound analgesia and is an ideal analgesic for injuries where opiates alone may not be enough. It is described in more detail later in the chapter.

INHALATIONAL AGENTS

The inhalational agents used in the management of trauma patients are *Entonox®* and *methoxyflurane*. Entonox is a 50:50 mixture of oxygen and nitrous oxide. It is usually carried in cylinders with a mouthpiece for inhalation. Entonox is particularly useful for early analgesia while other agents are being prepared as it has a rapid onset (and offset) of action. It is contraindicated in patients with suspected pneumothorax and patients with decompression illnesses, as the nitrous oxide increases the volume of any gaseous space. In cold temperatures (usually below 6°C) Entonox separates into its component parts: administration of only nitrous oxide causes hypoxaemia. Therefore, if stored in cold temperatures, the cylinder must be inverted several times before use to remix the gases.

Methoxyflurane is an inhalational analgesic widely used in Australia which has recently been licensed for use in adults in the UK. The main concerns regarding its use have included potential nephrotoxicity associated with its use in anaesthetic doses. There seems very little evidence to suggest that this is a significant concern in pre-hospital practice. Methoxyflurane appears to be a safe and efficacious drug in smaller (analgesic) doses (9,10). It shows particular promise in remote or mountain medicine and may be self-administered through a Penthrox® inhaler which, due to the colour and appearance of the device, is often referred to as the *'green whistle'*. Reasonable analgesia is available on intermittent use of one inhaler for a period of about one hour and the onset is rapid. Methoxyflurane, unlike Entonox, is not contraindicated in peumothorax or other conditions which involve air-filled spaces within the body.

New Ideas

Methoxyflurane (Penthrox®) is an inhalational analgesic agent for self-administration with potential advantages for use in pre-hospital care.

LOCAL ANAESTHETICS (LAs)

Like opioids, local anaesthetics (LAs) vary in their onset and duration of action (see Table 15.3). They are used for subcutaneous injection, and nerve blocks as topical creams to reduce cannulation pain, and very occasionally for intravenous field analgesia.

Table 15.3 Common local anaesthetic agents

Local anaesthetic	Maximum dose (SC injection)	Onset	Duration
Lidocaine	3 mg/kg 7 mg/kg when combined with adrenaline	5 minutes	30 minutes
Prilocaine	6 mg/kg	5 minutes	1–1.5 hours
Bupivacaine/ levobupivacaine	2 mg/kg	10–20 minutes	5–16 hours

Note: Each agent comes in different concentrations presented as a percentage. Care should be taken to check the concentration before calculating the volume of injection.

Local anaesthetics affect neuronal cell membrane sodium channels, blocking action potential transmission. Used correctly they are safe and very effective. However, due to the nature of their use, inadvertent nerve damage and intravascular injections are potential complications. Intravascular injection can lead to cardiovascular collapse, seizures and cardiac arrest. This must be recognised quickly, as early administration of a lipid solution (Intralipid®) acts to reduce toxicity. Ideally, Intralipid should be available in all areas where local anaesthetics are used (11), but following pre-hospital use, rapid transfer to hospital is likely to be more appropriate.

New Ideas

Intralipid® is a mixture of soya oil, glycerol, egg phospholipids and phosphate designed for parenteral feeding. In the event of LA toxicity, 1.5 mLs/kg of Intralipid should be administered IV over 1 minute followed by an infusion of 15 mLs/kg/hr. After 5 minutes if the first bolus has not restored cardiac stability or if the patient deteriorates, two further boluses should be given, each over a minute and 5 minutes apart followed by an infusion of 30 mLs/kg/hr. The maximum cumulative dose is 12 mL/kg.

There are numerous nerve, compartment and field blocks that provide local anaesthesia to different parts of the body. A guide to the simpler nerve blocks is given later, but the clinician will still need training to perform them in order to to achieve safety and efficacy. Frequent practice is required in order to remain competent in the performance of these techniques.

Topical LA is very useful in young children and patients with needle phobia but generally takes too long to work to be of value in pre-hospital trauma care. *EMLA cream* (eutectic mixture of local anaesthetics) contains lidocaine and prilocaine and can be applied to intact skin to achieve topical anaesthesia. The full effect is usually achieved in about 1 hour. *Ametop®* (tetracaine gel) is similar to EMLA but has a quicker onset of anaesthesia. *TAC* (tetracaine, adrenaline and cocaine) and *LET* (lidocaine, epinephrine and tetracaine) are two mixtures that can be used on open wounds. They have been successfully used to suture wounds in children (12,13).

Haematoma block is used for fractures of the wrist. Local anaesthetic (usually up to 20 mLs of 1% lignocaine without adrenaline) is directly injected into the haematoma that surrounds the fracture. The injection is inserted through the dorsal aspect of the wrist to minimise inadvertent arterial injection after the skin has been cleaned. LA is then injected into the haematoma under sterile conditions to enable fracture reduction. Haematoma block is inferior to a Biers block in terms of wrist fracture reduction rates but is popular due to the ease and speed of use (14). It theoretically converts a closed fracture into an open one, but rates of infection are extremely low. This block is very rarely performed before the patient arrives in hospital, as simple splintage is usually adequate for pain control. It may be considered if circumstances require the correction of an obvious deformity, and evacuation is likely to be very delayed.

Femoral nerve block (Figure 15.1 and Box 15.1) is used for fractures of the femur and can significantly reduce the need for opiate anaesthesia and allow a pain-free reduction of fracture. The related *fascia iliaca* block provides improved analgesia specifically for fractured necks of femur but requires a specific needle and longer acting local anaesthetic and is probably best reserved for the emergency department.

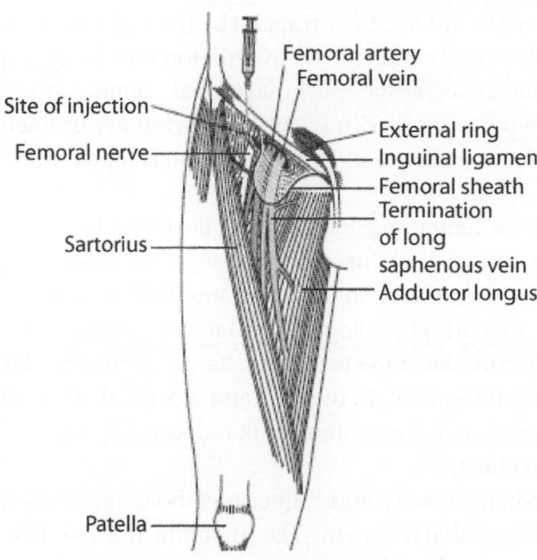

Figure 15.1 Landmarks for a femoral nerve block.

Digital nerve blocks (ring blocks) are used for anaesthetising digits on the hand or feet. They are not often performed in pre-hospital care, but may sometimes be needed, for example to allow the release of trapped digits from machinery. The technique is described in Box 15.2.

Although the use of local anaesthetic with adrenaline as a vasoconstrictor is usually avoided because of the risk of digital ischaemia, there is some recent evidence that shows this may not be a significant risk (15). It is still best avoided and especially in those peripheral vascular diseases such as Raynaud's disease.

BOX 15.1: Femoral Nerve Block Technique

- LA is injected around the femoral nerve as it passes below the inguinal ligament deep to the fascia lata in the groin.
- The nerve lies about 1 cm lateral to and slightly deeper than the femoral artery (remember *nerve–artery–vein–Y fronts: NAVY*) at a depth from the skin of about 2 to 3 cm.
- Having located the correct insertion point, check that the needle is not in a vessel by withdrawing the plunger.
- Inject 10–15 mLs of lignocaine.
- If the patient experiences a shooting pain or paresthesia during the needle insertion, the needle has touched the nerve and should be withdrawn.

BOX 15.2: Digital (ring) Block Technique

- The digits have two dorsal and two palmar nerves accompanying the digital vessels.
- 1–2 mL of anaesthetic is injected on either side of the digit to block these nerves.
- If the thumb or great toe is being blocked, additional local anaesthetic should be injected across the dorsum of the digit.
- LA with vasoconstrictors (adrenaline) should not be used for these blocks.

SEDATION

The wide variety of multimodal analgesic techniques will provide excellent pain relief for most trauma patients but in some cases, due to the nature of the injury or the procedures undertaken, or both, commonly employed techniques are inadequate to achieve or maintain effective pain relief. *Sedation in addition to analgesia* is frequently employed in these situations.

The patient with a fracture–dislocation of the ankle who is trapped by the foot and requires extrication from a vehicle offers an example of a situation in which sedation may be appropriate. Reassurance, strong opioid intravenous anaesthesia and inhalational agents are highly likely to provide good analgesia whilst the patient is in situ in the vehicle but are unlikely to be inadequate for dynamic analgesia when attempts are made to move the trapped limb and the patient.

Procedural sedation must be considered a temporary intervention designed to achieve a specific goal within the duration of effect of the drugs used. The dose of the chosen agent will be determined by the patient's clinical state, age, weight and pre-morbid medical status. Caution is required in frail patients and those with physiology altered to compensate for their injuries. The increased risk of cardiorespiratory decompensation exists on administration of sedating drugs due to decreased physiological reserves. In the frail and elderly, there is a significant likelihood of interaction with existing medications; as a result reduced doses should be used and these must be carefully titrated to effect.

In children, the smaller functional residual capacity and higher metabolic rate leads to a greater risk of hypoxaemia with respiratory embarrassment. The anatomical differences in children's airways (proportionally larger tongue plus narrow airway) make obstruction more likely (16).

Sedation is a pharmacologically affected state of consciousness described by various gradation scores including sequential depths of sedation up to general anaesthesia plus dissociative sedation (Table 15.4) (17,18).

Whilst sedation can be described using discrete levels, in practice it is not an easily compartmentalised phenomenon; rather there is a continuum, and inadvertent progression to deep sedation or general anaesthesia can, and does, occur.

The potential for apnoea, loss of airway protective reflexes and cardiovascular compromise require the precautions and considerations discussed later (19). Pre-oxygenation then continued administration of oxygen during procedural sedation reduces the incidence of hypoxaemia.

PRACTICE POINT

Sedation is not an easy option: It requires the same care and attention as general anaesthesia and a plan B in the event of airway compromise.

Capnography must be available whenever pre-hospital sedation is to be undertaken, and may provide early warning of changes in ventilation that could lead to hypoxaemia (20,21). Electrocardiogram (ECG), non-invasive blood pressure (NIBP) (cycling) and pulse oximetry should be monitored during sedation as must the level of consciousness. Ongoing multimodality monitoring is expected; assessment of the motor component of the Glasgow Coma Scale (GCS) has been validated as effective and safe during sedation (22,23).

Advanced airway equipment, suction and emergency drugs are essential in order to allow reversal of the sedation or conversion to general anaesthesia in the event of problems arising. Airway management techniques are discussed in Chapter 8. Pre-hospital sedation must not be undertaken by those who do not have the necessary skills to proceed to the induction of anaesthesia, including a full range of airway techniques up to and including surgical airway. Two practitioners must be present during induction and maintenance of sedation. Ideally the patient should have fasted for at least 4 hours (24,25), although this is unlikely to be the case in pre-hospital care. Just as in hospital practice, consent should be sought for the sedation as well as the procedure: in pre-hospital care, this is likely to be witnessed verbal consent (26).

Table 15.4 Levels of sedation

Level of sedation	Responsiveness	Airway	Spontaneous ventilation	Cardiovascular function
Anxiolysis	Normal (increased pre-procedural compliance)	Unaffected	Unaffected	Unaffected
Minimal	Normal response to verbal stimulation	Unaffected	Unaffected	Unaffected
Moderate	Purposeful response to verbal/ tactile stimuli	Unaffected	Adequate	Usually maintained
Deep	Purposeful response following repeated or painful stimulation	Intervention may be required	May be inadequate	Usually maintained
General anaesthesia	Nil	Intervention required	Likely to be apnoeic; ventilator support usually required	Often affected
Dissociative Sedation	May respond to verbal stimuli	Retention of protective airway reflexes	Generally adequate	Usually maintained

Source: Chudnofsky CR, Lozon MM, Sedation and analgesia for procedures, in *Rosen's Emergency Medicine: Concepts and Clinical Practice*, 5th ed., JA Marx, RS Hockberger, RM Walls (eds.), St. Louis, MO: Mosby, 2002, 2578–2590; American Society of Anesthesiologists, Continuum of depth of sedation: Definition of general anaesthesia and levels of sedation/analgesia, 2009.

For the safe sedation of children, SOAP ME, an acronym from the American Academy of Pediatrics, is a useful aid which neatly summarises the required elements of preparation (Box 15.3) (27).

BOX 15.3: Considerations for Safe Sedation in Children

S (Suction)	Appropriately sized and functioning suction device with attachments
O (Oxygen)	Sufficient oxygen supply with flow meters and appropriate delivery devices
A (Airway)	Patient-sized airway equipment
P (Pharmacy)	Correctly dosed drugs. Sufficient oxygen supply with flow for sedation, relevant antidotes and resuscitative drugs
M (Monitoring)	Pulse oximetry, ECG, BP, capnography
E (Equipment)	Specialist equipment depending upon each case requirement, e.g. paediatric compatible defibrillator

DRUGS FOR SEDATION

The relief of pain and anxiety and minimalisation of distressing recall in a way best tolerated by the patient are achieved with a range of drug classes and combinations. The evidence base and safety profiling of drugs beyond standard benzodiazepine and opioid combinations is expanding.

Entonox has rapid onset and offset of action. The time to peak effect is approximately one lung–brain circulation time (approximately 30 seconds); it takes approximately 60 seconds to wear off. It can be used on its own for various purposes such as anxiolysis in the needle averse, analgesia in simple reductions, or used concurrently with other agents to aid sedation (28–30).

Midazolam, a benzodiazepine, has a very short onset of action (1–2 minutes) and can last 30–60 minutes when administered IV/IO. The duration of action is similar to morphine and together they are a common procedural sedation combination.

Ketamine is a phencyclidine derivative, a dissociative anaesthetic with analgesic properties. The mechanism of action is multifactorial but mainly via N-methyl-D-aspartate (NMDA) receptor antagonism. In sub-anaesthetic doses of 0.25–0.5 mg/kg IV/IO there is profound analgesia with dissociation. It is an ideal analgesic for painful procedures in the trauma patient. Ketamine causes an increase in heart rate and blood pressure via sympathetic stimulation, respiration is not usually depressed, and although consciousness is altered, it is often not lost. It is relatively cardiostable and can be used in hypovolaemic patients. These properties make it an ideal analgesic and sedative in the pre-hospital phase during extrication or fracture reduction (31).

Ketamine has been associated with an emergence phenomenon in its recovery period characterised by hallucinations, nightmares and psychological distress. This is unusual after analgesic doses and its incidence is probably overstated (32). Co-administration of a small dose of benzodiazepine may settle this phenomenon. Patients who have been given ketamine should be allowed to recover in as quiet and restful an atmosphere as possible.

Propofol is lipophilic, sedative and hypnotic and normally used for general anaesthesia. It causes central nervous system depression via the GABAa receptor agonism. The onset of effect is rapid at 30–45 seconds and lasts up to 10 minutes. The duration of action is dose dependent. Propofol is metabolised in the liver, excreted by the kidneys and protein bound. It should be used with caution if pathology affects these pharmacokinetic factors. Dosages beyond a sedative dose (0.1 mg/kg/min) can result in deep anaesthesia where laryngeal reflexes and respiratory drive are lost, putting the patient at risk of aspiration and hypoxaemia. In addition propofol can cause significant hypotension, which may complicate the management of the seriously injured casualty (33). As propofol confers no analgesic effect, a concomitant analgesic, such as fentanyl, is required.

Reversal agents provide an additional level of safety during sedation. *Flumazenil* is very occasionally used to reverse adverse benzodiazepine effects including cardiorespiratory depression (34). It has a rapid onset of action but the half-life is considerably shorter than the shortest acting benzodiazepine. Caution is necessary when treating patients with a low seizure threshold like those with epilepsy, head injury or those on tricyclic antidepressants.

Naloxone (35) is an opioid reversal agent that, like flumazenil, has a short half-life. Its duration of effect can be prolonged by intramuscular administration. It should be noted that naloxone also reverses the analgesic effect of opioids; careful titration is needed in these cases. Both flumazenil and naloxone must be available before pre-hospital sedation is carried out.

PRE-HOSPITAL EMERGENCY ANAESTHESIA

Anaesthesia for the ill or injured patient is indicated for a number of reasons including the provision of ongoing treatment, safe transfer and facilitation of urgent investigations. In trauma the likelihood of other concurrent physiological compromise is high, and the incidence of serious airway complications in this patient group in these environments is significantly higher than during elective anaesthetic practice (36).

PREPARING FOR ANAESTHESIA

In pre-hospital care it is essential to ensure that the scene is safe and will stay safe for the duration of the procedure. Adequate (360°) access to the patient is essential. Every effort must be made to pre-oxygenate the patient: adjuncts, sedation and assisted ventilation may all be required. Effective pre-oxygenation significantly increases the time before desaturation occurs during the period of hypopnoea and apnoea. In the injured patient, it is impossible to predict the duration of safe apnoea and the aim must be to bring the patient's SpO_2 as close to 100% as possible and to de-nitrogenate the functional residual capacity (FRC) of the lungs before anaesthesia is induced. This will maximise the lung oxygen reservoir. Failure to achieve an SpO_2 >95% before tracheal intubation predicts a higher likelihood of desaturation during intubation with increased potential for harm.

Adequacy of pre-oxygenation is determined by technique but also by patient positioning, and physiology (chronic impairment and acute changes due to injury or illness). Head-up tilt is ideal but rarely possible in the pre-hospital environment. Whenever possible, 100% oxygen should be administered via a tight-fitting mask for at least 3 minutes, an acceptable pre-oxygenation period assuming normal tidal volumes and respiratory rate. However, the ill or injured patient may not be adequately pre-oxygenated with this technique. A low respiratory rate precludes sufficient alveolar ventilation to replace nitrogen in the functional residual capacity with oxygen, and lung pathology whether acute or chronic causes shunt physiology resulting in alveoli being perfused but not ventilated.

An SpO_2 <95% after 3 minutes of tidal volume breathing with a high FiO_2 source is evidence of shunting. Increasing FiO_2 will not improve this; assisted ventilation (low volume, low pressure and reasonably slow) is required. If the patient requires assisted ventilation before induction, this should continue after administration of the induction drug whilst waiting for the onset of complete paralysis.

Critically ill and injured patients are frequently agitated and this may affect delivery of effective care, including pre-oxygenation. Small boluses of sedation may be given (often the induction drug to be used for emergency anaesthesia) to achieve patient compliance and facilitate pre-oxygenation and other pre-anaesthesia preparations. This technique is known as *delayed sequence induction*. Forgoing optimal pre-oxygenation due to agitation and proceeding directly to general anaesthesia is unacceptable due to the associated higher risk of hypoxaemia and harm.

New Ideas

APNOEIC OXYGENATION

Continued delivery of oxygen to the alveoli during apnoea will occur if the airway is patent, for example during laryngoscopy. At pre-oxygenation, nasal cannula placed under mask and set at 15 L/min will significantly increase the time before desaturation.

Intravenous access must be available and working (flushed or with a running intravenous infusion). Intraosseous access is an effective alternative to multiple unsuccessful attempts to place an intravenous cannula. Monitoring standards should follow AAGBI (Association of Anaesthetists of Great Britain and Ireland) recommendations (wherever RSI performed) (37) and include ECG, SpO_2 and blood pressure monitoring (NIBP set to 2–3 minute auto cycles or intra-arterial BP). Using the capnograph during pre-oxygenation confirms that it is working.

BOX 15.4: Suggested Anaesthetic Regimes

		Option 1	Option 2	Option 3	Option 4	Option 5
		CVS 'stable'	CVS 'less stable'	CVS 'unstable'	Agonal or peri-arrest	Anticipated difficult intubation
a.	**Induction**	2 mg/kg ketamine	1 mg/kg ketamine	0.5 mg/kg ketamine	Omit	1–2 mg/kg ketamine
b.	**Adjunct**	2 mcg/kg fentanyl	1 mcg/kg fentanyl	Omit	Omit	Omit
c.	**Paralysis**	1 mg/kg rocuronium	1 mg/kg rocuronium	1 mg/kg rocuronium	1 mg/kg rocuronium	2 mg/kg suxamethonium

There is no ideal drug for emergency anaesthesia, although in the sick and injured the safety profile of some drugs appears to be far better than others. Ketamine is widely used for this reason both in and out of hospital and is recommended as the drug of choice for pre-hospital induction of anaesthesia (38) (Box 15.4). When preparation is completed, and with ongoing pre-oxygenation, an emergency anaesthesia checklist should be completed, with active engagement of the whole team. Safe practice means that all members of the team have a role in assisting with and monitoring the process. Fatalities have resulted from the erroneous belief that determination of correct placement is the responsibility of the intubator alone. Other members of the team, who will be less task centred, are ideally placed to identify errors and problems on induction of and during anaesthesia.

Precalculated doses of induction and neuromuscular blocking drugs are then administered (IV/IO). Ideally, if the likelihood of use justifies it, anaesthetic drugs should be drawn up and labelled at the beginning of each shift.

Ketamine is recommended for pre-hospital induction of anaesthesia. Doses of 0.5 to 2 mg/kg should be used, titrated to the haemodynamic state of the patient. Typically 2mg/kg will be a suitable dose for the very stable patient; 1mg/kg is used in a less responsive and/or more unstable patient. In very unstable patients the dose should be reduced further to 0.5 mg/kg.

Ketamine is relatively haemodynamically stable and has a wide therapeutic margin; as a result, a small overdose is unlikely to cause significant problems (a fact which is relevant in a working environment where the patient's weight is only estimated). There is considerable experience of the use of ketamine as an induction agent for the whole spectrum of injury patterns. In particular ketamine is now accepted to be safe for traumatic brain injury and for patients who may be fitting.

Ketamine is best avoided in patients with significant cardiac disease or post ROSC from a predominantly cardiac cause of an arrest. Induction with 1 to 3 mcg/kg of fentanyl with or without a small dose of midazolam and a normal dose of rocuronium offers an acceptable alternative in these patients.

ADJUNCTS

If the patient is haemodynamically stable, fentanyl can be given in addition to the induction agent ketamine. This will prevent a hypertensive response to laryngoscopy. As well as optimising the physiology of the patient. This is particularly useful in head-injured patients. The dose given must be altered according to the patient's cardiovascular status and relative size.

In cardiovascularly unstable patients the fentanyl should be omitted. A suitable dose is 2 mcg/kg in a stable patient, 1 mcg/kg if the patient is less stable, or none if they are unstable.

MUSCLE RELAXANTS

Rocuronium (1 mg/kg) should be used as the standard muscle relaxant in patients where difficult intubation is not anticipated. It has been demonstrated that a *'quick-look assessment'* often identifies the group of patients in which most difficult laryngoscopies are likely to be encountered. If a difficult laryngoscopy is anticipated, then 2 mg/kg of suxamethonium should be used, and fentanyl must be omitted. Ongoing muscle relaxation is subsequently achieved with 0.6 mg/kg of rocuronium.

POST-INTUBATION MAINTENANCE OF ANAESTHESIA

Ongoing sedation of the ventilated patient will be maintained with boluses of sedatives depending on the cardiovascular status of the patient. Signs of awareness include lacrimation and a strong bounding pulse with a rise in heart rate and blood pressure. If a weak, thready tachycardia is present, then hypovolaemia should be excluded as a cause, and end tidal CO_2 can be used as a surrogate cardiac output monitor.

In a patient with a good blood pressure who is tachycardic, boluses of 25 to 50 mcg of fentanyl and 1 mL of midazolam are appropriate for maintenance anaesthesia. In a patient who is hypotensive but requiring further sedation, then boluses of 10 to 20 mg of ketamine are appropriate. In a stable patient a combination of the above can be used as guided by the blood pressure and heart rate.

PAEDIATRIC ANAESTHESIA

Pre-hospital anaesthesia of small children is very rarely required. In many cases the risks of pre-hospital emergency anaesthesia outweigh the potential benefits. Where airway compromise cannot be overcome with simple airway manoeuvres, the risk–benefit equation may change and drug-assisted intubation may become appropriate. The experience of the pre-hospital team attending the child may also influence the risks and benefits.

CONCLUSION

Analgesia and anaesthesia are essential components of pre-hospital care. Many, perhaps the majority of, patients will require analgesia, some will need sedation, and a relatively small number will need general anaesthesia. Where anaesthesia is contemplated, the indications should be clear and the procedure should be performed in the full awareness of the associated risks. Clear protocols and governance are essential.

REFERENCES

1. Subcommittee on Taxomony. Pain terms: A list with definitions and notes on usage. *Pain* 1979;6:249–252.
2. *Oxford Advanced Learner's Dictionary of Current English*. 6th ed. Analgesia. Oxford University Press, 2000.

3. Albrecht E, Taffe P, Yersin B, Schoettker P, Decosterd I, Hugli O. Undertreatment of acute pain (oligoanalgesia) and medical practice variation in prehospital analgesia of adult trauma patients: A 10 year retrospective study. *British Journal of Anaesthesia* 2013;110(1):96–106.
4. Weisman SJ, Bernstein B, Schechter NL. Consequences of inadequate analgesia during painful procedures in children. *Archives of Pediatrics and Adolescent Medicine* 1998;152(2):147–149.
5. Breivik EK, Bjornsson GA, Skovlund E. A comparison of pain rating scales by sampling from clinical trial data. *Clinical Journal of Pain* 2000;16(1):22–28.
6. Hicks CL, Von Baeyer CL, Spanfford PA, Van Korlaar I, Goodenough B. The faces pain scale-revised: Toward a common metric in pediatric pain measurement. *Pain* 2001;93:173–183.
7. Ong CK, Seymour RA, Lirk P, Merry AF. Combining paracetamol with nonsteroidal anti-inflammatory drugs: A qualitative systemic review of analgesic efficacy for acute postoperative pain. *Anesthesia and Analgesia* 2010;110(4):1170–1179.
8. Craig M, Jeavons R, Probert J, Benger J. Randomised comparison of intravenous paracetamol and intravenous morphine for acute traumatic limb pain in the emergency department. *Emergency Medicine Journal* 2012;29(1):37–39.
9. Coffey F, Wright J, Hartshorn, Hunt P, Locker T, Mirza K, Dissmann P. STOP!: A randomised double-blind, placebo-controlled study of the efficacy and safety of methoxyflurane for the treatment of acute pain. *Emergency Medicine Journal* 2014;31(8):613–618.
10. Buntine P, Thom O, Babl F, Bailey M, Bernard S. Prehospital analgesia in adults using inhaled methoxyflurane. *Emergency Medicine Australasia* 2007;19(6):509–514.
11. Association of Anaesthetists of Great Britain and Ireland. Management of severe local anaesthetic toxicity.
12. Comparison of topical anaesthetic agents for minor wound closure in children. *Emergency Medicine Journal* 2012;29(4):339–340.
13. Zempsky WT, Karasic RB. EMLA versus TAC for topical anaesthesia of extremity wounds in children. *Annals of Emergency Medicine* 1997;30(2):163–166.
14. www.bestbets.org
15. Mohan PP, Cherian PT. Epinephrine in digital nerve block. *Emergency Medicine Journal* 2007;24(11):789–790.
16. Bauman BH, McManus JG. Pediatric pain management in the emergency department. *Emergency Medicine Clinics of North America* 2005;23(2):393–414.
17. Chudnofsky CR, Lozon MM. Sedation and analgesia for procedures. In *Rosen's Emergency Medicine: Concepts and Clinical Practice*, 5th ed., JA Marx, RS Hockberger, RM Walls (eds). St. Louis, MO: Mosby, 2002, 2578–2590.
18. American Society of Anesthesiologists. Continuum of depth of sedation: Definition of general anaesthesia and levels of sedation/analgesia. 2009.
19. AAGBI Safety Statement: The use of capnography outside the operating theatre. Association of Anaesthetists of Great Britain and Ireland, 2011.
20. Deitch K, Miner J, Chudnofsky CR, Dominici P, Latta D. Does end tidal CO2 monitoring during emergency department procedural sedation and analgesia with propofol decrease the incidence of hypoxic events? A randomized controlled trial. *Annals of Emergency Medicine* 2010;55:258–264.
21. Sivilotti MLA, Messenger DW, van Vlymen J, Dungey PE, Murray HE. A comparative evaluation of capnometry versus pulse oximetry during procedural sedation and analgesia on room air. *Canadian Journal of Emergency Medicine* 2010;12:397–404.

22. Godwin SA, Caro DA, Wolf SJ, Jagoda AS, Charles R, Marett BE, Moore J. Clinical policy: Procedural sedation and analgesia in the emergency department. *Annals of Emergency Medicine* 2005;45:177–196.
23. Royal College of Anaesthetists and College of Emergency Medicine. Safe sedation of adults in the emergency department.
24. Practice guidelines for preoperative fasting and the use of pharmacological agents to reduce the risk of pulmonary aspiration: Application to healthy patients undergoing elective procedures: A report by the American Society of Anesthesiologist Task Force on Preoperative Fasting. *Anaesthesiology* 1999;90:896–905.
25. Thorpe RJ, Benger J. Pre-procedural fasting in emergency sedation. *Emergency Medicine Journal* 2010;27(4):254–261.
26. Department of Health (UK). Reference guide to consent for examination or treatment. 2009.
27. American Academy of Pediatrics, Committee on Drugs. Guidelines for monitoring and management of pediatric patients during and after sedation for diagnostic and therapeutic procedures: Addendum. *Pediatrics* 2002;110(4):836–838.
28. Entonox. Anaesthesia UK. Retrieved from http://www.anaesthesiauk.com/ on April 10, 2009.
29. Ahlborg G, Axelsson G, Bodin L. Shift work, nitrous oxide exposure and spontaneous abortion among Swedish midwives. *Occupational and Environmental Medicine* 1996;53:374–378.
30. Branptom P. Review of Toxicological Data on nitrous oxide. MGC 153/08. European Industrial Gases Association (EIGA). 2008.
31. Porter K. Ketamine in prehospital care. *Emergency Medicine Journal* 2004;21:351–354.
32. Treston G, Bell A, Cardwell R, Fincher G, Chand D, Cashion G. What is the nature of emergence phenomenon when using intravenous or intramuscular ketamine for paediatric procedural sedation? *Emergency Medicine Australasia* 2009;21(4):315–322.
33. https://www.medicinescomplete.com/mc/bnf/current/PHP8521-propofol-non-proprietary.htm.
34. https://www.medicinescomplete.com/mc/bnf/current/PHP8653-flumazenil.htm.
35. https://www.medicinescomplete.com/mc/bnf/64/PHP8656-naloxone-hydrochloride.htm.
36. Cook TM, Woodhall N, Frerk C (eds). 4th National Audit Project (NAP4): Major complications of airway management in the UK. Royal College of Anaesthetists and Difficult Airway Society. 2011.
37. Association of Anaesthetists of Great Britain and Ireland (AAGBI). Recommendations for standards of monitoring during anaesthesia and recovery. February 14, 2007.
38. Sehdev RS, Symmons DA, Kindl K. Ketamine for rapid sequence induction in patients with head injury in the emergency department. *Emergency Medicine Australasia* 2006;18(1):37–44.

16 The injured child

OBJECTIVES

After completing this chapter the reader will

- Be aware of the differences in pre-hospital trauma care between children and adults
- Be aware of the challenges posed by pre-hospital paediatric trauma care
- Be able to assess and treat the injured child in the pre-hospital setting

INTRODUCTION

Paediatric trauma can present a significant challenge to the pre-hospital practitioner. Many practitioners lack experience in managing children as well as the knowledge required to do so and consequently are not confident when dealing with the injured child. Recognising the acutely sick or injured child can be difficult without experience, and management can be technically challenging, especially in very small children, and complex due to the variations in size between neonates at one end of the spectrum and adolescents at the other. In addition, there is undoubtedly a sense of higher emotional engagement when dealing with children.

The amount of serious paediatric trauma continues to decline. In the year 2000 there were 5011 seriously injured children (<18 years) and 191 deaths as a result of road traffic accidents in the UK. By 2014 this had fallen to 2519 seriously injured and 83 deaths (4.7% of all road deaths) (1). The 2012 Trauma Audit & Research Network (TARN) data contains 737 children with an Injury Severity Score (ISS) of >15, of which over 90% was blunt in mechanism (2). Trauma accounted for just 2.4% of all unplanned paediatric intensive care unit (PICU) admissions in 2014 (3). These figures are a great success story but as a result many pre-hospital practitioners will have limited exposure to serious paediatric trauma. Consequently practitioners must seek knowledge of the key differences in assessing and treating children, and must develop a structure which will enable them to successfully manage the injured child in the pre-hospital environment. That said, the pre-hospital practitioner can be confident that much of their adult trauma skill and experience is directly transferable to children.

Most of the anxiety surrounding emergency paediatric care is heightened by self-perceived lack of ability and fear of the consequences of error in caring for seriously injured children. This is not always justifiable and practitioners should be confident that they can provide good immediate care. Whilst children may be different from adults in certain ways, and the favourite phrase 'they're not just little adults' is too often used; children are still little human beings and have much in common with older patients.

INITIAL ASSESSMENT

<C>ABCDE

The framework for assessing and treating the injured child is exactly the same as that for an adult, namely <C>ABCDE. Generally speaking children sustain the same injuries and require the same pre-hospital management as adults, albeit in a modified form. Because of their size, anatomy and physiology, children are more likely to be multiply injured (4), and significant injury can easily go unrecognised or be underestimated. Practitioners must be aware of the normal ranges of physiological parameters at different ages (Box 16.1) (5). Other obstructions to assessment include the non-verbal or distressed and uncooperative child. This section will highlight key differences in the assessment of the injured child (also see Table 16.1).

BOX 16.1: Normal Paediatric Vital Signs

Age (years)	Heart rate	Respiratory rate	Systolic B/P
<1	110 – 160	30–40	70–90
1–2	100–150	25–35	80–95
2–5	95–140	25–30	80–100
5–12	80–120	20–25	90–110
>12	60–100	15–20	100–120

CATASTROPHIC HAEMORRHAGE

Peripheral, immediately life-threatening haemorrhage is rarely seen in civilian pre-hospital practice, but when present, the control of catastrophic haemorrhage takes immediate priority, as in adults. Limb tourniquets can be used on almost any size of child, but some pelvic splints may not fit smaller children and improvisation may be required. Haemostatic agents can be used in junctional haemorrhage in the same manner as in adults.

AIRWAY

Careful assessment of the paediatric airway is required. The paediatric larynx is higher and more anterior than in adults (C3/4 versus C6/7) and is more pliable and therefore less susceptible to cartilage fracture, but there may be injury without anatomical disruption or crepitus. However, the small diameter of the paediatric airway means oedema or haematoma will lead to obstruction more quickly than in adults.

Table 16.1 Key anatomical and physiological differences of children

	Key differences	Relevance
Catastrophic haemorrhage	Higher mL/kg blood volume	Rapid exsanguination
	Smaller total circulating volume	
	Higher cardiac index	
Airway	Higher, more anterior larynx with floppy epiglottis	Miller (straight) laryngoscope blades and different technique
	Narrow airway	More rapid obstruction with oedema or swelling
	Soft neck/airway tissues	Easy to compress and occlude with handling or swelling
	Changing anatomy with age	Different positions of the open airway
		Changing equipment and technique requirements
Breathing	Compliant chest wall	Thoracic injury without external evidence or rib fracture
	High, anterior ribs	Diaphragmatic breathing
		No or less thoracic abdominal organ protection
	Diaphragmatic breathing	Respiratory failure when diaphragmatic movement is impaired by injury or gastric distension
	Lower functional residual capacity and high oxygen consumption	Rapid de-saturation following pre-oxygenation and reduced laryngoscopy time
	Changing respiratory rate with age	Failure to recognise the injured child
Circulation	Changing pulse rate and blood pressure with age	Failure to recognise the injured child
	Difficulty accessing veins	Reliance on alternative routes of drug and fluid delivery
		Task focus and scene delay
	Less stroke volume variation	High significance of tachycardia in response to hypovolaemia
	Increased cardiovascular compensation for hypovolaemia	Hypotension occurs later and considered a peri-arrest finding
Disability	Low glycogen stores and high metabolic rate	Propensity for hypoglycaemia
	More permeable blood brain barrier	Never use hypotonic/hyponatremic fluids for resuscitation, risk of cerebral oedema
Exposure	Higher surface body area to weight ratio	Propensity for hypothermia

Signs of airway injury or obstruction are given in Box 16.2

Airway obstruction will require immediate resolution and possibly advanced airway management. This should be performed by clinicians competent in paediatric advanced airway management (see Chapter 15). Basic airway management can be tricky, in particular for infants, since small movements can obstruct the airway and constant vigilance and repositioning is required. Maintaining an airway in order to provide bag–valve–mask (BVM) ventilation with the two-person technique is particularly useful in children. Appropriately sized airway adjuncts must be carried to assist in basic airway management.

BOX 16.2: Signs of Airway Injury or Obstruction

- Snoring/gurgling
- Stridor
- Voice disturbance
- Cough/bark
- Surgical emphysema
- Tracheal shift
- Palpable disruption
- Crepitus
- Loss of landmarks (swelling)
- Respiratory distress
- Hypoxia
- Visible penetrating wounds with bubbling/sucking

CERVICAL SPINE

A detailed understanding of the mechanism of injury is required in order to assess the likelihood of cervical spine injury. The cervical spine should be assessed for pain, tenderness and restricted range of movement. In addition the child must be assessed for signs of neurological deficit. If any of these are present in the context of trauma, immobilisation should be considered (see Chapter 13).

BREATHING

An increased rate and effort of breathing is an early sign and should always raise suspicion of chest injury or hypovolaemia. It should be actively sought. It is vital to inspect the chest, bearing in mind that external signs of injury may be absent. Signs of increased effort of breathing and respiratory compromise are given in Box 16.3.

BOX 16.3: Signs of Increased Effort of Breathing and Respiratory Compromise

- Tachypnoea
- Nasal flaring
- Intercostal or subcostal recession
- Tracheal tug
- Accessory muscle use and posturing
- Grunting
- Cyanosis
- Agitation
- Altered consciousness

It is important to remember that exhaustion and bradypnoea are peri-arrest signs, and if they are present, immediate support is required. Careful palpation may reveal evidence of rib injury and abnormal chest movement. Percussion and auscultation may add valuable information but are often not practical in the pre-hospital environment where assessment may be limited to a 'look and feel'. The respiratory rate and oxygen saturation should be measured using an appropriately sized paediatric or infant oxygen saturation probe and recorded.

If there is a breathing problem requiring BVM ventilation, it is important to maintain an open airway and not to insufflate the stomach which will lead to diaphragmatic splinting and respiratory failure and ultimately cardio-respiratory arrest. This is very easily done in the heat of the moment in small sick children and some degree of gastric insufflation is practically unavoidable. When arriving at a scene where a child is receiving assisted ventilation, an assessment should be performed for gastric distension and consideration given to decompressing the stomach with a gastric tube if insufflation is suspected and evacuation likely to be delayed.

If BVM ventilation is being provided for anything but a brief period, a nasogastric or orogastric tube in the case of head injury will need to be be inserted to allow periodic decompression of the stomach. Active suction on the gastric tube may be necessary.

CIRCULATION

A common and serious pitfall is the failure to recognise shock in children. Children compensate exceptionally well for volume loss but progress rapidly to cardiac arrest when decompensation occurs. Paediatric cardiac arrest has a very poor outcome, and pre-hospital practitioners must pay particular attention to identifying hypovolaemia in trauma in order to prevent deterioration to the point of arrest. For many years measuring blood pressure in children was not encouraged, however, all injured children should have their blood pressure recorded. To achieve this, appropriately sized non-invasive blood pressure cuffs must be available. When assessing circulation the pre-hospital practitioner should record:

- Pulse (site, rate and volume)
- Capillary refill time
- Blood pressure
- Skin colour
- Skin temperature of peripheries
- Respiratory rate
- Consciousness

In infants the radial pulse is difficult to palpate, and the brachial pulse should be used instead to record the presence and rate of peripheral pulses.

In the presence of any of the signs listed in Table 16.2 together with a mechanism suggesting significant injury, hypovolaemia must be suspected and managed.

DISABILITY

All injured children require a blood glucose measurement (BM stix® or similar). Children are at particular risk of hypoglycaemia at times of physiological stress. This has the potential to cloud assessment by altering consciousness and cardiorespiratory observations.

Table 16.2 Signs of shock in children

Signs of hypovolaemia/shock in children	Pitfalls
Tachycardia	Also caused by pain, fear and hypoxia; where there is a mechanism for injury, always assume the cause is hypovolaemia
Delayed central capillary refill time (greater than 2 seconds)	Check centrally, e.g. the chest; ambient temperature may effect refill time
Weak or absent peripheral pulses	Brachial pulse in infants, radial in older children
Pallor	May be affected by ambient temperature, pain and fear
Cold peripheries	May be affected by ambient temperature
Tachypnoea	Also caused by chest injury, pain and fear
Altered consciousness	Also caused by hypoxia, hypoglycaemia intoxication and head injury
Measured hypotension	Age-/size-specific reference ranges; hypotension is a late and pre-arrest sign

Careful examination for head injury is required. Any fall from over a metre should be considered significant in addition to high-energy injury such as being struck by a vehicle. Significant features in the child's history which must be sought include an increased risk of bleeding (for example from haemophilia; children are rarely on anticoagulant or antiplatelet drugs but a few, such as cardiac patients, are) and previous cranial neurosurgery. The child must be carefully examined for signs of head injury (Box 16.4).

BOX 16.4: Signs and Symptoms of Head Injury

- Haematoma
- Abrasion or lacerations
- Deformity/depression
- Fluid or blood from the nose or ears
- Distended or tense anterior fontanelle
- Pupil abnormalities
- Abnormal eye movement
- Abnormal limb tone, power and reflexes
- Abnormal gait
- Irritability
- Respiratory depression/apnoea
- Altered consciousness

EXPOSURE

Injured children require a brief but full exposure to identify all injuries. Handling and movement should be kept to a minimum to preserve formed clots and prevent pain. Hypothermia mitigation and if possible warming are required for all trauma patients including in the warmer months. Hypothermia contributes to coagulopathy in trauma victims and its associated increased mortality. Once assessment and emergency treatment is complete, the child should be wrapped with blankets, including covering their head. In more severe conditions, an active warming device with heat packs should be used.

INJURIES AND THEIR MANAGEMENT

AIRWAY

Airway injuries are uncommon in children and account for less than 0.5% of trauma presentations (6). Management of the compromised airway follows the same stepwise approach used for adults beginning with opening manoeuvres and progressing to advanced airway techniques. Airway and ventilation equipment must be appropriately sized, including tube holders, capnography, ventilation circuits and rescue devices such as supraglottic airway devices. Instrumentation and insertion of airway devices should be done under direct vision to avoid injury to the soft tissues. Children are particularly susceptible to vagal stimulation, especially if they are hypovolaemic. Over-instrumentation of the oropharynx can cause bradycardia and arrest.

Oedema or compression of the airway due to swelling will cause rapid airway obstruction, particularly in younger children. In certain circumstances such as burns, 'elective' advanced management may be required prior to transfer if it is felt that the airway may become obstructed in transit.

It is taught that cricothyroid surgical airway insertion is not to be attempted in children under 12 years old. The anatomical changes of puberty make surgical airway insertion possible. If a surgical airway is being considered in a child, careful assessment of the laryngeal anatomy is required. Needle cricothyroidotomy can provide some oxygenation in extremis but not ventilation. This is still practically difficult, and equipment to attempt this should be preassembled in the bag. Nevertheless, a child must *never* be allowed to die of an obstructed airway because a surgical airway has not been performed: do a cricothyroidotomy. Complications such as tracheal stenosis can be dealt with later in a live child.

HEAD INJURY

Head injury is the most common traumatic cause of immediate death in children, and head injury (both isolated and in multiple injuries) is associated with the highest mortality rates amongst children (2,4), more than doubling the mortality rates of isolated chest and abdominal injuries. National Institute for Health and Care Excellence (NICE) guidance on head injuries includes pre-hospital assessment and describes the predictor variables for significant head injury. Hospital assessment will be required in any high-energy mechanism, and for children with a history of cranial neurosurgery, bleeding disorder, anticoagulation (or antiplatelet medication) and any suspicion of non-accidental injury. Children with any of the signs or symptoms in Box 16.5 will also require hospital assessment.

BOX 16.5: Symptoms and Signs in Head Injury Which Mandate Hospital Assessment

- Altered consciousness
- Altered behaviour/irritability
- Focal neurology
- Seizure
- Vomiting
- Amnesia
- Persistent headache
- Significant soft tissue injury
- Clinical signs of skull fracture
- Suspected penetrating injury
- Intoxication

Children with an obviously minor injury who are asymptomatic may be considered for discharge from scene within local and national guidance. However, the carers of the children must receive careful head injury advice.

AVPU is a useful rapid assessment of consciousness but pre-hospital clinicians must be competent in the application of the paediatric and infant Glasgow Coma Scales (Table 16.3).

Table 16.3 The paediatric Glasgow Coma Scale

	>1 Year		<1 Year	Score
Eye opening	Spontaneously		Spontaneously	4
	To verbal command		To shout	3
	To pain		To pain	2
	No response		No response	1
Motor response	Obeys		Spontaneous	6
	Localises to pain		Localises to pain	5
	Flexion withdrawal from pain		Flexion withdrawal from pain	4
	Flexion abnormal to pain		Flexion abnormal to pain	3
	Extension to pain		Extension to pain	2
	No response		No response	1
	>5 Years	**2–5 Years**	**0–23 Months**	
Verbal response	Orientated	Appropriate words/phrases	Smiles/coos appropriately	5
	Disorientated/ confused	Inappropriate words	Cries but consolable	4
	Inappropriate words	Persistent cries and screaming	Persistent inappropriate crying and/or screaming	3
	Incomprehensible sounds	Grunts	Grunts, agitated and restless	2
	No response	No response	No response	1
	TOTAL PAEDIATRIC GLASGOW COMA SCORE (3–15):			

If sedation or pre-hospital anaesthesia is required, the best pre-sedation/induction GCS and the state of the pupils should be recorded.

Patients with severe head injury are likely to require critical care including intubation and ventilation. The aims of pre-hospital critical head injury care in children are to maintain normal ventilation (oxygenation and carbon dioxide elimination), cerebral perfusion and normoglycaemia.

Good analgesia, sedation and paralysis are essential to prevent awareness, gagging and ventilatory difficulty, all of which raise intracranial pressure. Compression of the neck with tube ties, tube holding devices, cervical collars or dressings should be avoided and if at all possible a 30-degree head up position should be maintained. If there is clinical evidence of raised intracranial pressure, it is essential to ensure all the above are being achieved and consider hypertonic fluids if available (mannitol or hypertonic saline, both of which can be given to children).

SPINAL INJURY

Spinal injuries in children are uncommon. In children up to 14 years of age 82% of spinal injuries are cervical, the majority of which are in the upper cervical spine (7). The most common causes of spinal injury are motor vehicle collisions, sports and falls. The majority of spinal injuries are isolated but nearly 40% are associated with head injury (8).

Cervical spine immobilisation in children is a challenge. Children are less likely to cooperate with restrictive control measures and thus create more movement around the cervical spine if this is attempted. The rigid application of 'triple immobilisation' has been de-emphasised and very importantly C-spine immobilisation must never be prioritised over any life-saving intervention or critical care. Cervical spine collars are no longer recommended for children and should not be used for immobilisation. Spinal immobilisation should only be considered when

- There is peripheral neurological deficit.

or

- There is a mechanism consistent with cervical spine injury or clinical findings suggestive of potential injury:
  - Neck pain
  - Reduced range of movement/torticollis
  - Injury above the clavicle

And

- The child is not fully alert and cooperative.

Or

- The child has undergone pre-hospital anaesthesia.
- There is a reduced level of consciousness.

Fully conscious children with potential injury but no neurological deficit do not require cervical spine immobilisation and can maintain their own cervical spine control during transfer to hospital.

If immobilisation is required this should initially be manual. Co-operative children can have head blocks and tape applied or can be immobilised using a vacuum mattress. In the rare occurrence of penetrating cervical spine injury, immobilisation is not required.

Like adult patients, children should never be transported on spinal boards; these are appropriate for extrication only. Scoop stretchers and vacuum mattress devices can be used to transport and transfer children.

Table 16.4 Summary of chest injuries in children

Injury	Signs	Pre-hospital interventions
Pneumothorax	Tachypnoea Hypoxia Unilateral breath sounds	Oxygen
Open pneumothorax	Penetrating wound Tachypnoea Hypoxia Reduced breath sounds	Chest seal dressing
Tension pneumothorax	Tachypnoea Hypoxia Signs of shock	Oxygen Chest decompression
Massive haemothorax	Tachypnoea Signs of shock Unilateral breath sounds Dull to percussion	Oxygen Volume replacement Chest drainage
Flail chest	Paradoxical chest wall movement Tachypnoea Hypoxia	Analgesia Oxygen (Ventilatory support)
Cardiac tamponade	Signs of shock Penetrating wound	Oxygen Volume replacement (Thoracotomy)

CHEST INJURY

Chest injury accounts for approximately 20%–30% of paediatric major trauma (9) (Table 16.4). It is the second leading cause of death following head injury (2). The paediatric chest wall is highly compliant leading to significant energy transfer to the thoracic cavity without external signs of injury. Rib fractures occur in only 1%–2% of chest injuries, however if present they are associated with a very high risk of other system injuries (10). Chest injuries should be suspected where there is a consistent mechanism or signs of injury, respiratory distress or hypovolaemia.

Children sustain the same chest injuries as adults, but because of their size are more likely to be multiply injured. Most children with a chest injury will have injuries in another body area (4).

Pre-hospital chest decompression may be required. It is essential that appropriately sized equipment is available and that providers are familiar with procedures in children. 'Finger thoracostomy' may not be possible in small children, as the rib spaces can be too narrow; a pair of forceps should be used. For emergency decompression of a tension pneumothorax, a cannula may well provide temporary resolution because of the thin and less muscular chest wall.

ABDOMINAL INJURY

Children are more susceptible to intra-abdominal injury than adults. Because of their size, thinner and less muscular abdominal wall and less thoracic and pelvic protection, there is more energy transfer to the intra-abdominal structures. Splenic and then hepatic injuries are the commonest intra-abdominal injuries (11,12).

Abdominal pain is almost always seen in significant injury but signs of peritoneal irritation on examination are frequently absent (13). In studies of children presenting to level 1 trauma centres, over 50% of children with a direct blow to the abdomen, for example from cycle handlebars, had a significant abdominal injury. Any similar mechanism should heighten suspicion of intra-abdominal injury. Positive findings on abdominal examination (tenderness, abrasions or contusion) are associated with significantly increased chance of intra-abdominal injury (14,15). These children should have hospital assessment.

MUSCULOSKELETAL INJURY

PELVIS

Pelvic fractures are far less common in children than adults with an incidence of around 50% that of adults (16), accounting for 1%–3% of pelvic fractures seen by orthopaedic surgeons (17). Additionally life-threatening haemorrhage is less likely in children, possibly due to the pliability of the immature pelvis and more effective vasoconstriction of healthy vessels. Exsanguination is more likely to be from organ injury: the incidence of gastrointestinal and solid organ injury is similar in the adult and paediatric populations (16,18). There is conflicting evidence regarding differences in mortality between adults and children whose reported mortality is up to 25% (19). The principles of clot preservation should still apply, namely stabilisation and minimal handling. Around 10% of fractures are unstable (19). Pelvic stabilising devices should still be applied in the pre-hospital setting and maintained until imaging is obtained, if the mechanism and clinical findings suggest pelvic fracture, but they must be appropriately sized and applied.

EXTREMITIES

Pre-hospital clinicians should be aware of the different pattern of fractures seen in children. In every case the joint above and below the injury must be examined, as localisation of injuries can be difficult (particularly in non-verbal children) and pain is quite often referred. Causing pain during examination only increases the child's level of distress. Assessment and examination must always start with the uninjured limb. The examination should be limited to the minimum required and adequate analgesia should be provided as soon as possible. Limbs should be splinted and elevated where practical. Neurovascular status distal to the injury should be recorded.

In the upper limb, supracondylar fractures of the humerus are common in younger children. Scaphoid injuries are very rarely seen in young children but begin to appear when approaching puberty. Distal radial and radial head injuries are more likely.

PRACTICE POINT

A long leg box splint or vacuum splint provides an effective transport and immobilisation device for an infant.

In the lower limb, *toddler's fractures* (spiral fractures of the tibia) are a very common fracture in children. The typical presentation is a non-weight bearing child complaining of lower limb pain following what is often a very minor mechanism of injury. They typically occur in ambulatory children up to 3 years old. In older children an injury not to be missed is a *slipped upper femoral epiphyses (SUFE)*. It should be excluded in any episode of trauma, minor or otherwise, leading to limp, hip, thigh or knee pain, and pain or restricted movement on hip examination in a child approaching puberty or older (10–17 years). Hospital referral should therefore be considered for any child who is not weight bearing.

BURNS

Each region of the United Kingdom has a nominated paediatric burns centre and there will be local guidelines on referral and transfer as well as access to burns treatment advice via telephone.

Paediatric burns are common. It must be remembered that blunt trauma may accompany burns: signs of hypovolaemia in a patient with burns in the pre-hospital phase are unlikely to be due to the burn. Burns may occur as a result of safeguarding issues or non-accidental injury, and the pre-hospital practitioner must be vigilant for evidence of concern at the scene. The criteria for paediatric burns referral are given in Box 16.6.

BOX 16.6: Criteria for Referral to a Paediatric Burns Centre

- All burns greater than 1% total body surface area (the size of the child's palm)
- Circumferential burns
- Burns involving the face, hands, perineum or chest
- Burns with inhalational injury including smoke or gas
- Electrical, chemical or radiation burns
- Neonatal burns of any size
- Burns where there are safeguarding concerns
- Burns in a systemically unwell child
- Old or infected burns

Fluids resuscitation is only required if there are signs of shock. If the presentation is delayed, then fluids should be calculated using the Parklands Formula.

Burns are extremely painful and thus the burned child will be distressed and difficult to manage. Vascular access can be difficult if burns are extensive and in these patients intramuscular ketamine may be particularly useful (see analgesia section). All burns should be covered to prevent airflow over the injury.

VASCULAR ACCESS AND FLUID RESUSCITATION

ACCESS

Intravenous (IV) access in most children is perfectly achievable, but in toddlers, infants and shocked children it can be technically difficult if the practitioner is not well practised in paediatric cannulation. In the event of a seriously injured child requiring emergency fluids or drugs, multiple attempts at cannulation can lead to unnecessary delays in treatment and extended time at scene. If the initial attempt to cannulate is unsuccessful, then the practitioner should move straight to intraosseus (IO) access. Practitioners who are not skilled in the cannulation of smaller or unwell children should consider using an intraosseus needle device as the first route of access. The preferred site for IO access is the tibia, however, there are several alternatives including the distal femur and proximal humerus. Care should be taken to site needles away from epiphyses, although this is practically impossible if the proximal humerus is chosen. The evidence suggests that significant consequences as a result of epiphyseal damage are exceptionally rare. The pain of flushing and infusion can be considerable and the use of a slow bolus of lidocaine is often advocated. This is at the discretion of the practitioner and may not be warranted if the child is very unwell. If it is considered , great care must be taken in drawing up the correct dose. Once IO access is established, all fluids and drugs must be actively infused using a syringe and not left to passively infuse.

PRACTICE POINT

In critical trauma, after one failed attempt at intravenous access, insert an intraosseus line.

FLUID RESUSCITATION

Hypotension in children represents cardiovascular decompensation as a result of prolonged hypovolaemia, acidosis and hypoxia. This will be rapidly and potentially irretrievable. As a consequence hypotension cannot be used as a safe end point for resuscitation. When there are signs of hypovolaemia (Table 16.2) in the context of trauma it should be assumed that the child requires fluid resuscitation and the low blood pressure must not be written off as a result of pain or distress.

Resuscitation with blood products is best, however, not all pre-hospital services currently carry blood and most still rely on crystalloid fluids for volume replacement. Whichever fluid is used, children should receive boluses of 5 mL/kg repeated after reassessment and to the target end point. A reasonable end point is the presence of an *easily palpable* radial pulse (brachial in infants). If non-invasive blood pressure monitoring with an appropriate sized cuff is available it should be used. A reasonable measured end point following fluids would be the lower end of the age-specific normal systolic blood pressure range.

TRAUMATIC CARDIORESPIRATORY ARREST

Traumatic cardiorespiratory arrest (TCRA) in children requires expert coordinated treatment to identify and very rapidly correct reversible causes of arrest (Table 16.5).

It may be difficult to distinguish arrest from an extremely low cardiac output state, but both conditions require the same rapidly applied steps:

- Intubation and end tidal carbon dioxide monitoring
- Oxygenation and ventilation
- Bilateral thoracostomies
- Volume replacement
- Reassessment
- Consideration of thoracotomy if there is no return of output

Outcomes in paediatric thoracotomy are similar to those in adults (20). Thoracotomy in children is indicated in low velocity penetrating chest trauma and cardiac arrest. Its role in other causes of traumatic arrest in children, including blunt trauma has not yet been fully established.

Table 16.5 Causes of TCRA and interventions

Cause	Intervention
Catastrophic haemorrhage and hypovolaemia	Control external haemorrhage, splint the pelvis Replace volume
Hypoxia	Open and secure airway Ventilate
Tension pneumothorax	Perform bilateral thoracostomy (see text)
Cardiac tamponade	Perform thoracotomy and pericardial release
High spinal injury	Provide advanced life support

ANALGESIA

Excellent pain control is an essential and basic standard in the management of injured children. Analgesia will reduce tachycardia and bleeding, reduce distress and result in a calmer, more cooperative child. Not only will it settle the child, enabling further assessment, but it will also calm parents and carers, enabling a better patient–parent–provider therapeutic dynamic. The essential steps in achieving this are first, recognition of the problem and second, a comprehensive knowledge of the agents and routes available to the pre-hospital practitioner. Full dosing information can be found in Box 16.7 and Tables 16.6 and 16.7.

BOX 16.7: Calculating a Child's Weight

An estimation of the child's weight will be required for fluid and drug prescription. A carer may know the child's weight and it is worth remembering to ask. Recently new weight formulae have been published to reflect the increasing weight of Western paediatric populations (21). The traditional formula

$$\text{Weight in kg} = (\text{Age} + 4) \times 2$$

is simple to remember and for drugs and fluids in the pre-hospital setting is not likely to cause harm. However the older the child, the more the potential underestimation (22). There are new formulae adjusted to age (21).

1 to 12 months	(0.5 × Age months) + 4
1 to 5 years	(2 × Age years) + 8
6 to 12 years	(3 × Age years) + 7

Pounds to kilogram conversion:

$$\text{Weight in kg} = \text{Weight in pounds}/2.2$$

Table 16.6 Intranasal diamorphine dosing table (using 10 mg vial of diamorphine; a worked example is given in Box 16.8)

Weight (kg)	Volume saline added (mL)	Notes
15	1.3	1. Estimate weight or weigh to nearest 5 kg
20	1.0	2. Add weight specific volume of 0.9% sodium Chloride to 10mg vial of diamorphine powder
25	0.8	
30	0.7	
35	0.6	3. Draw up 0.2 mL of the solution
40	0.5	
50	0.4	
60	0.3	

Source: Kendal LM et al., *BMJ* 2001;332:261–265.
Note: Once drawn up, administer into nostril using a mucosal atomiser device. This will deliver 0.1 mg/kg of diamorphine.

Table 16.7 Paediatric drug doses

Drug	Route[a]	Dose	Cautions
Paracetamol	Oral Rectal Intravenous	15 mg/kg (maximum 1g) QDS 15 mg/kg (maximum 1g) QDS Over 10kg 15mg/kg (maximum 1g) QDS Under 10kg 7.5 mg/kg QDS (Maximum 30mg/kg/day)	Always check if paracetamol has been administered by carers.
Ibuprofen	Oral only	5 mg/kg (maximum 400 mg) TDS	May exacerbate asthma; avoid in renal disease, gastric ulceration and bleeding disorders
Diclofenac	Oral Rectal	1 mg/kg (max 50 mg) TDS 1 mg/kg (max 50 mg) TDS	May exacerbate asthma; avoid in renal disease, gastric ulceration and bleeding disorders
Codeine[b]	Oral only	1 mg/kg (maximum 60 mg) QDS	Contraindications below
Tramadol	Oral Intravenous	1 mg/Kg (max 50 mg) QDS 1 mg/Kg (max 50 mg) QDS	Serotonergic side effects
Oramorph	Oral only	1–3 months, 50–100 mcg/kg, 4 hourly 3–6 months, 100–150 mcg/kg, 4 hourly 6–12 months, 100–200 mcg/kg, 4 hourly Over 1 year, 200–300 mcg/kg, 4 hourly	Respiratory and CNS depression. Nausea and vomiting
Morphine	Intravenous only	50 mcg/kg boluses up to 200 mcg/kg titrated to pain	Respiratory and CNS depression. Nausea and vomiting
Fentanyl	Intravenous Intranasal	0.25 mcg/kg in boluses up to 1 mcg/kg titrated to pain 1 mcg/kg atomised into nostril(s)	Respiratory and CNS depression. Nausea and vomiting If >0.4 mL, divide between nostrils
Diamorphine	Intravenous Intranasal		Respiratory and CNS depression. Nausea and vomiting
Ketamine (sedation and analgesia)	Intravenous Intramuscular Intranasal	0.25–0.5 mg/kg 2–4 mg/kg 3 mg/kg	Dysphoria Consider small dose of benzodiazepine
Ketamine (induction of anaesthesia)	Intravenous Intramuscular	1–2 mg/kg 5–8 mg/kg	Adjust dose to physiological status

(Continued)

Table 16.7 (Continued) Paediatric drug doses

Drug	Route[a]	Dose	Cautions
Midazolam (sedation)	Intravenous	0.1 mg/kg	Respiratory and CNS depression, particularly with opiates
Suxamethonium	Intravenous	1–2 mg/kg	
Rocuronium	Intravenous	0.6–1.2 mg/kg	
Mannitol (20%)	Intravenous	1.25–2.5 mL/kg	
Hypertonic saline (3%)	Intravenous	1–2 mL/kg	

[a] All IV doses apply to intraosseus route.
[b] Codeine is now contraindicated in all children less than 12 years of age and children 12 to 18 years of age who are post-tonsillectomy or -adenoidectomy with a history of sleep apnoea. Alternatives to codeine are dihydrocodeine, oral morphine solution and tramadol.

ORAL ANALGESIA

Oral analgesics include paracetamol, ibuprofen and opioids.

Codeine is now contraindicated in all children less than 12 years of age and children 12 to 18 years of age who are post-tonsillectomy or -adenoidectomy with a history of sleep apnoea.

BOX 16.8: Intranasal Morphine Dose: Worked Example

Estimated weight 20 kg
Add 1.0 mL to 10 mg vial of diamorphine powder
Draw up 0.2 mL
Dose given equals 4 mg (0.1 mg/kg)

RECTAL ANALGESIA

Rectal administration is a useful route in distressed or vomiting infants. Both paracetamol and diclofenac can be administered via the rectal route.

INTRAVENOUS ANALGESIA

Titrated intravenous opiates remain the gold standard for the control of severe pain. However, intravenous access can be difficult to achieve and cause distress for the child. It can also be a cause of unacceptable scene delay. For most children, pain will be controlled by alternative routes. Analgesics suitable for IV administration include paracetamol, morphine, fentanyl and ketamine.

INTRAMUSCULAR ANALGESIA

Intramuscular ketamine is a rapid and effective route for delivering good pain control. It is particularly useful in burns where the patient is both very distressed and is difficult to cannulate. Whilst analgesic, sedative and anaesthetic doses are quoted, the reality is that the distinction can be difficult to achieve. Practically, any ketamine use in children will produce some altered consciousness. Monitoring, equipment and safety requirements should reflect those of sedation.

INTRANASAL

Intranasal is a particularly useful route for achieving effective and rapid analgesia. Ketamine, fentanyl and diamorphine are all well absorbed through the nasal mucosa. Diamorphine is commonly used in UK emergency departments for burns and fracture analgesia. Initially piloted in the 1990s it is acceptable to patients and staff, is extremely well tolerated and very safe (21). The drugs need to be in a low volume, and volumes above 0.4 mL should be divided between nostrils. At volumes above 0.4 mL efficacy may be lost. The drugs should be administered using a 1 mL syringe and a mucosal atomiser device (MAD). Doses for intranasal drugs are detailed in Tables 16.6 and 16.7.

INHALED ANALGESIA

Older children, essentially those of school age and above, will be able to used inhaled agents such as nitrous oxide and oxygen mix (Entonox®). This will provide temporary but not definitive pain relief. The child is likely to be more cooperative once some analgesia or sedation secondary to the nitrous oxide is achieved. This may allow the practitioner to gain IV access, dress or splint the injury, and provide further pain relief.

NON-PHARMACOLOGICAL PAIN RELIEF

One should never underestimate the powers of the *'magic bandage'*. Children in pain need reassurance and comfort – be nice! Dressing wounds will reduce pain. All injured limbs should be placed in a sling or splinted and elevated. Wherever possible, parents should be allowed to stay with their children unless parental anxiety is sufficient to complicate management.

SEDATION AND ANAESTHESIA

PRINCIPLES

Around 8% of severely injured children are intubated prior to arrival at hospital (2). Clinicians undertaking pre-hospital emergency anaesthesia (PHEA) and intubation in children must be trained and competent in induction of anaesthesia and advanced airway management. The indications for pre-hospital anaesthesia and intubation are

- To secure and protect and airway
- Neuroprotection in head injury
- Respiratory failure
- To facilitate the humane provision of emergency care
- To facilitate safe transfer (particularly air transport)

Pre-hospital clinicians are likely to be less experienced in PHEA in children than in adults. It is important that regular team training in paediatric PHEA scenarios is undertaken to minimise risk and maximise success. All team members should be familiar with the correct sizing of equipment and drug dosing in children (Boxes 16.7 and 16.9 and Tables 16.6 and 16.7).

Most pre-hospital critical care units have moved now to using cuffed endotracheal tubes in children of term age and over. It is vital that the practitioner is familiar with the sizing and correct inflation of cuffed tubes. It is also vital that it is very clearly handed over on arrival to hospital by the pre-hospital team and acknowledged by the receiving team that a cuffed tube has been used.

Aside from endotracheal tubes the clinician will also require paediatric sized and specific equipment including

- Endotracheal tube holder
- Catheter mount
- Paediatric colorimetric end tidal carbon dioxide indicator

- Correctly sized straight and curved laryngoscope blades
- Introducer
- Bougie

Sedation of children may be required to facilitate extraction or packaging, and for procedures such as fracture or joint reduction when there is immediate concern regarding neurovascular status. Practitioners who undertake sedation must be prepared to take over the airway and thus should be trained and competent in paediatric pre-hospital anaesthesia. Children who are sedated must have full monitoring including end tidal carbon dioxide.

BOX 16.9: Paediatric Airway Sizes

Endotracheal tube internal diameter in mm

Cuffed = (Age/4 + 4) – 0.5

Uncuffed and microcuff = Age / 4 + 4

Endotracheal tube oral length in cm

Age/2 + 12

Supraglottic Airway Device Sizing

LMA		I-gel	
Weight/kg	Size	Weight/kg	Size
<5	1.0	2–5	1.0
5–10	1.5	5–12	1.5
10–20	2.0	10–25	2.0
20–30	2.5	25–35	2.5
30–50	3.0	30–40	3.0

PREPARATION

The assessment and treatment of children often causes heightened anxiety because of lack of experience and familiarity. Practitioners can mitigate this by being thoroughly prepared to treat children when it is required. Appropriately sized equipment must be available and fit for purpose. Practitioners must be familiar with its use, and aide memoires will help with fluid and drug calculations and are readily available in paper and electronic form. Pre-hospital unit training and clinical governance activity must regularly include paediatric topics. Access to senior paediatric advice may be available and relevant phone numbers should be carried.

SAFEGUARDING

In the TARN report, 10% of children under 2 years old were injured non-accidentally (2). Information from the scene of injury and on the observed nature of presentation and family dynamics can be vital to enable community and secondary care health care professionals to make decisions regarding safeguarding children. Pre-hospital clinicians will have the advantage of seeing the child in the community setting and possibly in the home. Any such observations and concerns must be documented and passed on to the relevant organisations. The injury mechanism must be correlated with the injuries seen, and the child's behaviour and interaction with clinicians and family members observed. Any delay in accessing health care and inconsistencies in history should be noted and passed on. Smaller children, particularly non-ambulatory children, with injuries should have a full examination whenever possible, particularly if discharge at the scene is being considered. Cause for concern forms or similar notifications of concern to social workers can be completed and returned. When there are concerns surrounding safeguarding, it is essential to enquire about other children in the household. Immediate child safety concerns should be reported to the police who have dedicated safeguarding officers. Advice can usually be obtained from community paediatricians or by contacting the local paediatric emergency department. All pre-hospital clinicians should be trained to the correct safeguarding children level.

DESTINATIONS

Around 45% of severely injured children in the TARN report were taken to a major trauma centre (MTC) as the first admitting hospital. Most of these were taken to either a children's or adult and children's MTC. Currently there are only 5 children's MTCs and 11 adult and children's MTCs out of a total of 26 MTCs in England. UK-based evidence to show improved outcomes at children's MTCs is not yet available. Pre-hospital practitioners should apply local trauma network criteria to choose their destination. Unstable children should be taken to the nearest unit and should not bypass emergency facilities.

SUMMARY

Managing children who have been victims of trauma requires attention to detail and a knowledge of paediatric anatomy and physiology and how it changes with age. However, the principles of management are essentially the same in children as in adults. Practice as a team reduces anxiety and improves care in this vulnerable group of patients.

REFERENCES

1. Department for Transport (UK) statistics, Reported casualties by road user type, age and severity, Great Britain, 2014.
2. The Trauma Audit & Research Network. Severe Injury in Children 2012.
3. PICANet annual report, 2015.
4. Bayreuther J, Wagener, Woodford M, Edwards A, Lecky F, Bouamra O, Dykes E. Paediatric trauma: Injury pattern and mortality in the UK. *Archives of Disease in Childhood: Education and Practice Edition* 2009;94:37–41.
5. Advanced Life Support Group. *Advanced Paediatric Life Support: The Practical Approach (APLS).* 5th ed. Blackwell, 2005.
6. Mandell DL. Traumatic emergencies involving the paediatric airway. *Clinical Pediatric Emergency Medicine* 2005;6:41–48.
7. Brown R, Brunn MA, Garcia V. Cervical spine injuries in children: A review of 103 patients treated consecutively at a level 1 pediatric trauma center. *Journal of Pediatric Surgery* 2001;36:1107–1114.
8. Cirak B, Ziegfield S, Knight VM, Chang D, Avellino AM, Paidas CN. Spinal injuries in children. *Journal of Pediatric Surgery* 2004;39:607–612.
9. Deasy C, Gabbe B, Palmer C, Bevan C, Crameri J, Butt W, Fitzgerlad M, Judson R, Cameron P. Paediatric and adolescent trauma within and integrated trauma system. *Injury* 2012;43:2006–2011.
10. Kessel B, Dagan J, Swaid F, Ashkenazi I, Olsha O, Peleg K, Givon A, Israel Trauma Group, Alfici R. Rib fractures: Comparison of associated injuries between pediatric and adult population. *American Journal of Surgery* 2014;208:832–834.
11. Lynn KN, Werder GM, Callaghan RM, Sullivan AN, Jafri ZH, Bloom DA. Pediatric blunt splenic trauma: A comprehensive review. *Pediatric Radiology* 2009;39:904–916.
12. Potoka DA, Saladino RA. Blunt abdominal trauma in the pediatric patient. *Clinical Pediatric Emergency Medicine* 2005;6:23–31.

13. de Jong WJ, Stoepker L, Nellensteijn DR, Groen H, El Moumni M, Hulscher JB. External validation of the Blunt Abdominal Trauma in Children (BATiC) score: Ruling out significant abdominal injury in children. *Journal of Trauma and Acute Care Surgery* 76:1282–1287.
14. Hynick N, Brennan M, Schmit P, Noseworthy S, Yanchar NL. Identification of blunt abdominal injuries in children. *Journal of Trauma and Acute Care Surgery* 2014;76:95–100.
15. Holmes JF, Lillis K, Monroe D, Borgialli D, Kerrey BT, Mahajan P, Adelgais K et al. Identifying children at very low risk of clinically important blunt abdominal injuries. *Annals of Emergency Medicine* 2013; 62:107–116.
16. Ismail N, Bellemare JF, Mollitt DL, DiScala C, Koeppel D, Tepas JJ 3rd. Death from pelvic fracture: Children are different. *Journal of Pediatric Surgery* 1996;31:82–85.
17. Holden C. Paediatric pelvic fractures. *Journal of the American Academy of Orthopaedic Surgeons* 2007;15:172–177.
18. Demetriades D, Karaiskakis M, Velmahos GC, Alo K, Murray J, Chan L. Pelvic fractures in pediatric and adult trauma patients: Are they different injuries? *Journal of Trauma* 2003;54:1146–1151.
19. Fractures of the pelvis in children: A review of the literature. *European Journal of Orthopedic Surgery and Traumatology* 2013;23:847–861.
20. Easter JS, Vinton DT, Haukoos JS. Emergent pediatric thoracotomy following traumatic cardiac arrest. *Resuscitation* 2012;83:1521–1524.
21. Kendal LM, Reeves BC, Latter VS. Multicentre radomised controlled trial of nasal diamorphine for analgesia in children and teenagers with clinical fractures. *BMJ* 2001;332:261–265.
22. Luscombe MD, Owens BD, Burke D. Weight estimation in paediatrics: A comparison of the APLS formula and the formula 'Weight=3(age)+7'. *Emergency Medicine Journal* 2001;28:590–593.

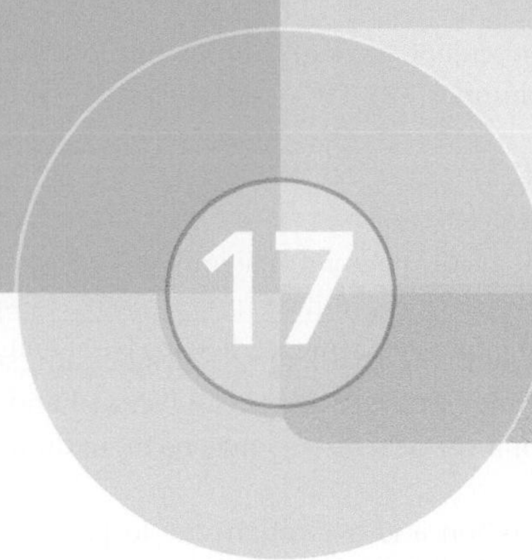

17 Trauma in pregnancy

OBJECTIVES

After completing this chapter the reader will

- Understand the anatomical and physiological changes which occur in pregnancy
- Understand the obstetric complications of trauma
- Understand the principles of pre-hospital management of the pregnant trauma patient

INTRODUCTION

The possibility of pregnancy needs to be considered in all female trauma patients of child-bearing age (between puberty and the menopause). Although the practitioner may be concerned that there are two patients to manage, the outcome of a viable foetus is reliant on the optimal resuscitation of the mother (1). In pregnant women, trauma may not infrequently be the consequence of domestic violence or psychiatric conditions which may make management more complex.

MECHANISMS OF INJURY

The *Centre for Maternal and Child Enquiries* (CMACE) report reviewing all maternal deaths in the UK from 2006 to 2008 identified 30 deaths in pregnant women involving trauma, from a total of 261 patients (11%) (2). Life-threatening trauma in pregnant women is therefore fortunately rare.

In the CMACE report the most common cause of death from trauma in pregnant women was a road traffic collision as a passenger or pedestrian. This accounted for 15 deaths. Failure to wear a seat belt and failure to position the seat belt in the correct position were common factors. Domestic violence is still distressingly common and the CMACE study identified eight pregnant women who were murdered by violent methods. Between 2006 and 2008, six pregnant women committed suicide by traumatic means (including hanging, jumping from height, setting themselves alight or stabbing).

ANATOMY AND PHYSIOLOGY IN PREGNANCY

AIRWAY

Management of the airway in pregnant women is potentially challenging. Weight gain, soft tissue oedema and enlarged breasts may impede laryngoscopy. A bougie and short-handled laryngoscope must be available (3). The landmarks for a surgical airway may be more difficult to identify.

Pregnant women are at increased risk of regurgitation and aspiration due to pregnancy hormones relaxing the gastro-oesophageal sphincter, delayed gastric emptying, and increased intra-gastric pressure from upward pressure on the diaphragm from the gravid uterus. If advanced airway manoeuvres are required, intubation with a cuffed endotracheal tube is preferred over a laryngeal mask airway, with the use of cricoid pressure during induction of anaesthesia and early decompression of the stomach with a naso- or orogastric tube.

BREATHING

Pregnancy leads to increased oxygen consumption and reduced functional residual capacity. Oxygen should be given to all pregnant women, irrespective of their recorded SpO_2. Rapid desaturation will occur during intubation and it may be useful to administer 15 L via nasal cannula throughout the procedure as well as ensuring an adequate period of pre-oxygenation via a mask. The tidal volume increases by 20% at 12 weeks and up to 40% at term. Hyperventilation is normal, with the result that the pregnant patient should be running a low-normal end tidal CO_2. During pregnancy the thorax is less compliant due to breast enlargement and increased intra-abdominal pressure, so bag–valve–mask ventilation may be more difficult. The diaphragm rises by up to 4 cm as the uterus enlarges. This means any thoracostomy or chest drain insertion will need to be performed higher (3rd or 4th intercostal space) to avoid intra-abdominal incision.

CIRCULATION

In the supine position the gravid uterus will cause compression of the inferior vena cava reducing venous return and therefore cardiac output. This can occur from 20 weeks or earlier (4): if there is a visible 'bump', then the supine position should be avoided. Even if a woman is asymptomatic lying flat, the foetus may be compromised. If a pregnant woman is found to be hypotensive, it is important to check that she is lying in a 'left lateral tilt' position.

Heart rate is increased by 10–15 beats per minute by the third trimester. Blood pressure falls by 10–15 mmHg in the second trimester and returns to near normal by term. Circulating blood volume increases by up to 50% in the third trimester. This means that significant haemorrhage can occur (more than 1.5 litres) before signs of hypovolaemic shock become evident. Shunting of uterine and placental blood into the maternal circulation may mask maternal shock. The foetus may be in hypovolaemic shock even if the mother *appears* normovolaemic.

The uterine circulation is directly dependent on maternal blood pressure. Once the mother develops hypotension from hypovolaemia, peripheral vasoconstriction will reduce uterine blood flow further. It is likely that with a maternal systolic blood pressure of 90 mmHg or a palpable radial pulse the foetus will still be perfused adequately. Therefore the principles of permissive hypotension (fluids titrated to a radial pulse, an alert (A) conscious level or systolic blood pressure of 90 mmHg) are still appropriate in pregnancy. In late pregnancy the uterus displaces the abdominal viscera making patterns of injury and abdominal examination less reliable, and there is increased vascularity of the pelvis which means pelvic fractures may easily cause life-threatening haemorrhage (Box 17.1).

BOX 17.1: Anatomical and Physiological Changes in Pregnancy

Airway

- Soft tissue oedema and enlarged breasts may make intubation more difficult.
- Surgical airway may be more difficult as landmarks may be more difficult to identify.
- There is an increased risk of regurgitation and aspiration.

Breathing

- Increased oxygen consumption.
- Reduced functional residual capacity.
- Rapid desaturation may occur during rapid sequence intubation.
- Tidal volume increases by 20% at 12 weeks and to 40% at term.
- Hyperventilation is normal.
- The thorax is less compliant.
- The diaphragm rises by up to 4 cm.

Circulation

- The gravid uterus will cause compression of the inferior vena cava reducing venous return and therefore cardiac output.
- Heart rate is increased by 10–15 beats per minute by the third trimester.
- Blood pressure falls by 10–15 mmHg in the second trimester and returns to near normal by term.
- Blood volume increases by up to 50% in the third trimester.

Other

- In late pregnancy the uterus displaces the abdominal viscera making patterns of injury and abdominal examination less reliable.
- Increased vascularity of the pelvis means pelvic fractures may easily cause life-threatening haemorrhage.

OBSTETRIC COMPLICATIONS FOLLOWING TRAUMA

PLACENTAL ABRUPTION

Placental abruption is the premature separation of the placenta from the uterine wall. It may occur after relatively minor trauma and can also present late, up to 3–4 days after the initial incident (5). Haemorrhage occurs between the placenta and the uterine wall and is commonly concealed with little or no external bleeding from the vagina.

Placental abruption will normally cause severe abdominal pain and premature contractions may develop. There is tenderness over the uterus with classically a tense, hard, woody feeling to the uterus on palpation, and the fundal height may be higher than expected if the gestation is known. There may be vaginal bleeding which is commonly dark in colour, and as discussed earlier, the amount does not correlate with the severity of bleeding. Significant separation of the placenta will result in intra-uterine death.

PLACENTA PRAEVIA

Placenta praevia is where the placenta is abnormally located in the lower part of the uterus, near to, or over the cervix. Placenta praevia is diagnosed on routine antenatal scans so the mother should be aware of this diagnosis. In the presence of placenta praevia, separation of the placenta is likely to result in significant vaginal bleeding which is bright red in colour. In contrast to a placental abruption, the patient may not be in pain and the uterus will not be tender to palpation. However, the bleeding may cause uterine irritation and provoke premature contractions which *will* cause intermittent pain.

In both placental abruption and placenta praevia the mother may demonstrate signs of hypovolaemic shock. In both cases this is a life-threatening condition for both the mother and the foetus.

UTERINE RUPTURE

A uterine rupture is a tear in the uterus. This may be caused by blunt trauma to the abdomen and is usually associated with later gestation with an expanded uterus and a previous caesarean section scar (3). The patient presents with severe abdominal pain and may exhibit hypovolaemic shock from concealed major haemorrhage. The top of the fundus may be difficult to distinguish and extra-uterine foetal parts may be palpated. Uterine rupture is a life-threatening emergency for both the mother and the foetus.

PREMATURE LABOUR

Trauma to the uterus may injure the myometrium causing cells to release prostaglandins that stimulate uterine contractions. With significant uterine damage and a greater gestational age this may progress to premature labour. In the majority of cases contractions resolve without treatment.

FOETAL DEATH

Direct foetal injury is rare. Indirect injury may occur due to hypoxia or hypotension in the mother, the conditions described earlier, or a placental or cord injury. Attempts to diagnose foetal death in the pre-hospital environment are unnecessary, as this will not change management. After diagnosis at hospital the mother will go on to have an induced vaginal delivery of the deceased foetus if there are no significant maternal injuries.

FOETO-MATERNAL HAEMORRHAGE

Even minor trauma may cause trans-placental haemorrhage from the foetus to the maternal circulation. A Kleihauer test should be performed at hospital on all Rhesus D negative women to estimate the amount of foetal blood cells present in the maternal circulation. All Rhesus negative mothers who are more than 12 weeks pregnant will require anti-D IgG injection within 72 hours of injury (6).

PRACTICE POINT

Women who are more than 12 weeks pregnant will require anti-D IgG injection within 72 hours of injury.

PENETRATING INJURY TO THE UTERUS

As pregnancy progresses, the uterus acts as a shield for the maternal abdominal organs, although this means a potentially poor prognosis for the foetus. The uterine muscle and amniotic fluid reduce energy transfer from higher energy missiles. Penetration of the umbilical cord or placenta may cause placental abruption or life-threatening haemorrhage.

INITIAL ASSESSMENT

HISTORY

In addition to the standard AMPLE history (**A**llergies, **M**edications, **P**ast medical history, **L**ast ate or drank, **E**vents [what happened]), an obstetric history should be obtained from the pregnant patient or her relatives. In the UK, the patient usually has her own antenatal records which will provide useful information.

The additional questions which should be asked of the pregnant trauma victim are

- How many weeks pregnant are you or when was the last menstrual period (LMP; the first day of their last menstrual period)?
- Is it a singleton pregnancy or a multiple birth?
- Have any problems been identified in this pregnancy (for example a low lying placenta)?
- How many previous pregnancies and deliveries have occurred? Were they normal vaginal deliveries or caesarean sections, and were there any complications with these? This information can be recorded as *gravidity* (the total number of pregnancies including this one) and *parity* (the total number of births), for example G2 P1.
- When did you last feel the baby move and is it moving normally? (Unfortunately, a dead foetus may be felt to move as it floats in amniotic fluid, conversely the absence of foetal movements does not mean foetal death.)
- Have you had any contractions or abdominal pain?
- Have you had any vaginal bleeding or discharge?

PRACTICE POINT

Optimal assessment and management of the maternal injuries will lead to the best prognosis for the foetus.

EXAMINATION

The standard <C>ABCDE approach should be adopted for the management of the pregnant trauma patient. In addition to this it will be necessary to make a more detailed assessment of the abdomen. This can be described as <C>ABCDEFG with the F standing for *fundus* and the G for *go to a hospital or major trauma centre with obstetric* capability (5).

ASSESSING FUNDAL HEIGHT

Fundal height can be used to estimate the gestation in an unconscious woman. The first method is using anatomical landmarks to give a gross estimation of the gestational age. At

12–14 weeks the uterus becomes palpable out of the pelvis, at 20–22 weeks the uterus is at the level of the umbilicus, and by 34–36 weeks the uterus reaches the costal margin (see Figure 17.1).

After 24 weeks gestation the fundal height measurement can be made by identifying the upper border of the symphysis pubis and the uterine fundus and measuring the distance between with a tape measure. The measurement in centimetres should then correspond to the gestation in weeks, with an allowance of ±2 centimetres difference. This is less practical in the pre-hospital environment.

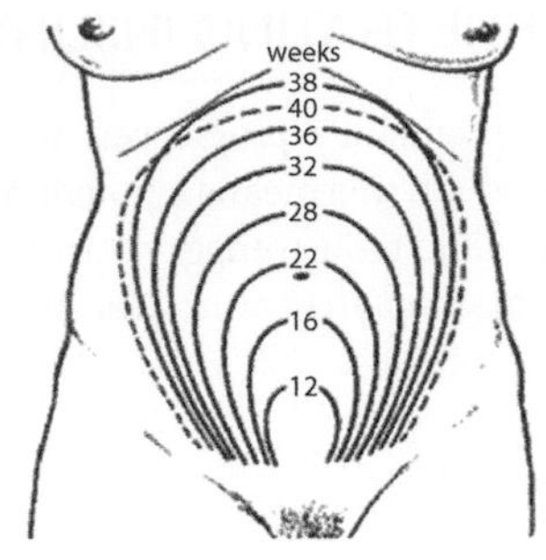

Figure 17.1 Fundal height and gestation.

PRACTICE POINT

A fundal height below the umbilicus is probably the most useful measure as it suggests that emergency caesarean section will not influence the survival of the mother or foetus.

ASSESSMENT OF THE ABDOMEN

The presence of a Pfannenstiel scar from a previous caesarean section should be noted; this is found as a transverse scar just above the mons pubis.

The abdomen should be palpated for any tenderness or rigidity. Contractions or foetal movements may be palpable.

External blood loss from the vagina must be identified with an assessment of the amount and the presence of any clots or active bleeding. There may also be clear fluid if the membranes have ruptured or a yellow-green fluid suggesting meconium staining. There is no indication for a pre-hospital vaginal examination. Verbal consent must be obtained from conscious patients and information provided to the patient and relatives about the need for inspection. The patient's dignity and modesty must be maintained at all times and another health care practitioner should be used as a chaperone when possible. The patient may refuse or may request a female member of staff.

FOETAL ASSESSMENT

Foetal well-being is extremely difficult to assess in the pre-hospital environment. Foetal heart sounds may be heard with a standard stethoscope or pre-hospital ultrasound, if available, can be used to view the foetal heart. However, neither are reliable; they may delay transport and do not influence the pre-hospital management of the patient. This means that foetal assessment is not indicated in the pre-hospital setting but will need to be performed on arrival to hospital.

MANAGEMENT

CATASTROPHIC HAEMORRHAGE CONTROL

Catastrophic haemorrhage is exceptionally rare, but where necessary, exsanguinating external bleeding should be controlled using the techniques described in Chapter 7.

AIRWAY AND CERVICAL SPINE CONTROL

The standard assessment of the airway will be made with consideration that any intubation may be difficult and there is a high risk of regurgitation so cricoid pressure should be applied.

BREATHING

High-flow oxygen must be given to all pregnant women who have suffered trauma. Because of the anatomical changes described earlier, thoracostomy needs to be performed at a higher level (3rd or 4th intercostal space) than on the non-pregnant patient.

CIRCULATION

The gravid uterus must be displaced to the left as soon as possible in order to reduce aortacaval compression and increase venous return. This can be done by manual displacement (see Figure 17.2). If the patient is on a scoop stretcher, padding can be placed under the stretcher on the right side to give a left lateral tilt of 15 to 30 degrees (5). This will allow in-line spinal immobilisation to be maintained. Padding placed directly under the right side of the patient is not advisable following blunt trauma as this will cause rotation of the spine, but may be used in penetrating trauma when spinal immobilisation is not required.

The traditional principles of permissive hypotension for fluid resuscitation and titrating fluids to a radial pulse apply equally to pregnant women (7). There is a fine balance between increasing the blood pressure by fluid resuscitation, which will improve perfusion of the foetus and vital organs and the risk of disrupting clots and increasing haemorrhage. It is assumed that the foetus will be adequately perfused with a maternal systolic blood pressure of 90 mmHg. Pregnant patients with a suspected pelvic injury should have a pelvic splint applied.

Pregnancy is not a contraindication to using tranexamic acid and this should be given to all patients showing signs of hypovolaemia or who have suspected internal haemorrhage following trauma (8). For patients with difficult vascular access or injuries to the upper limbs, cannulation in the lower limbs should ideally be avoided, as flow may be affected by vena caval compression from the gravid uterus (9).

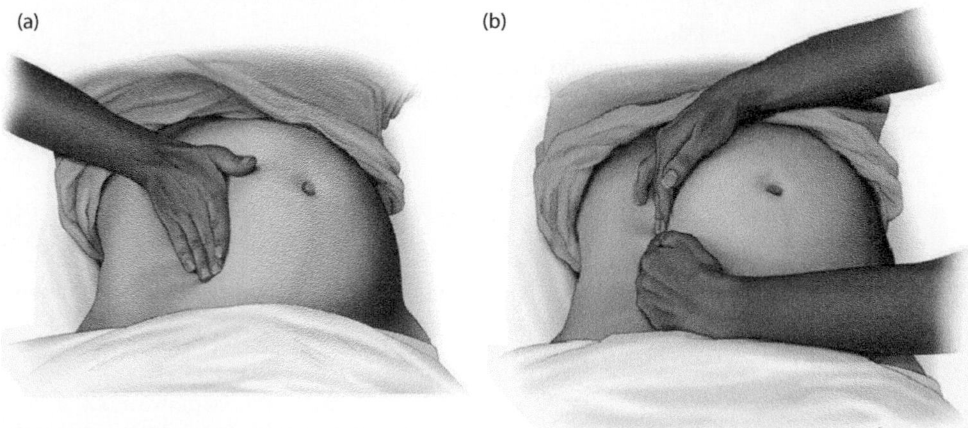

Figure 17.2 Manual displacement of the uterus to the left with (a) operator on right side of patient and (b) operator on left side of patient.

New Ideas

Tranexamic acid should be given to pregnant patients following significant trauma

DISABILITY AND EXPOSURE

There are no major differences in management during pregnancy. The patient's modesty must be maintained during examinations and they must be kept warm. Any drugs administered must be safe in pregnancy. For analgesia, Entonox®, paracetamol, morphine and ketamine can be considered.

CHOICE OF DESTINATION

Determining the most appropriate hospital may involve a complex decision-making process. For the pregnant major trauma patient the gold standard will be to transfer to a major trauma centre (MTC) with on-site senior obstetric clinicians and theatres as well as neonatal and paediatric support. For the time-critical patient in which there is a long transfer time to the gold standard, but a shorter transfer to an MTC without obstetric support on-site is possible, the latter may be the only option. Trauma networks should discuss these eventualities so it is clear what the options might be in different locations.

For the time-critical pregnant major trauma patient, a pre-alert is essential in order to ensure that senior obstetric, anaesthetic and neonatal/paediatric staff (when there is a gestation >24 weeks) are ready for the patient's arrival. Where there are short transfer times to the receiving hospital (<20 minutes) or the trauma occurs out of hours it may be advisable to ask ambulance control to contact the hospital before the full pre-alert message to allow time for mobilisation of resources.

Pregnancy >20 weeks is frequently used as an indicator on pre-hospital major trauma triage tools that the patient may benefit from being transported to a MTC regardless of vital signs, mechanism of injury or injury patterns. However, studies show that pregnancy alone is not an independent predictor of the need for trauma team activation by the receiving department (10,11).

PRACTICE POINT

The patient with minor injuries or who is apparently uninjured following an RTC or abdominal trauma should be taken to the local emergency department with obstetric facilities for further assessment of the foetus.

MATERNAL CARDIAC ARREST FOLLOWING TRAUMA

In the event of a maternal cardiac arrest following trauma, resuscitation should be commenced immediately and continued during transfer to hospital.

Following the diagnosis of cardiac arrest the immediate management is

- Basic life support
- Left lateral tilt if the patient is secured on an orthopaedic scoop stretcher (or long spinal board) or manual lateral displacement of the uterus to the left by a team member
- Rapid assessment of fundal height or bystander confirmation of gestational age

Chest compressions will need to be performed slightly higher on the sternum to allow for the elevation of the diaphragm and abdominal contents caused by the gravid uterus (9). Defibrillation pads may be difficult to apply over large breasts and with a left lateral tilt in place.

If the fundal height is below the umbilicus, there are no obstetric interventions which will improve outcome, so the focus is on the standard management of a traumatic cardiac arrest (12). This includes intubation and ventilation; bilateral thoracostomies; reduction and splintage of long bone fractures and pelvic fractures; arrest of major external haemorrhage and intravenous or intraosseous access with fluid resuscitation, ideally blood. It also includes consideration of a resuscitative thoracotomy in the case of penetrating chest trauma (13).

If the fundal height is above the umbilicus, a resuscitative caesarean section or *emergency hysterectomy* is indicated if the patient fails to respond to initial resuscitation. At 20–24 weeks, the primary role of the procedure is to save the life of the mother by improving cardiac output and it is unlikely that the foetus will survive. Above 24 weeks the aim is to attempt to save both the mother and foetus (9).

This procedure should start after 4 minutes of unsuccessful cardiopulmonary resuscitation, as the neurological outcome of the foetus and success of return of spontaneous circulation in the mother will decline with time. Nevertheless, foetal and maternal survival has been reported even when perimortem caesarean section was performed after 30 minutes of arrest (14).

If the pre-hospital practitioner has the required training, skills and governance support within their organisation to perform a pre-hospital emergency hysterotomy, the procedure may take place on scene. Organisations should have their own standard operating procedures for this situation written in conjunction with local obstetricians. If no such policy is in place, the patient should be rapidly transported to the nearest emergency department with senior obstetric staff on site, with a clear pre-alert message communicating the resources required on arrival.

The technique of performing an emergency hysterectomy will require multiple personnel to undertake the following tasks (15):

- Management of the cardiac arrest (intubation, thoracostomies, etc.)
- Performance of the hysterectomy
- Resuscitation of the foetus (if >24 weeks of pregnancy)

Practitioners should undergo simulation training with obstetric colleagues in order to prepare for such an event.

SUMMARY

Death from trauma in pregnancy in the UK population commonly results from the mechanisms of RTC or domestic violence or is associated with psychiatric disorders. The main principle of the management of trauma in pregnancy is that the resuscitation of the mother facilitates resuscitation of the foetus. All visibly pregnant women should be placed in a left lateral tilt or should have manual displacement of the uterus to avoid aortocaval compression.

Obstetric complications such as placental abruption or uterine rupture may present as hypovolaemic shock after even relatively minor trauma, and the resuscitating team must be aware of this possibility. Assessment of fundal height is essential if the gestational age is not known from the history, but *all* pregnant women should be conveyed to hospital after any form of blunt trauma.

Emergency hysterotomy should be considered for all pregnant women in cardiac arrest who have a fundal height above the umbilicus and in whom there has been no response to 4 minutes of CPR.

REFERENCES

1. Barraco RD, Chiu WC, Clancy TV, Como JJ, Ebert JB, Hess LW, Hoff WS et al. Practice management guidelines for the diagnosis and management of injury in the pregnant patient: The EAST Practice Management Guidelines Work Group. *Journal of Trauma* 2010;69(1):211–214.
2. Centre for Maternal and Child Enquiries (CMACE). Saving Mothers' Lives: Reviewing maternal deaths to make motherhood safer: 2006–08. The Eighth Report on Confidential Enquiries into Maternal Deaths in the United Kingdom. *BJOG* 2011;118(Suppl 1):1–203.
3. Campbell TA, Sanson TG. Cardiac arrest and pregnancy. *Journal of Emergencies, Trauma, and Shock* 2009;2(1):34–42.
4. Ueland K, Novy MJ, Peterson EN, Metcalfe J. Maternal cardiovascular dynamics, IV: the influence of gestational age on the maternal cardiovascular response to posture and exercise. *American Journal of Obstetrics and Gynecology* 1969;104:856–864.
5. Advanced Life Support Group. *Pre-Hospital Obstetric Emergency Training: The Practical Approach*. Wiley Blackwell, 2010.
6. Royal College of Obstetricians and Gynaecologists (RCOG). Rhesus D prophylaxis, The use of anti-D immunoglobulin for (Green-top Guideline 22). March 2011.
7. Joint Royal Colleges Ambulance Liaison Committee. UK Ambulance Services Clinical Practice Guidelines 2013. Association of Ambulance Chief Executives (AACE), 2013.
8. Roberts I, Perel P, Prieto-Merino D, Shakur H, Coats T, Hunt BJ, Lecky F, Brohi K, Willett K. Effect of tranexamic acid on mortality in patients with traumatic bleeding: Prespecified analysis of data from randomized control trial. *BMJ* 2012;345:e5839.
9. American Heart Association. Cardiac arrest associated with pregnancy. *Circulation* 2005;112:IV-150–IV-153.
10. Greene W, Roninson L, Rizzo AG. Sakran J, Hendershot K, Moore J, Weatherspoon K, Fakhry SM. Pregnancy is not a sufficient indicator for trauma team activation. *Journal of Trauma* 2007;63(3):550–554.
11. Aufforth R, Edhayan E, Dempah D. Should pregnancy be a sole criterion for trauma code activation: A review of the trauma registry. *American Journal of Surgery* 2010;199(3):387–389.
12. Soar J et al. European Resuscitation Council Guidelines for Resuscitation 2010. Section 8. Cardiac arrest in special circumstances. *Resuscitation* 2010;81:1421–1424.
13. Lockey DJ, Lyon RM, Davies GE. Development of a simple algorithm to guide the effective management of traumatic cardiac arrest. *Resuscitation* 2013;84(6):738–742.
14. Einav S, Kaufman N, Sela HY. Maternal cardiac arrest and perimortem caesarean delivery: Evidence or expert-based? *Resuscitation* 2012;83(10):1191–200.
15. Carley S. Perimortem C-section at St. Emlyn's. http://stemlynsblog.org/peri-mortem-c-section-at-st-emlyns/. Accessed December 10, 2013.

18 Trauma in the elderly

OBJECTIVES

After completing this chapter the reader will

- Understand the particular challenges of managing the elderly trauma patient
- Understand the potential importance of past medical history and drug history in how an elderly patient responds to trauma
- Recognise the possibility of significant injury following apparently minor trauma

INTRODUCTION

Management of trauma in patients of advanced years provides many challenges for clinicians. In the context of ageing populations the incidence of traumatic injuries amongst the elderly is rising throughout the world. Differences in injury profiles compared to younger victims of trauma, combined with the physiological and pharmacological effects of advanced age and the treatment of existing medical co-morbidities necessitate an approach to the management of trauma in the elderly that is specifically tailored to the clinical needs of these patients. Problems may range from obvious issues such as mobility to more subtle issues such as difficulty communicating with the deaf in noisy environments or with partially sighted patients. Each phase of patient management from the point of injury through to rehabilitation must be carefully considered when formulating an appropriate holistic approach to the management of traumatic injuries in the elderly. However, many of the techniques used in managing the older patient form part of good medical practice in the management of trauma patients of all ages.

THE EPIDEMIOLOGY OF TRAUMA IN THE ELDERLY

In Western countries the term *elderly* has for many years been defined as an age equal to or in excess of 65 years (1). Changing population demographics and patterns of health in individuals of this age have meant that more recently care of the elderly services around the United Kingdom have pushed this transition to 70 or even 75 years old. Patients in their nineties, once uncommon in emergency departments, now represent a significant part of the emergency workload. Elderly patients have consistently been shown to be more vulnerable to injury than their younger counterparts, have higher rates of mortality and spend longer in hospital following injuries of comparable severity (1–5). Elderly victims of trauma consume greater amounts of healthcare resources per injury, suffer a greater number of complications and have poorer long-term outcomes (6,7).

As a consequence of increased longevity, especially in Western societies, the incidence of trauma amongst elderly populations is increasing (8). As many in the elderly population are living longer and experiencing healthier, more active and, in many cases, more adventurous lifestyles, they are in fact becoming more exposed to a greater risk of trauma than previously (9). There is growing consensus that the traditional definition of *elderly* requires refinement given the changes in overall health and life expectancy that have been observed in many countries (10). Trauma outcomes in patients of advanced years have been reported to deteriorate with each 1-year increase in age resulting in a 6% increase in the probability of death (11). Notable increases in mortality amongst older trauma patients have been identified after the age of 75 (12–13), and there is an emerging trend to divide older victims of trauma into *older age* (aged 65–75), *elderly* (aged 75–85) and *extreme old age* (aged >85) groups (14–17). A better indication of physiological age can be made by using the term *frailty* for which validated scoring systems exist, although these have limited utility in the pre-hospital environment.

In contrast to trauma cases involving younger patients in which there is a higher incidence amongst males, elderly victims of trauma are more likely to be female (18–20). This is likely to be multi-factorial and to mirror the overall demographics of elderly populations in many Western countries in which life expectancy for women exceeds that of men (10,18). In contrast, however, males have been shown to be more likely to suffer traumatic brain injuries than females (20) and are more commonly injured as a result of road traffic collisions (RTCs) (21), probably reflecting the increased incidence of driving amongst elderly males compared to females.

Trauma in the elderly is a complicated, multifaceted area that requires a detailed understanding amongst healthcare professionals involved in the provision of trauma care. The incidence of reported traumatic injury in the elderly population is rising commensurate with the proportional increase in the ageing population (18).

MECHANISM OF INJURY IN ELDERLY TRAUMA

The vast majority of elderly patients present with blunt traumatic injuries and the most common mechanism of injury is falls from less than 2 metres (9,22–24). The elderly are most likely to be injured in their own home, reflecting the high incidence of falls as the mechanism of injury. Approximately 1 in 10 people over the age of 65 visit an emergency department each year following a fall-related injury (25) but only 25% require admission (26). The physiological changes of ageing and decreases in bone mass, reaction time and balance have all been identified as predisposing factors to falls in elderly people (27). Ten percent of falls in older people result in significant injuries (28). Falls prevention is therefore an important and expanding area of geriatric care in many countries in an attempt to reduce the incidence and limit the complications from this type of injury (29).

Following falls, RTCs are the next most common mechanism of injury amongst the elderly population (29–34). Traditionally, elderly patients injured in an RTC were more likely to be pedestrians struck by vehicles (35–36), however, with greater numbers of older adults retaining driving licences, over the last two decades an increasing proportion of RTCs have involved elderly patients as drivers or passengers (37,38). The risk factors for greater mortality and injury in RTCs involving elderly road users and pedestrians include vision problems, slower reflexes, co-morbid conditions, cognitive impairment, decreased bone density, and alcohol and medication use (9,37–39).

Injuries to older adult pedestrians have been shown to be more severe than those to younger pedestrians involved in similar accidents (39,40). Injury profiles amongst drivers and passengers involved in RTCs are also different in elderly patients compared to younger counterparts involved in similar accidents (34,41,42). Elderly patients are more likely to suffer long bone and pelvic fractures following RTCs than their younger counterparts, probably due to the effects of osteoporosis (43). There is a higher incidence of chest wall injuries with rib fractures and haemopneumothorax in elderly patients with abdominal injuries which require laparotomy being more common amongst younger drivers (43,44). It is postulated that this observation is due to changes in the way forces are distributed throughout the body through seat belts and airbags in older and younger patients (45,46). Decreased muscle mass and chest wall compliance in the elderly have been identified as possible causative factors for the observed higher incidence of chest wall injuries in this group (43). Chest injuries amongst elderly patients are of great importance, as those that sustain blunt chest wall injury with rib fractures have been shown to have twice the mortality and morbidity of younger patients with similar injuries (47). For each additional rib fracture in the elderly, mortality increases by 19% and the risk of pneumonia by 27% (47).

After falls and road traffic collisions, trauma following attempted suicide is the next most common cause of injury in adults aged over 65 (48). In countries with ready access to fire arms, self-inflicted gunshot wound is the most common method of suicide and accounts for a notable proportion of reported penetrating injury amongst elderly patients (8). Older adults in urban settings are more likely to hang themselves or jump from a height as their method of attempting suicide, possibly due to ease of access, high lethality and an association with a high likelihood of polytrauma (40). In older adults, male gender, chronic pain and illness, social isolation and depression have been identified as risk factors for attempted suicide (49). The possibility of deliberate abuse of the elderly, especially those who are forgetful, deaf or suffering dementia, should always be considered and if necessary appropriate safeguarding steps taken.

PRACTICE POINT

Always consider the possibility of deliberately inflicted injury in the elderly.

PHYSIOLOGICAL RESPONSE TO TRAUMA IN THE ELDERLY

Decreased cardiovascular and respiratory reserves and the effects of pre-existing co-morbidities in elderly patients can adversely affect the physiological response of elderly victims of trauma (34,50). This may present clinicians with a diagnostic quandary in identifying patients who have suffered significant injuries in the early phases of their care.

Age-related insufficiency in cardiac output results in a state of hypoperfusion that adversely affects end organ perfusion following severe injury (2). In some elderly patients cardiac output can remain stable at rest, but due to reduced physiological reserves, they are unable to compensate for the stress caused by physical injury as effectively as younger victims of trauma (51).

As many as a third of patients who were identified as 'stable' in the resuscitation room following trauma, with heart rate and blood pressure readings in the normal range, suffered cardiac arrest within 24 hours of admission to hospital. Impaired cardiac output in elderly victims of trauma has been shown to be related to poorer outcomes and increased mortality in this patient group (52–54).

A high index of suspicion is required to identify hypoperfusion states in elderly trauma victims and the initial assessment in such cases should be tailored appropriately. Both serum lactate and arterial base deficit levels can be utilised as markers of poor perfusion, identifying patients that may benefit from intensive resuscitation and monitoring early in the hospital phase of their care (55–57). Normal base deficit levels in patients with an Injury Severity Score (ISS) ≥16 have been shown to have a lower negative predictive value for death in patients aged >55 years than in younger cohorts (40% versus 60%) (58). Moderate elevation of base deficit (−6 to −9) is associated with mortality rates of up to 60% in elderly trauma victims and of patients with severely elevated levels (>10) up to 80% die.

Whilst elevated serum lactate levels are associated with states of hypoperfusion, with rate of clearance directly correlating with mortality in both young and old patients (59), elderly patients have been shown to tolerate such states less effectively. In elderly patients, a serum lactate level of greater than 2.4 mmol/L for over 12 hours has been shown to be associated with increased mortality (60). In the pre-hospital environment this means that every effort must be made to ensure adequate perfusion and that ideally blood products should be used as the resuscitation fluids. Every attempt must therefore be made, by effective and prompt pre-hospital intervention, to avoid tissue hypoperfusion and acidosis.

New Ideas

Point of care pre-hospital lactate analysis is being trialled by a number of UK pre-hospital providers.

PAST MEDICAL HISTORY AND DRUG HISTORY

The majority of the elderly who are involved in trauma will be taking regular medication. In some cases their medication history will be very complex; in the majority of cases it is unlikely to be known to those treating them in the pre-hospital environment. However, when it is known, the drug history may offer a rapid means of establishing the patient's co-morbid conditions. It may even, for example with diabetic or ischaemic heart disease medication, suggest the possibility that the trauma was itself secondary to a medical problem. The most important drugs and elements of the past medical history which affect the response of a patient to trauma or may indicate a cause for an accident are listed in Box 18.1.

BOX 18.1: Drugs and Medical Conditions in Trauma

Trauma may occur secondary to

- Ischaemic heart disease
- Diabetes
- Epilepsy
- Instability poor balance, postural hypotension
- Confusion
- Depression
- Drowsiness (may be secondary to drugs including hypnotics)

Drugs which affect the physiological response to trauma or its management include

- Digoxin, beta-blockers, other anti-arrythmics
- Insulin, metformin, other hypoglycaemic agents
- Anticoagulants
- Sedatives and anxiolytics
- Anti-epileptics

THE EFFECT OF AGE ON SURVIVAL AND OUTCOME IN ELDERLY TRAUMA PATIENTS

Mortality rates following traumatic injuries are higher in patients aged >65 years (8,61,62), with mortality in some studies of up to 10% (32). Mortality has been shown to increase from the age of 40 years (63), even amongst those with moderate injuries (ISS 9 to 24). Even within the elderly trauma population, advanced age is associated with an increased likelihood of death (7,62,64,65). Advancing age has also been shown to be a predictor of late mortality in trauma victims. Being over the age of 65 has been shown to confer a 2.46-fold increase in the likelihood of death within 24 hours and 4.64-fold increase in the likelihood of death after 24 hours (34).

In addition to an increased likelihood of death following major trauma, elderly patients have been shown to suffer greater rates of complications and require longer periods of time in hospital than younger patients (1). Higher rates of pulmonary and infectious complications are reported in elderly trauma victims (50,61). This trend is observed in survivors even after discharge from hospital (48).

The incidences of cardiac, pulmonary and septic complications have been shown to be independent predictors of poor outcome in non-survivors in elderly trauma populations (2,42,66). The effect of complications on the likelihood of death following major trauma in elderly patients appears to be cumulative: (5.4% with no complications, 8.6% with a single complication, 30% with more than one complication). Complications have been shown to directly contribute to death in elderly trauma patients in up to a third of cases, with almost two-thirds of deaths being due to multi-organ failure (62).

THE EFFECT OF PRE-EXISTING MEDICAL CONDITIONS IN ELDERLY TRAUMA PATIENTS

Due to a higher incidence of pre-existing conditions in the elderly trauma population it has proved challenging to clearly separate the effects of age and premorbidity on mortality following significant injury. An added complication is the heterogeneous nature of pre-existing medical problems within patient populations.

A number of studies have identified the presence of pre-existing conditions as predicting poor outcome in elderly trauma victims (51,53,67,68). The effect of pre-existing conditions on mortality following trauma is more pronounced in middle-aged patients with moderate ISS but after 65 years of age, chronological age becomes the predominant predictor of death (63). As patients progress through 'old age' (65–74 years) to 'elderly' (>75 years), mortality rates have been shown to increase following a similar trend irrespective of the presence of pre-existing conditions (69).

The number and severity of pre-existing conditions suffered by individual patients appears to correlate with poorer outcome and increased mortality, but more data is required to fully understand this relationship (70).

INJURY SCORES AND MORTALITY IN ELDERLY TRAUMA PATIENTS

Whilst injury scores have been shown to be effective in predicting mortality in young patients, their use in an elderly population is less clearly defined (71). Discrepancies in the observed mortality rates between young and elderly cohorts with similar Injury Severity Scores have been identified (51,53,67,68). Mortality rates have been shown to increase sharply in elderly patients with ISS >18, most notably in those aged >75 years. Combinations of ISS and APACHE II scores have been investigated to attempt to refine prognostication following major trauma in elderly populations, but the evidence is limited.

The difficulties in accurately predicting mortality in elderly trauma victims based on injury profiles reflects the heterogeneous make-up of such populations and is probably heavily influenced by the effects of age, abnormal physiology related to the ageing process, pre-existing co-morbidities and the increased incidence of complications.

TREATMENT STRATEGIES IN ELDERLY TRAUMA PATIENTS

The traditional view held for many years was that the need for general surgical interventions in elderly patients following traumatic injury was associated with significantly increased rates of mortality (6). In recent years treatment strategies in elderly trauma populations have begun to evolve.

Evidence now suggests that early decisions to perform general surgery on elderly trauma patients can improve outcome (6) combined with aggressive and invasive monitoring to detect and correct states of hypoperfusion (72–74). Advanced age should never be the sole reason to withhold operative management in elderly trauma victims (75).

SUMMARY

Trauma in older people is becoming increasingly common. Inevitably, as more people survive into old age, their medical co-morbidities increase and they take more medication. Thus aging is associated with confounding factors which adversely affect outcomes compared to younger patient with the same injuries. In addition, factors such as deafness, poor hearing and confusion, although not invariably present, may in many cases make managing these patients more challenging. Optimum survival rates, therefore, for elderly trauma victims can only be achieved by application of the highest standards of care and scrupulous attention to detail. There is no place for half-hearted care for the elderly.

REFERENCES

1. Champion HR, Copes WS, Buyer D, Flanagan ME, Bain L, Sacco WJ. Major trauma in geriatric patients. *American Journal of Public Health* 1989;79(9):1278–1282.
2. Chang WH, Tsai SH, Su YJ, Huang CH, Chang KS, Tsai CH. Trauma mortality factors in the elderly population. *International Journal of Gerontology* 2008;(2):11–17.
3. National Safety Council. *Accident Facts,* 1986 ed. Chicago: NSC, 1986.
4. Baker SP, O'Neill B, Kapuf RS. Overview of injury mortality. In *The Injury Fact Book.* Lexington Books, 1984.
5. Snipes GE. Accidents in the elderly. *American Family Physician* 1982;26:117–122.
6. Tornetta P 3rd, Mostafavi H, Riina J, Turen C, Reimer B, Levine R, Behrens F, Geller J, Ritter C, Homel P. Mortality and morbidity in elderly trauma patients. *Journal of Trauma* 1999;46(4):702–706.

7. van Aalst Ja, Morris JA Jr, Yates HK, Miller RS, Bass SM. Severely injured geriatric patients return to independent living: A study of factors influencing function and independence. *Journal of Trauma* 1991;31:1096–1101.
8. Smith D, Enderson B, Maull K. Trauma in the elderly: Determinants of outcome. *Southern Medical Journal* 1990;83:171–177.
9. Labib N, Nouh T, Winocour S, Deckelbaum D, Banici L, Fata P, Razek T, Khwaja K. Severely injured geriatric population: Morbidity, mortality and risk factors. *Journal of Trauma* 2011;71(6):1908–1914.
10. Macninven, D. *Scotland's Population 2009. The Registrar General's Annual Review of Demographic Trends.* 155th edition. Scottish Government, Edinburgh, Scotland, 2009.
11. Grossman MD, Miller D, Scaff DW, Arcona S. When is an elder old? Effect of pre-existing conditions on mortality in geriatric trauma. *Journal of Trauma* 2002;52(2):242–246.
12. Richmond TS, Kauder D, Strumpf N, Meredith T. Characteristics and outcomes of serious traumatic injury in older adults. *Journal of the American Geriatrics Society* 2002;50:215–222.
13. Aitken LM, Burmeister E, Lang J, Chaboyer W, Richmond TS. Characteristics and outcomes of injured older adults after hospital admission. *Journal of the American Geriatrics Society* 2010;58(3):442–449.
14. Cagetti B, Cossu M, Pau A, Rivano C, Viale G. The outcome from acute subdural and epidural intracranial haematomas in very elderly patients. *British Journal of Neurosurgery* 1992;6:227–231.
15. Meldon SW, Reilly M, Drew BL, Manusco C, Fallon W. Trauma in the very elderly: A community based study of outcomes at trauma and nontrauma centers. *Journal of Trauma* 2002;29:494–497.
16. Bulpitt CJ, Peters R, Staessen JA, Thijs L, De Vernejoul MC, Fletcher AE, Beckett NS. Fracture risk and the use of diuretic (indapamide SR) +/– perindopril: A substudy of the Hypertension in the Very Elderly Trial (HYVET). *Trials* 2006;7:33.
17. Peters R, Beckett N, Burch L, de Vernejoul MC, Liu L, Duggan J, Swift C, Gil-Extremera B, Fletcher A, Bulpitt C. The effect of treatment based on a diuretic (indapamide) +/– ACE inhibitor (perindopril) on fractures in the Hypertension in the Very Elderly Trial (HYVET). *Age and Ageing* 2010;39(5):609–616.
18. O'Neill S, Brady RR, Kerssens JJ, Parks RW. Mortality associated with traumatic injuries in the elderly: A population based study. *Archives of Gerontology and Geriatrics* 2012;54(3):e426–e430.
19. Oyetunji TA, Ong'uti SK, Bolorunduro OB, Gonzalez DO, Cornwell EE, Haider AH. Epidemiological trend in elderly domestic injury. *Journal of Surgical Research* 2012;173(2):206–211.
20. Shinoda-Tagawa T, Clark DE. Trends in hospitalization after injury: Older women are displacing younger men. *Injury Prevention* 2003;9:214–219.
21. Langolis JA, Rutland-Brown W, Thomas KE. Traumatic brain injury in the United States: Emergency Department visits, hospitalisations and deaths. National Center for Injury Prevention and Control, Atlanta, GA, 2004.
22. Gates S, Fisher JD, Cooke MW, Carter YH, Lamb SE. Multifactorial assessment and targeted intervention for preventing falls and injuries among older people in community and emergency care settings: Systematic review and meta-analysis. *BMJ* 2008;336:130–133.
23. Peel NM. Epidemiology of falls in older age. *Canadian Journal of Ageing* 2011;15:1–13.

24. Inci I, Ozcelik C, Nizam O, Eren N. Thoracic trauma in the elderly. *European Journal of Emergency Medicine* 1998;5(4):445–450.
25. King MB. Falls. In *Principles of Geriatric Medicine and Gerontology*, 5th ed. W Hazzard, JP Blass, JB Halter (eds.). New York: McGraw-Hill, 2003, pp. 1517–1529.
26. National Center for Injury Prevention and Control. www.cdc.gov/ncipc/wisqars.
27. Wolf ME, Rivara FP. Nonfall injuries in older adults. *Annual Review of Public Health* 1992;13:509–528.
28. Thompson HJ, McCormick WC, Kagan SH. Traumatic brain injury in older adults: Epidemiology, outcomes, and future implications. *Journal of the American Geriatrics Society* 2006;54(10):1590–1595.
29. Gowing R, Jain MK. Injury patterns and outcomes associated with elderly trauma victims in Kingston, Ontario. *Canadian Journal of Surgery* 2007;50(6):437–444.
30. Kent R, Funk J, Crandall J. How future trends in societal ageing, air bag availability, seat belt use and fleet composition will affect serious injury risk and occurrence in the United States. *Traffic Injury Prevention* 2003;4:24–32.
31. de Souza JA, Igelsias AC. Trauma in the elderly. *Revista da Associacao Medica Brasileira* 2002;48:79–86.
32. McCoy GF, Johnston RA, Duthrie RB. Injury to the elderly in road traffic accidents. *Journal of Trauma* 1989;29:494–497.
33. McMahon DJ, Schwab CW, Kauder D. Comorbidity and the elderly patient. *World Journal of Surgery* 1996;20:1113–1119.
34. Perdue PW, Watts DD, Kaufmann CR, Trask AL. Differences in mortality between elderly and younger adult trauma patients: Geriatric status increases risk of delayed death. *Journal of Trauma* 1998;45:805–810.
35. Kong LB, Lekawa M, Navarro RA, McGrath J, Cohen M, Margulies DR, Hiatt JR. Pedestrian-motor vehicle trauma: An analysis of injury profiles by age. *Journal of the American College of Surgeons* 1996;182(1):17–23.
36. Peng RY, Bongard FS. Pedestrian versus motor vehicle accidents: An analysis of 5000 patients. *Journal of the American College of Surgeons* 1999;189(4):343–348.
37. National Highway Traffic Safety Association. Traffic Safety Facts 2002: Older Population. National Center for Statistics and Analysis, Washington DC, 2004.
38. Ekleman BA, Mitchell SA, O'Dell-Rossi P. Driving and older adults. In *Functional Performance in Older Adults*, BWM Bonder (ed.). Philadelphia: FA Davis, 2001, pp. 448–476.
39. Binder S. Injuries among older adults: The challenge of optimising safety and minimising unintended consequences. *Injury Prevention* 2002;8(Suppl 4):iv2–iv4.
40. Demetriades D, Murray J, Martin M, Velmahos G, Salim A, Alo K, Rhee P. Pedestrians injured by automobiles: Relationship of age to injury type and severity. *Journal of the American College of Surgeons* 2004;199(3):382–387.
41. Schiller WR, Knox R, Chleborad W. A five year experience with severe injuries in elderly patients. *Accident Analysis and Prevention* 1995;27:167–174.
42. Osler T, Hales K, Baack B, Bear K, Hsi K, Pathak D, Demarest G. Trauma in the elderly. *American Journal of Surgery* 1988;156:537–543.
43. Malik AM, Dal NA, Talpur KAH. Road traffic injuries and their outcome in elderly patients 60 years and above. Does age make a difference? *Journal of Trauma and Treatment* 2012;1(4). doi: 10.4172/2167-1222.100012.
44. Victorino GP, Chong TJ, Pal JD. Trauma in the elderly patient. *Archives of Surgery* 2003;138:1093–1098.

45. Bergeron E, Lavoie A, Clas D, Moore L, Ratte S, Tetreault S, Lemaire J, Martin M. Elderly patients with rib fractures are at greater risk of death and pneumonia. *Journal of Trauma* 2003;54:478–485.
46. Martinez R, Sharieff G, Hooper J. Three point restraints as a risk factor for chest injury in the elderly. *Journal of Trauma* 1994;37:980–984.
47. Bulger EM, Arneson MA, Mock CN, Jurkovich GJ. Rib fractures in the elderly. *Journal of Trauma* 2000;48:1040–1046.
48. Johnson CL, Margulies DR, Kearney TJ, Hiatt JR, Shabot MM. Trauma in the elderly: An analysis of outcomes based on age. *American Surgeon* 1994;60:899–902.
49. Demetriades D, Sava J, Alo K, Newton E, Velmahos GC, Murray JA, Belzberg H, Asensio JA, Berne TV. Old age as a criterion for trauma team activation. *Journal of Trauma* 2001;51:754–757.
50. Finelli FC, Jonsson J, Champion HR, Morelli S, Fouty WJ. A case control study for major trauma in geriatric patients. *Journal of Trauma* 1989;29:541–548.
51. Hossack KF, Bruce RA. Maximal cardiac function in sedentary normal men and women: Comparison of age-related changes. *Journal of Applied Physiology* 1982;53:799–804.
52. Oreskovich MR, Howard JD, Copass MK, Carrico CJ. Geriatric trauma: Injury patterns and outcome. *Journal of Trauma* 1984;24:565–572.
53. Horst HM, Obeid FN, Sorensen VJ, Bivins BA. Factors influencing survival of elderly trauma patients. *Critical Care Medicine* 1986;14:681–684.
54. Safih MS, Norton R, Rogers I, Gardener JP, Judson JA. Elderly trauma patients admitted to the intensive care unit are different from the younger population. *New Zealand Medical Journal* 1999;112:402–404.
55. Davis JW, Parks SN, Kaups KL, Gladen HE, O'Donnell-Nicol S. Admission base deficit predicts transfusion requirements and risk of complications. *Journal of Trauma* 1996;41:769–774.
56. Davis JW, Shackford SR, Holbrook TL. Base deficit as a sensitive indicator of compensated shock and tissue oxygen utilization. *Surgery, Gynecology and Obstetrics* 1991;173:473–476.
57. Dunham CM, Belzberg H, Lyles R, Weireter L, Skurdal D, Sullivan G, Esposito T, Namini M. The rapid infusion system: A superior method for the resuscitation of hypovolemic trauma patients. *Resuscitation* 1991;21:207–226.
58. Davis JW, Kaups KL. Base deficit in the elderly: A marker of severe injury and death. *Journal of Trauma* 1998;45:873–877.
59. McNelis J, Marini CP, Jurkiewicz A, Szomstein S, Simms HH, Ritter G, Nathan IM. Prolonged lactate clearance is associated with increased mortality in the surgical intensive care unit. *American Journal of Surgery* 2001;182:481–485.
60. Schulman AM, Claridge JA, Young JS. Young versus old: Factors affecting mortality after blunt traumatic injury. *American Surgeron* 2002;68:942–947.
61. Lonner J, Koval K. Polytrauma in the elderly. *Clinical Orthopaedics and Related Research* 1995;318:136–143.
62. Pellicane J, Byrne K, DeMaria E. Preventable complications and death from multiple organ failure among geriatric trauma victims. *Journal of Trauma* 1992;33:440–444.
63. Morris JA Jr, MacKenzie EJ, Damiano AM, Bass SM. Mortality in trauma patients: The interaction between host factors and severity. *Journal of Trauma* 1990;30:1476–1482.
64. Battistella FD, Din AM, Perez L. Trauma patients 75 years and older: Long-term follow-up results justify aggressive management. *Journal of Trauma* 1998;48:618–624.
65. Knudson MM, Lieberman J, Morris JA Jr, Cushing BM, Stubbs HA. Mortality factors in geriatric blunt trauma patients. *Archives of Surgery* 1994;129:448–453.

66. Shabot MM, Johnson CL. Outcome from critical care in the 'oldest old' trauma patients. *Journal of Trauma* 1995;39:254–259.
67. Broos PL, D'Hoore A, Vanderschot P, Rommens PM, Stappaerts KH. Multiple trauma in elderly patients. Factors influencing outcome: Importance of aggressive care. *Injury* 1993;24:365–368.
68. Broos PL, Stappaerts KH, Rommens PM, Louette LK, Gruwez JA. Polytrauma in patients of 65 and over. Injury patterns and outcome. *International Surgery* 1988;73:119–222.
69. Milzman D, Boulanger B, Rodriguez A, Soderstrom CA, Mitchell KA, Magnant CM. Pre-existing disease in trauma patients: A predictor of fate independent of age and Injury Severity Score. *Journal of Trauma* 1992;2:236–243.
70. Gubler KD, Davis R, Koepsell T, Soderberg R, Maier RV, Rivara FP. Long-term survival of elderly trauma patients. *Archives of Surgery* 1997;132:1010–1014.
71. Baker SP, O'Neill B, Haddon W Jr, Long WB. The injury severity score: A method for describing patients with multiple injuries and evaluating emergency care. *Journal of Trauma* 1974;14:187–196.
72. Nagy KK, Smith RF, Roberts RR, Joseph KT, An GC, Bokhari F, Barrett J. Prognosis of penetrating trauma in elderly patients: A comparison with younger patients. *Journal of Trauma* 2000;49:190–193.
73. Demetriades D, Karaiskakis M, Velmahos G, Alo K, Newton E, Murray J, Asensio J, Belzberg H, Berne T, Shoemaker W. Effect on outcome of early intensive management of geriatric trauma patients. *British Journal of Surgery* 2002;89:1319–1322.
74. Demetriades D, Sava J, Alo K, Newton E, Velmahos GC, Murray JA, Belzberg H, Asensio J, Berne T. Old age as a criterion for trauma team activation. *Journal of Trauma* 2001;51:754–756.
75. Godley CD, Warren RL, Sheridan RL, McCabe CJ. Nonoperative management of blunt splenic injury in adults: Age over 55 years as a powerful indicator for failure. *Journal of the American College of Surgeons* 1996;183:133–139.

19 Burns

OBJECTIVES

After completing this chapter the reader will

- Understand the initial priorities in the management of burns
- Recognise the association between burns and other injuries
- Understand that early shock in the burned patient implies the presence of unrecognised haemorrhagic trauma

INTRODUCTION

Burns are one of the most common injuries sustained by the general population, both at home and at work. However, the frequency of severe burns in the UK is fortunately relatively low. Over 13,000 burn injuries require hospital attention occur every year in England and Wales. Approximately 1000 patients suffer major burns each year, with 50% occurring in children under the age of 12 years old (1).

Severe burns are multi-system injuries which require advanced resuscitation and a multi-disciplinary approach in order to be managed effectively.

SCENE SAFETY

A burns patient is likely to have originated from a scene which is hostile to rescuers. There may be multiple hazards on scene which require skilful management. In the majority of situations, the primary responsibility for scene management and safety rests with the fire service. They have expertise in casualty extrication, firefighting and working in confined/smoke-filled environments wearing the necessary personal protective equipment (PPE).

Other hazards include the presence of noxious fumes associated with the burning of household objects, including cyanide and the risk of carbon monoxide poisoning. In cases of chemical exposure, specific PPE may be required depending on the chemical involved. Under no circumstances should clinicians enter hazardous areas requiring specific PPE unless they have previously been trained to use it.

SCENE SAFETY

The initial priority is to stop the burning process. The patient should be removed from the burning source and any burnt clothing should be removed from the patient as quickly and as safely as possible. Any materials adherent to the patient's skin may need to be left in place and not forcibly be removed unless there is an immediate threat to life or limb. Any jewellery should be removed, as swelling following the burn may make later removal difficult.

The majority of burns sustained domestically are likely to be superficial or partial thickness in nature, thus early effective first aid is likely to reduce the ongoing burning process, provide analgesia and promote healing. Cooling the burned skin under a running cold-water tap is a highly effective method and should be continued for a period of at least 20 minutes (2). The use of ice or ice water (<8°C) is not recommended (3).

Simultaneously the patient should be kept warm to maintain body temperature. Care should be taken not to render the patient hypothermic; cold and wet clothing should be removed and the patient should be wrapped in warm, dry blankets if possible.

TYPES OF BURN

A thermal burn caused by flame is the most common type of burn sustained in the adult population; these are often associated with inhalational airway burns and other traumatic injuries.

In paediatrics, burns due to scalding are much more common and typically affect the upper limbs and torso. All too commonly these are caused by the spilling of hot drinks or other liquids onto the child. The elderly population is also frequently injured by scald burns.

Contact burns occur when there is prolonged contact with a hot object or short contact against a very hot object. The typical example encountered in UK pre-hospital practice is when an elderly or otherwise infirm patient falls against a hot surface and is unable to move away from the object, for example a radiator, that is causing the burning.

Chemical and electrical burns both have specific characteristics which will be discussed later in this chapter.

A burn wound compromises the physiological functions of the skin, including its ability to control temperature, provide an effective barrier to infection, maintain fluid balance and offer sensory perception. The burn wound also can be aesthetically damaging to the skin's appearance and can cause significant psychological morbidity.

A burn wound displays three zones according to a model proposed by Jackson in 1953 (4). The central zone is the most severely damaged necrotic tissue and is known as the 'zone of coagulative necrosis'. This represents the primary burn injury and the damage is irreversible. The degree of necrosis is proportional to the duration of exposure and the temperature of the contact.

Surrounding this central zone is a potentially salvageable area of injury known as the 'zone of stasis'. In the zone of stasis the microcirculation of the dermis is compromised, and if the patient is inadequately fluid resuscitated or suffers further physiological insult, then this zone will progress to necrosis.

Finally the peripheral 'zone of hyperaemia' is caused by an increase in blood flow and the release of pro-inflammatory cytokines. In a severe burn (total burn surface area [TBSA] >20%) the local inflammatory response from the zone of hyperaemia is sufficient to cause systemic inflammatory response syndrome (SIRS).

BURN DEPTH

Burns are conventionally divided according to their depth, into

- Simple erythema
- Partial thickness
- Full thickness

Simple erythema results from a very superficial burn without skin loss. The affected area is pink and painful but with normal looking skin, such as occurs in sunburn.

Partial thickness burns involve the epidermis and dermis. The extent of burn into the dermis determines the appearance and healing potential of the burn. Superficial partial thickness burns involve a thin layer of dermis and are characterised by blisters. Deep dermal burns destroy the deep dermal plexus of nerves and capillaries. Therefore the burn has a mottled red appearance, does not blanch to pressure and has decreased sensation. Mid-dermal burns will show features of both superficial and deep dermal burns.

In *full thickness burns* the skin is entirely destroyed and deeper structures may be involved. The burn appears leathery, waxy, firm and dry. On pinprick examination the burn may be insensate and does not bleed. This burnt skin is called an *eschar.*

Burn injuries are rarely homogenous and a burn wound may encompass varying degrees of depth of injury. In the pre-hospital environment, differentiation between the different depths of partial thickness burns is difficult and of limited immediate value. Repeated examination over the first 48 hours post burn injury is often required to accurately judge the depth of a burn, but its relevance is in terms of long-term healing and it does not impact specifically on the pre-hospital management. It is, however, important to distinguish simple erythema from partial and full thickness burns since simple erythema is not included when calculating burn size.

ASSESSMENT OF BURN SIZE

A number of different methods are available for estimating burn depth. Accurate assessment of *total burn surface area (TBSA)* is important in order to direct initial fluid management and also to triage patients in need of specialist burn care. It is not essential to work out precise fluid replacement calculations in the pre-hospital arena unless this time is likely to be very prolonged. When estimating TBSA it should be remembered that only partial and full thickness burns should be included in the calculation. The methods commonly used for assessing TBSA are described next.

WALLACE RULE OF NINES

The Wallace Rule of Nines is the traditional method of assessing burns in adults (Figure 19.1) (5). The arms account for 9% each, each leg 18%, the head and neck 9%, the abdomen and thorax 18% front and 18% back, and the remaining 1% is the genitalia and perineum. Due to the changing proportions of a child's head and limb size relative to the total body surface area, the standard Rule of Nines should not be used in children.

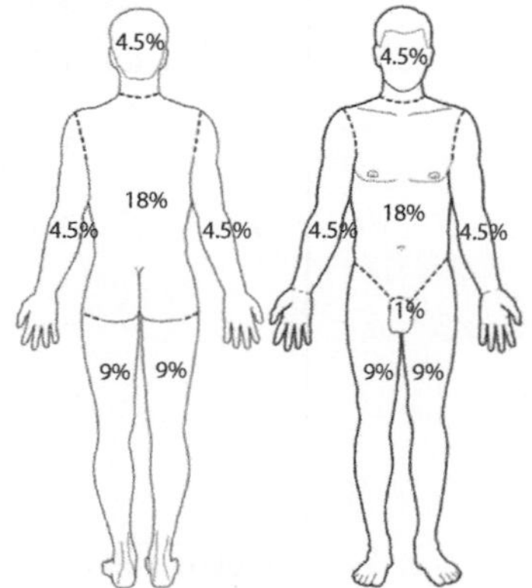

Figure 19.1 The Rule of Nines in adults.

SERIAL HALVING

Another quick technique suitable to the pre-hospital environment is that of serial halving. Begin by looking to see if the TBSA is more or less than 50% burnt. If less than 50% TBSA, then estimate whether they are more or less than 25% burnt. Continue halving until a burn size is estimated.

HAND SURFACE

It is estimated that the patient's palm (including the adducted fingers) can be used as 1% TBSA (6). Therefore the number of patient's handprints that would be required to cover the burns can estimate the total burn size. It is accurate for burns up to 15% TBSA, it can also be used for assessing greater than 85% TBSA by measuring the unburnt skin using the same method. For burns between 15% and 85% TBSA it is thought to be inaccurate.

LUND AND BROWDER CHART

This method allows for a simultaneous recording and assessment of TBSA (7). The areas of the body burnt are given a weighted percentage dependent on the age of the patient. The percentage allocated to head and leg areas change with age to reflect the changes in body surface area with age. The Lund and Browder chart is appropriate for calculations in both adults and children, and is the preferred method for in-hospital assessment (Figure 19.2). Small pre-laminated charts are available for pre-hospital use. Once completed the chart should remain with the patient.

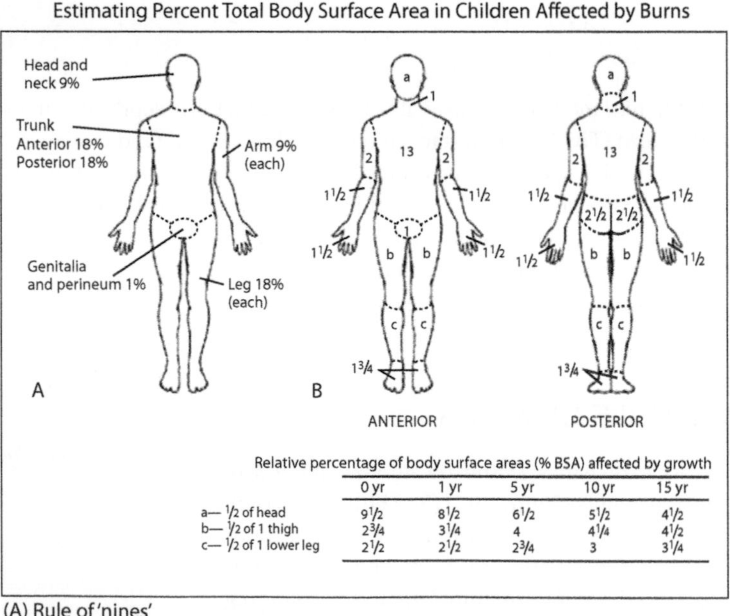

Relative percentage of body surface areas (% BSA) affected by growth

	0 yr	1 yr	5 yr	10 yr	15 yr
a— ½ of head	9½	8½	6½	5½	4½
b— ½ of 1 thigh	2¾	3¼	4	4¼	4½
c— ½ of 1 lower leg	2½	2½	2¾	3	3¼

(A) Rule of 'nines'
(B) Lund-Browder diagram for estimating extent of burns

Figure 19.2 The Lund and Browder Chart.

New Ideas

A further way of estimating the area of burn is by using a smart phone or tablet with an appropriate app. The area of burn can be coloured in on an outline of a patient figure using the touchscreen interface, with the device then offering a suggested percentage area of the burn. An example app is Mersey Burns (see http://merseyburns.com/) (8).

PRE-HOSPITAL ASSESSMENT AND MANAGEMENT OF THE BURNED PATIENT

All burned patients should be initially managed following current trauma protocols, particularly when there is risk that the patient may have fallen (for example to escape a burning building) or have been involved in an explosion where they have been thrown as part of the effects of the blast.

Whilst the burn may be a distracting injury, it should not be allowed to draw attention from undertaking an assessment of both the scene and the patient to determine the presence of other injuries that could pose a greater or more immediate threat to life.

INITIAL HISTORY TAKING

Where possible, an initial *AMPLE (Allergies, Medication, Past medical history, Last ate or drank, Events)* and tetanus immunisation history should be taken. It may be the case that the pre-hospital provider may be the only person able to obtain a first-hand history if the patient later develops airway oedema and requires intubation.

The exact mechanism, events surrounding the burn and nature of the burn exposure should be recorded if possible. It is important to note any treatment received prior to the arrival of trained providers.

An accurate witness account should be recorded in cases of paediatric burns; this will usually come from a parent/guardian. The initial account will become particularly important if there is a suspicion of non-accidental injury (NAI).

INITIAL ASSESSMENT

AIRWAY

A high index of suspicion should be maintained for the risk of inhalation injury leading to potential airway compromise. Risk factors for inhalational injury include flame burns to the face and prolonged exposure to heat in a confined environment. The signs listed in Box 19.1 should be actively sought as evidence of a potential airway burn (9).

BOX 19.1: Signs Suggestive of Airway Burns

- Full thickness facial burns
- Stridor
- Respiratory distress
- Evidence of swelling on laryngoscopy
- Smoke inhalation
- Singed nasal hairs

Any evidence of the signs in Box 19.1 should alert the pre-hospital provider to the presence of a potential airway burn. This can quickly progress to airway oedema and the airway may become compromised within a relatively short timeframe. However, reports of very rapid airway obstruction are uncommon, and in most cases intubation can wait until arrival in hospital if conditions at the scene make inhibation hazardous or difficult. These patients should be rapidly transported to a major trauma centre or burns centre as per local protocols. Instrumentation of the airway should be avoided in order to prevent worsening oedema and causing airway compromise. A hospital pre-alert should include the concern/presence of airway burns in order to ensure senior airway specialists are present to receive the patient in the emergency department.

If the skills to provide pre-hospital emergency anaesthesia (PHEA) on scene are available, consideration may be given to securing the airway on scene, particularly if there is evidence of airway burns or established airway compromise. Persistently hypoxic patients may also require PHEA and invasive ventilation. The ability and equipment to secure a surgical airway should be immediately available if considering PHEA in this situation.

BREATHING

Burns patients should be given high flow oxygen through a non-rebreathing mask. This may be omitted if the burn is very localised (i.e. <5% TBSA) and no inhalational component is suspected.

Ventilation may become compromised in the presence of circumferential deep dermal or full thickness burns affecting the chest and limiting adequate expansion. This may require escharotomies (surgical incision into the burnt skin) to be performed to relieve the restriction. These are rarely if ever required in the pre-hospital environment and is only indicated for circumferential (or near circumferential eschar) with impending/established respiratory compromise due to thoraco-abdominal burns.

If there is clinical suspicion of a blast injury, pre-hospital providers should be aware of the risk of blast lung, which can impair ventilation. There is also the possibility of barotrauma causing a pneumothorax and/or lung contusions. These injuries should be managed as per local trauma protocols with rapid transfer to a major trauma centre.

CIRCULATION

Following a significant burn intravascular fluid is lost locally into the burn wound and systemically into the interstitial space. Although hypovolaemic shock can occur in large burns, this is unusual in the very early stages, and if present mandates a thorough search for a cause of haemorrhage.

PRACTICE POINT

Early shock suggests the presence of a haemorrhage from an associated injury.

Cannulation should be attempted, ideally through areas of unburnt skin. Intraosseous (IO) is an alternative route for fluid replacement. Intravenous fluid should be started for all burns of >20% TBSA, and/or when transport to definitive care is likely to exceed 1 hour. In the pre-hospital environment, crystalloid fluid should be used as fluid replacement. Ideally fluid given should be warmed to prevent worsening hypothermia.

A calculation of initial fluid requirements can be made using the Parkland formula (Box 19.2) (10). It is essential to remember that this formula (and every other burns formula) does not take into account fluid loss from other injuries.

BOX 19.2: The Parkland Formula

Fluid requirement for first 24 hours

- 2 to 4 mL crystalloid × % TBSA × Weight (kg)
- 50% in first 8 hours (from time of burn)
- 50% in next 16 hours

Higher volumes should be used for inhalational injuries and electrical burns (up to 9 mL/kg may be needed).

In paediatrics, normal maintenance fluid requirements should be added to any resuscitation fluid calculation.

In pre-hospital practice where transfer times may be short, an alternative fluid regimen for burns >20% TBSA (10% in children) is

- Adults = 1000 mL
- 10 to 15 years = 500 mL
- 5 to 10 years = 250 mL
- <5 yrs = No fluids

Care should be taken not to overinfuse, especially if the patient is elderly or has left ventricular failure. Patients with associated traumatic injuries should receive fluid therapy based on local guidelines for trauma resuscitation.

Circumferential limb burns can cause significant reduction in distal perfusion and ischaemia. However, escharotomies carry significant risk of complications, including iatrogenic neurovascular injury. They are not indicated to performed in the pre-hospital environment, except in prolonged field care situations.

DRESSINGS

The application of dressings will help to keep the wound clean and provide analgesia. The ideal dressing should be non-adherent and allow the burn wound to be visualised without unnecessary and painful removal of dressings. The use of a cellophane wrap is ideal for this task. It should be applied in strips and layers, and must not be wrapped around a limb, which can result in a constrictive effect as the wound and surrounding tissue swells.

The use of hydrogel dressings is not recommended unless no other alternative is available. There is no evidence for the benefit of hydrogel dressings in pre-hospital care for wound healing (11). Cooling temperatures to aid healing are not effectively achieved and such dressings must remain uncovered to allow air movement so as to facilitate cooling (12). Prolonged use should be monitored to avoid inducing hypothermia in patients.

ANALGESIA

The application of effective dressings will usually provide good levels of analgesia for patients with mild to moderate burns. Some patients will require intravenous analgesia and an intravenous opioid can be titrated as required. Patients may require ketamine for analgesia. In children the intranasal route can be used for the administration of both diamorphine and ketamine.

HYPOTHERMIA MITIGATION

Once the thermoregulatory capability of the skin has been lost through the burning process, significant heat loss can occur. This can be compounded by aggressive cooling of the burn and surrounding skin associated with excessive evaporative heat losses. Once a burnt patient has become hypothermic it is very difficult for them to be rewarmed and this has a detrimental effect on wound healing and survival.

Any wet clothing should be removed and the patient should be wrapped in warm, dry blankets once the burn wounds have been appropriately dressed. The use of bubble wrap and warming blankets will help to reduce heat loss. The ambient temperature within the ambulance should be increased if possible. If transporting the patient by aircraft, care should be taken to exclude any draughts. If the patient is anaesthetised, an oesophageal temperature probe may be used to monitor core body temperature.

ANTIBIOTICS

The use of prophylactic antibiotics is not recommended for the majority of burns; only in rare cases of gross contamination would pre-hospital antibiotics be warranted. Some patients will require a tetanus immunisation booster, but this will be given in hospital.

CARBON MONOXIDE AND CYANIDE

Carbon monoxide (CO) is produced when incomplete combustion occurs. The symptoms of CO poisoning vary from mild malaise to coma and death. Standard pulse oximetry will not detect the presence of CO. All patients at risk of being exposed to CO should be given high-flow oxygen until arrival at hospital when arterial oxygen and CO concentrations can be measured. It is worth noting that CO levels are now routinely measured pre-hospital by the hazardous area response team (HART).

Cyanide is present as hydrogen cyanide gas in most domestic fires. No test is available for the diagnosis of cyanide poisoning, and the symptoms and signs are non-specific. There is a failure of oxygen utilisation by the tissues, which occurs despite high-inspired oxygen concentrations. The specific treatment for cyanide poisoning in the pre-hospital environment is hydroxocobalamin.

CHEMICAL BURNS

Chemical burns usually occur as a result of industrial accidents. In such industrial locations, chemicals information and specific treatments may be available. Where possible the chemical that the patient has been exposed to should be recorded. Initial management is to irrigate the area with copious amounts of water. Care should be taken to avoid washing the chemical onto unaffected skin or the exposed skin of rescuers.

Hydrofluoric acid is a common chemical used in glass etching and in the manufacture of printed circuit boards. Exposure to even 1% TBSA can be fatal due the systemic effects of fluoride ions, dependent upon the concentration strength. Calcium gluconate can be used to neutralise the acid and prevent continued injury.

ELECTRICAL BURNS

Electrical current can cause contact burns if it passes through the body or flash burns if it arcs close to the body. The degree of tissue damage is proportional to the voltage.

In domestic, low voltage burns, there may be local burns at the entry and exit points but minimal damage along the tract through which the current has travelled. The alternating nature of domestic electricity can lead to arrhythmias, especially if the tract is across the thorax.

In high voltage (>1000 V) burns, there is significant tissue damage between entry and exit points despite the skin potentially appearing normal. Extensive deep damage to the muscles can lead to rhabdomyolysis and renal failure. These burns require aggressive fluid resuscitation.

A flash burn can occur when high voltage electricity arcs close to a patient and causes a thermal burn to the skin but does not lead to damage to deeper structures as current does not pass through the body. The ECG should be monitored for arrhythmias during transport if there is evidence or suspicion of electrical injury.

TRIAGE AND TRANSFER

Local protocols vary as to whether direct triage to a burns centre is possible. Patients with suspicion of concomitant trauma should initially be managed in a centre that can deal with the possible injuries; this is likely to be a major trauma centre in the UK.

Guidelines from the British Burn Association and National Health Service (NHS) exist for the threshold to refer or discuss burn cases with specialist burn care.

- All burns ≥2% TBSA in children or ≥3% in adults.
- All full thickness burns and all circumferential burns.
- Any burn with suspicion of non-accidental injury should be referred to a burn unit/centre for expert assessment within 24 hours.
- Any burn >30% in adults or >15% in children, or any burn likely to need intensive care requires a burn centre.

The following cases should be discussed with a burns service as they may require transfer to specialist care:

- All burns to hands, feet, face, perineum or genitalia.
- Any chemical, electrical or cold burn injury.
- An unwell child with a burn or concerns of toxic shock syndrome.
- Concerns regarding burn injuries and co-morbidities that may affect treatment or any burn that has not healed in 2 weeks.

NON-ACCIDENTAL INJURY

Although the majority of burns are accidental, a small proportion of paediatric burns are as a result of non-accidental injury. Occasionally these injuries can present in the elderly and dependant adult populations also.

The role of the pre-hospital practitioner is to accurately record the history surrounding the event and to make an assessment of the scene. Any concerns should be passed on to the receiving hospital team. Local safeguarding policies should be followed in order to allow any concerns to be recorded and followed up.

SUMMARY

Burns are common; fortunately severe burns are rare. When severe burns do occur they are associated with great distress for the patient, and very often anxiety in the practitioner. Initial management is straightforward and the key is not to be distracted by the appearance of the burn wound. Simple attention to the <C>ABCDE process, exclusion (as far as is possible) of immediately life-threatening injury elsewhere, awareness of the context in which the injury has occurred, fluid replacement without recourse to complex formulas, covering the wound and providing analgesia are all that is required.

REFERENCES

1. Stylianou N, Buchan I, Dunn KW. A review of the international Burn Injury Database (iBID) for England and Wales: Descriptive analysis of burn injuries 2003–2011. *BMJ Open* 2015:5(2):e006184.
2. Bartlett N, Yuan J, Holland AJ, Harvey JG, Martin HC, La Hei ER, Arbuckle S, Godfrey C. Optimal duration of cooling for an acute scald contact burn injury in a porcine model. *Journal of Burn Care and Research* 2008;29(5):828–834.
3. Venter THJ, Karpelowsky JS, Rode H. Cooling of the burn wound: The ideal temperature of the coolant. *Burns* 2007;33(7):917–922.
4. Jackson DM. The diagnosis of the depth of burning. *British Journal of Surgery* 1953;40(164): 588–596.
5. Wallace AB. The exposure treatment of burns. *The Lancet* 1951;257(6653):501–504.
6. Nagel TR, Schunk JE. Using the hand to estimate the surface area of a burn in children. *Pediatric Emergency Care* 1997;13(4):254–255.
7. Lund CC, Browder NC. The estimation of areas of burns. *Surgery Gynecology and Obstetrics* 1944;79(352):8.
8. Barnes J, Duffy A, Hamnett N, McPhail J, Seaton C, Shokrollahi K, James MI, McArthur P, Pritchard Jones N. The Mersey Burns App: Evolving a model of validation. *Emergency Medicine Journal* 2015;32(8):637–641.
9. Sauaia A, Ivashchenko A, Peltz E, Schurr M, Holst J. Indications for intubation of the patient with thermal and inhalational burns. In *A42 ARDS: Risk, treatment, and outcomes.* American Thoracic Society, 2015, p. A1619.
10. Baxter CR, Shires T. (1968). Physiologic response to crystalloid resuscitation of severe burns. *Annals of New York Academy of Science* 1968;150:874–893.
11. Goodwin NS, Spinks A, Wasiak J. The efficacy of hydrogel dressings as a first aid measure for burn wound management in the pre-hospital setting: A systematic review of the literature. *International Wound Journal* 2016;13(4):519–525.
12. Coats TJ, Edwards C, Newton R, Staun E. The effect of gel burns dressings on skin temperature. *Emergency Medicine Journal* 2002;19(3):224–225.

FURTHER READING

Allison K, Porter K. Consensus on the prehospital approach to burns patient management. *Emergency Medicine Journal* 2004;21:112–114.

Palao R, Monge I, Ruiz M, Barret JP. Chemical burns: Pathophysiology and treatment. *Burns* 2010;36:295–304.

Rowan MP, Cancio LC, Elster E, Burmeister DM, Rose LF, Natesan S, Chan RK, Christy RJ, Chung KK. Burn wound healing and treatment: Review and advancements. *Critical Care* 2015;19(1):243.

Sheppard NN, Hemington-Gorse S, Shelley OP, Philp B, Dziewulski P. Prognostic scoring systems in burns: A review. *Burns* 2011;37:1288–1295.

Victoria Burns Management Guidelines, http://www.vicburns.org.au/index.html.

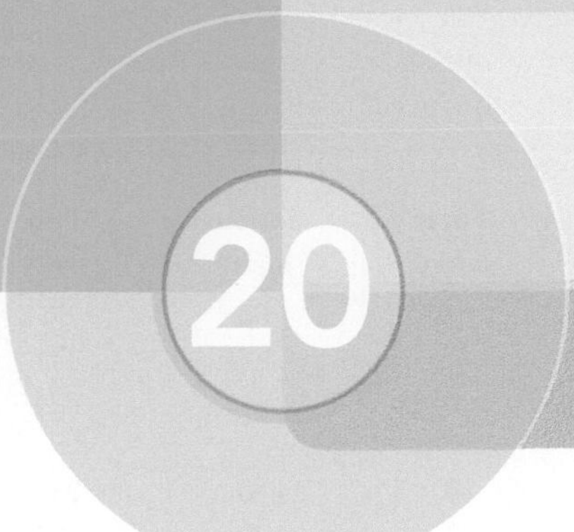

Firearms, ballistics and gunshot wounds

OBJECTIVES

After completing this chapter the reader will

- Understand the basic pathophysiology of gunshot wounds
- Understand the spectrum of injury arising from the use of firearms
- Be aware of the general principles of management of firearms injuries in the pre-hospital environment

INTRODUCTION

Throughout the history of conflict, human ingenuity has focused on methods of killing and injuring at a distance. With firearms, this is achieved by the transfer of chemical energy from the propellant into a projectile's kinetic energy (KE) and then the transfer of the projectile's KE into the tissues it strikes.

The use of chemical energy in the form of gunpowder to move projectiles had been around for centuries in Asia when Edward III used a cannon for the first time in Europe in 1346. The English used artillery to defeat Genoese crossbowmen fighting for King Philip VI during the Battle of Crećy (1). Over the following centuries, refinements in metallurgy and chemistry allowed the size of firearms to reduce to handguns, shotguns and rifles or *small arms*. This chapter will focus on the science underpinning these weapons, the injuries they produce and the strategy for treating casualties of firearms.

EPIDEMIOLOGY

The United Kingdom has one of the lowest rates of firearm assaults and homicides in the world (2). Table 20.1 shows characteristics of firearm offences and injuries over a 12-month period in England and Wales (3).

In 2011 the UK had 0.23 firearms-related deaths per 100,000 of the population. This compares to 10.64 in the United States (2013 figures) and 1.75 in Norway. No major European state has a lower rate than the UK. These figures include, murder, suicide and accidents.

Table 20.1 Firearms offences in England and Wales, 2011–2012

Weapon type	Firearm offences	Offences involving shots fired	Fatal injury	Serious injury	Minor injury
Shotguns	495	248 (50.1%)	16	56	36
Handguns	2651	332 (13%)	18	103	56
Imitation, BB or airsoft firearms	1377	1,053 (76%)	0	8	624
Rifles/others	1478	597 (40%)	8	48	313
Air weapons	3554	3160 (89%)	0	29	329
Total	9555	5388 (56%)	42	244	1358

Source: Office for National Statistics, Violent crime and sexual offences, 2011/12, *Statistical Bulletin*, London, 2013.
Note: Serious injury is defined as requiring hospital admission. BB/airsoft guns are very low velocity air weapons.

NOMENCLATURE AND CLASSIFICATION

The nomenclature of firearms is confusing with the use of metric and imperial measurements, and overlapping, synonymous terms.

BULLETS

A bullet is the projectile. Bullets are moved by the detonation of an explosive termed the *propellant*. The propellant is enclosed by a *casing* fixed to the back of the bullet and is ignited by a small impact sensitive explosive called the *primer* which is itself ignited when it is struck by the firing pin (Figure 20.1).

The classification of ammunition is complicated and not obviously logical. The diameter of the bullet is known as its calibre; this corresponds to the internal diameter of the gun barrel. Confusingly, this measurement is frequently given both in millimetres and fractions of an inch. For example, the same calibre round could be described as 5.56 mm or .223.

In the NATO system of classification, two numbers are used to describe a type of ammunition: the first refers to the calibre and the second to the length in millimetres. Commonly just the calibre is used, for example 5.56 × 45 mm ammunition is normally just referred to as '5.56 mm'.

However, different manufacturers make different lengths of bullets of the same calibre and similarly change the dimensions of the casing to allow different quantities of propellant. For example, bullets of 7.62 mm calibre are manufactured with lengths of 39 mm (AK-variant weapons), 51 mm (NATO) and 25 mm for handguns.

Some manufacturers use designations where the second number or word refers to the quantity of propellant. The term *magnum* implies a variant of standard ammunition with a greater quantity of propellant in a larger casing. An example of this is the .357 magnum round which has the same sized bullet as a .38 special but 11.5 grains of propellant compared to 6.7 in the original version.

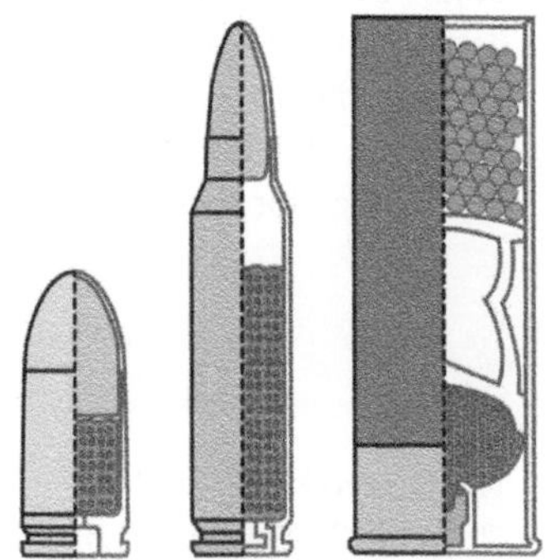

Figure 20.1 Schematic showing longitudinal cross section of 9 × 19 mm and 5.56 × 45 mm and shotgun cartridge.

FIREARMS

Guns are machines that convert the chemical energy in an explosive into the kinetic energy of a projectile and include mortars, artillery and firearms. A *firearm* is a portable gun that fires a projectile across a relatively flat trajectory. Firearms involve a controlled explosion in the *breech*, which then drives the bullet along the *barrel* and out of the gun.

The term 'firearm' describes both extremely large weapon systems, which must be transported mounted to vehicles, as well as those that can be carried by hand. These man-portable firearms are usually referred to as *small arms* and will be the focus of this chapter. However, for simplicity the term *firearm* will be used throughout.

Small arms are divided into handguns, rifles and shotguns. A *handgun* is a short-barrelled weapon that can be operated with one hand; handguns are further subdivided into pistols with rounds stored in a straight magazine or revolvers in which rounds sit in a revolving drum.

Rifles are long barrelled weapons that have to be held with both hands and typically rested against the shoulder. The term 'rifle' is misleading since both handguns and rifles are rifled (have spiral grooves on the inside of their barrels). Rifles can have heavier barrels able to withstand greater forces than handguns and therefore typically fire higher-energy rounds.

Shotguns are similar in appearance to rifles but instead of firing a single bullet, fire multiple small spherical projectiles called *shot* through an un-rifled barrel. Shotguns are described according to their calibre, known as *gauge* in the US and *bore* in the UK. Bores are numbered according to the size of a lead sphere made from a given fraction of one pound of lead which fits the internal diameter of the barrel. For example a 12-bore shotgun has a barrel diameter that fits a sphere of 1/12th of a pound of lead, and a 20-bore has a barrel diameter that fits a sphere of 1/20th of a pound of lead. Therefore a higher number indicates a smaller barrel. Shotgun ammunition can vary enormously according to the number and size of shot.

A simple, practical division of firearms is into 'long' and 'short' weapons. This can be readily understood by victims or bystanders of a firearm incident. Attempts to determine this by pre-hospital medics will be extremely useful in anticipation of the likely injury patterns and should be included in part of the ATMIST handover. Shotgun wounds are normally obvious clinically and unmistakeable on X-ray due to the large number of foreign bodies of uniform size, but differentiating between handgun and rifle wounds can be difficult and reliant on a thorough history from pre-hospital practitioners. Table 20.2 shows the comparative characteristics and wounding patterns of shotguns, rifles and handguns. Shotgun pellets spread from the muzzle of a gun in a conical shape with the result that the inflicted wounds become more separated the further the victim is from the weapon when it is fired. However at very short ranges, shotgun wounds can be devastating with massive soft tissue destruction as the mass of pellets will act, in effect, as a single massive projectile.

Table 20.2 Comparison of firearm types grouped according to 'long' or 'short'

	'Short'	**'Long'**	
Appearance of firing position	Held in one or two hands away from the body	Held with both hands, rested against the shoulder	
Weapon type	Handgun	Rifle	Shotgun
Example ammunition	9 × 19 mm	5.56 × 45 mm	Shot
Kinetic energy (joules)	550	1800	3200
Muzzle velocity (metres per second)	390	930	400
Projectile weight (grams)	7.5	4	40
Wounds	Permanent cavity	Permanent and temporary cavity	Wide but shallow wound*

* The wounding effect of a shotgun depends on the distance from muzzle to target.

FIREARMS IN THE UK

The UK has one of the tightest legal frameworks governing firearms in the world; their use is restricted by the 1997 Firearms Act and the 2006 Violent Crime Reduction Act. In practical terms, only rifles and shotguns (together with appropriate ammunition) may be legally owned by private citizens.

Police forces in the UK have access to a variety of firearms, and casualties from law enforcement and security operations may well require treatment. Typically police rely on handguns and sub-machine guns firing 9 × 19 mm ammunition, but increasing numbers of police forces are issuing firearms officers with rifles firing 5.56 × 45 mm rounds.

Police forces also occasionally use *Attenuating Energy Projectiles (AEPs)* during public order operations. The AEP replaces plastic or rubber bullets often called 'baton rounds' and is regarded as a less lethal form of firearm. AEPs are made from 98 g of polyurethane and are 37 × 100 mm in size. AEPs are slow (<100 ms^{-1}) and despite their large mass typically only possess around 250 joules of kinetic energy, depending on range. An AEP can cause significant blunt injuries and is theoretically life threatening but no fatalities have been reported following their use in the UK (4).

BALLISTICS

Ballistics is the science of projectiles and is divided into three areas. *Internal ballistics* deals with the behaviour of the projectile in the gun, *external ballistics* describes the flight of the projectile and *terminal ballistics* examines the transfer of energy from the projectile into its target.

INTERNAL BALLISTICS

The ignition of the propellant results in the extremely rapid conversion of a solid into a gas; this explosion occurs in the casing, held in the breech at the rear of the barrel. At the moment of ignition (detonation) the gas occupies a very small volume under enormous pressure. This pressure is released by forcing the bullet along the barrel. The bullet accelerates along the barrel as the propellant continues to burn and produce gaseous products. The rifling in the barrel is helical and either comprised of raised *lands* between *grooves* or more subtle 'hills and valleys' in polygonal rifling. Both forms cause the bullet to spin around its longitudinal axis, providing stability to the bullet in flight.

EXTERNAL BALLISTICS

The KE of the round is related to the velocity and is determined by the following equation:

$$KE = \frac{mv^2}{2}$$

where

KE is kinetic energy.
m is mass of the projectile.
v is velocity of the projectile.

It is important to note that the velocity is squared in this equation and therefore increases in velocity have a greater effect on the energy of the bullet than increasing its mass.

Projectiles are at their fastest when they leave the end of the barrel (the *muzzle*) hence *muzzle velocity*. From the point of leaving the muzzle, the projectile is slowed by the effect of drag as it passes through the air. Drag is complex and consists of two main components: *pressure drag* and *skin friction*. In supersonic bullets there is the additional factor of *wave drag*. These components of drag are simplified by combining them into the *drag coefficient*, which differs between projectiles. The *drag force* is the resultant retarding force on the bullet as it travels through the air and is given by the equation:

$$F_d = 1/2pv^2C_dA$$

where

F_d is the drag force acting to slow the bullet.
C_d is the drag coefficient.
p is the mass density of the air the bullet is passing through.
v is the velocity of the projectile.
A is the cross-sectional surface area of the projectile.

It is important to note that in this equation, as in the KE equation, velocity is squared; therefore higher velocity projectiles are subject to much greater drag.

The drag coefficient is dependent on multiple factors including the shape of the bullet. A 'sharper' bullet is less susceptible to drag. The sharpness of a bullet is quantified by the ratio of the calibre to the curve of the front of the bullet and is measured in ogives as shown in Figure 20.2. Bullets with higher ogives are 'sharper' and less susceptible to drag. Clearly if a projectile is unstable in flight, it presents a greater surface area as it tumbles. It is therefore subject to much greater drag and will slow rapidly.

The concept of drag is also relevant in the understanding of the transfer of kinetic energy into the tissues and will be revisited in the next section.

BULLET INSTABILITY

Despite the spinning effect conveyed to the bullet by the rifling, it does not travel with perfect stability along the axis of its trajectory. There are three main types of instability: yaw, precession and nutation.

Yaw is defined as the linear oscillation of the bullet around the axis of the trajectory and can be thought of as 'wobble'. *Precession* is the helical rotation or spiralling of the nose of the projectile around the axis of the trajectory. *Nutation* is the small oscillations of the nose from the rotational arc of precession. Of these types of projectile instability, the most significant is yaw (5). However, during the flight of modern bullets, yaw is negligible and is probably less than 2°. (Figure 20.3) (6).

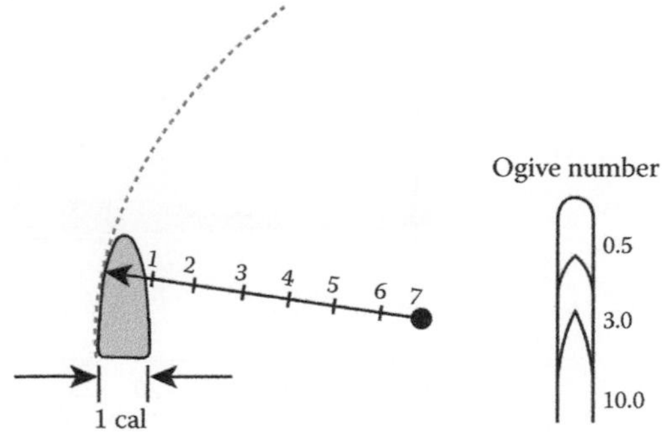

Figure 20.2 Schematic showing ogive arc calculations on the left and typical ogive values on the right.

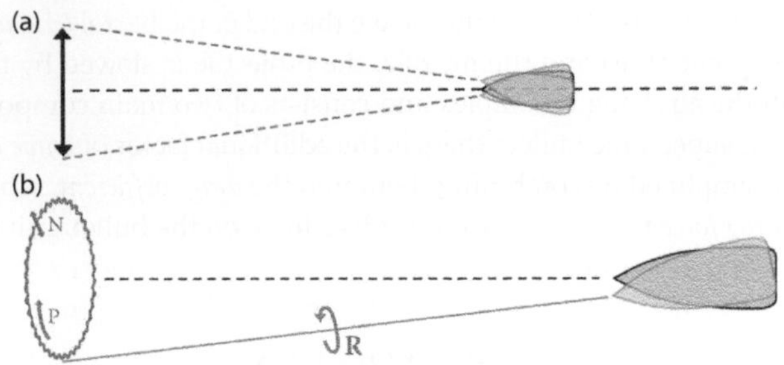

Figure 20.3 (a) Schematic showing yaw, or 'linear wobble'. This has been exaggerated for the purposes of illustration and is usually less than 2°. (b) Schematic showing precession (P) or rotation of the nose around the axis of flight, along with nutation (N), a rocking motion in the axis of rotation. Throughout these movements, the bullet spins (R) around its longitudinal axis, conveyed by the rifling of the barrel.

TERMINAL BALLISTICS

The most relevant area of ballistic physics to the trauma practitioner is *terminal* ballistics. This is concerned with the passage of the projectile into the casualty and the transfer of KE into the casualty's tissues. It is the 'work' done by the projectile as it transfers its KE that causes tissue damage. It is important to recognise that the action of a projectile as it passes through tissue is idiosyncratic and largely unpredictable. Unlike internal and external ballistics, which have clear laws of physics describing them, terminal ballistics describes a much more complex set of interactions and therefore offers few 'rules' that predict wounding patterns. Projectiles can ricochet within bodies, follow unpredictable paths and seemingly defy scientific expectations.

In the simplest sense, the KE transferred into tissues is simply the difference between the KE of the projectile as it strikes the body and that which remains when it exits tissue. If the projectile does not exit the tissues, all of its KE will be transferred into the body. Projectiles damage tissue via three mechanisms: *permanent cavity formation, temporary cavity formation* and generation of a *shock wave* as shown in Figure 20.4.

PERMANENT CAVITY

The projectile cuts and shears tissue as it passes through the casualty creating a tract that is the same diameter as the projectile. This tract, the *permanent* cavity, is typically a continuation

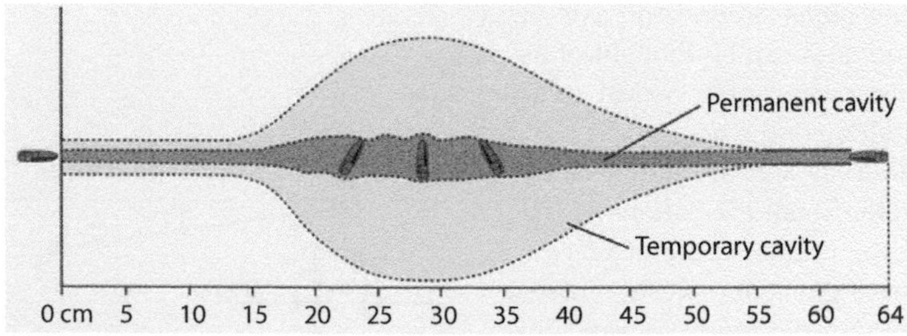

Figure 20.4 Schematic showing the three components of ballistic wounding: the permanent cavity directly behind the path of the bullet, the temporary cavity expanding radially away from the bullet tract and the shock wave.

of the trajectory of the projectile and is similar to that which would be created by a spear, arrow or stabbing weapon of the same diameter. If a round fragments, which can occur either in soft tissue or after bone strike, then each fragment will create a permanent cavity and possibly even a temporary cavity (see below), dramatically increasing tissue damage.

As has been previously stated, there are few rules in terminal ballistics. However, lower energy handgun projectiles (for example 9 × 19 mm bullets), normally only produce a permanent cavity. Gunshot wounds (GSWs) produced by these rounds usually involve damage limited to structures and organs lying in the path of the projectile. Therefore, in *through and through* injuries, where both entry and exit wounds exist, the structures damaged can be predicted with a fair degree of accuracy. However, it is important to recognise that higher energy handgun projectiles can form a temporary cavity (see later). Where the round has not been recovered or the weapon type is unknown, it is perilous to assume that damage from cavitation will not have been caused.

CAVITATION AND TEMPORARY CAVITY FORMATION

The formation of a temporary cavity is a feature of fluid dynamics. As the projectile travels through tissue, it creates momentary areas of very low pressure in its wake. The pressure can be so low that the tissue, acting as a liquid, can vaporise. It is important to note that this is an effect of low pressure, not increase in temperature. It is analogous to the phenomena that the boiling point of water decreases as altitude increases.

This newly created vapour expands radially from the path of the projectile, stretching tissues and causing tensile damage. Following expansion, the vapour rapidly returns to a liquid state, causing a subsequent drop in pressure. As the pressure drops the tissues return to their relaxed state. The ability of tissues to tolerate this temporary tensile damage will determine the amount of tissue destruction. For example, muscle and lung tissue are very elastic and tolerate this temporary stretching well: tissue damage is therefore minimal. Liver and brain tissue are inelastic and therefore relatively intolerant of cavitation, so tend to suffer devastating tissue damage. The size of the temporary cavity formed is related to the turbulence of the flow of the projectile. A stable, high ogive bullet will pass through tissue for some distance without creating much turbulent flow and therefore cause little cavitation.

An unstable, expanding or fragmenting round however, creates massive turbulent flow. As the projectile passes through tissue, the spin conferred upon it by the rifling is slowed, reducing its stability and increasing the yaw. This is combined with the likelihood that the projectile will not cross tissue interfaces perpendicular to them, causing further destabilisation. If the penetration distance through tissue is sufficient, or if it strikes bone, it is likely that the bullet will tumble. When its long axis is at 90° to its trajectory, the rate of energy transfer and cavitation is greatest, as shown in the Figure 20.5.

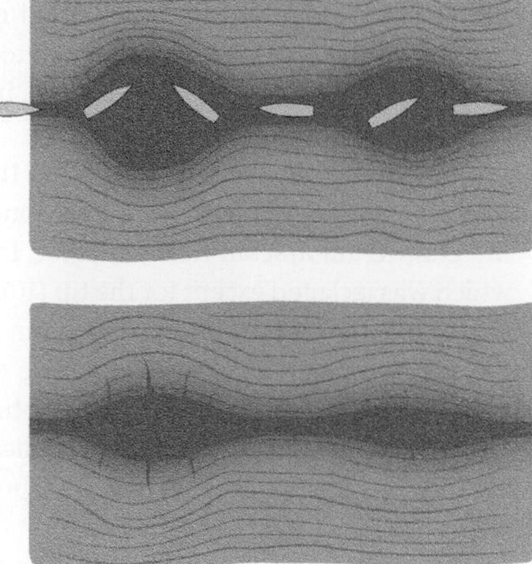

Figure 20.5 Schematic showing the formation and persistence of the temporary cavity, with maximal cavity formation at point where the projectiles tumble and turn through 180° to the direction of travel.

It is important to recognise the fact that cavitation does not necessarily occur throughout the wound tract: there will only be a large exit wound if significant cavitation occurs at the point the projectile leaves the body.

SHOCK WAVE

The shock wave is one of the most controversial areas of ballistics, as the significance of this component is not yet fully understood. It has long been recognised that when a projectile strikes tissue, a tiny region of very high pressure is generated. This propagates through the tissue at approximately the speed of sound in water (1434 ms^{-1}), typically faster and therefore ahead of the projectile (7).

Some investigators, particularly those examining actual shootings and animal models, believe a significant degree of the damage sustained can be attributed to the shock wave (8,9). However, other investigators discount the wounding potential of the shock wave and regard it as insignificant when compared to cavitation (6).

BULLET DESIGN AND ENERGY TRANSFER

Bullet design is of significant interest to the trauma practitioner due to the effect that it has on the wound pattern. As shown in the earlier equation, a projectile's kinetic energy increases in proportion to its mass; however, enlarging the surface area that the bullet presents to the air increases drag. Bullets have therefore traditionally been made from dense metals to reduce this effect. For centuries, lead formed the predominant component for both its density and softness. The softness means that it deforms and flattens when it strikes its target. The deformation leads to an increase, or expansion, in the advancing surface area only after striking the target, thus increasing the drag and the rate of energy transfer into the casualty's tissues.

Despite this, the softness of lead bullets has a disadvantage. The switch in propellants in the late 19th century from gunpowder to more powerful nitrocellulose significantly increased the velocity of bullets as they passed down the barrel. It was noted that at speeds above 300 ms^{-1} there was excessive damage to the bullet as it travelled down the barrel. To combat this, bullets were wrapped, or *jacketed*, in copper and became known as *full metal jacket (FMJ)* bullets.

It was noted in the late 1800s that the standard British army round, the FMJ Mk II .303, had less 'stopping power' than traditional lead bullets. To counter this, the superintendent of the Dum-Dum arsenal near Calcutta, India, Captain Neville Bertie-Clay, developed a round which was jacketed except for the tip (10). This protected the lead of the bullet core, but allowed the soft, exposed nose to expand on impact. The expanding effect was further enhanced by the addition of a hollow tip in the nose of the bullet in the Mk IV round. These semi-jacketed rounds were noted to produce devastating injuries when they were first used in the Battle of Omdurman in 1898. British Army soldiers issued with the old Mk II rounds reportedly cut off the tips to increase their expansion upon impact. The term *'Dum-Dum'* has been associated with expanding rounds ever since.

Expanding rounds have been shown to produce wounds an order of magnitude larger than comparable FMJ bullets (11). In 1899, the signatories to a Hague convention declared that in conflicts between them, they would 'abstain from the use of bullets which expand or flatten easily in the human body, such as bullets with a hard envelope which does not entirely cover the core, or is pierced with incisions'. Expanding bullets are permissible for security services

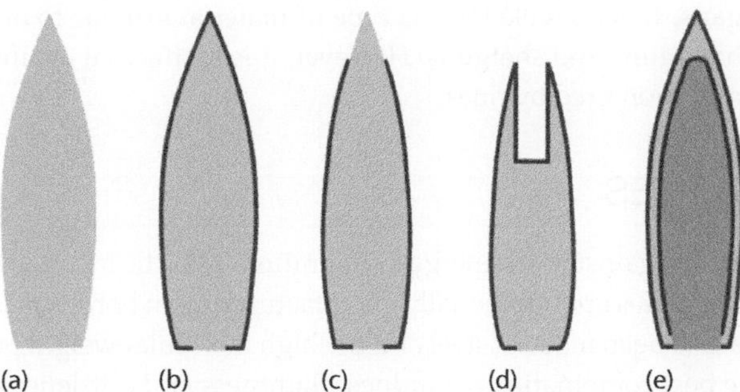

Figure 20.6 Schematic showing variations in bullet design. (a) is an un-jacketed, soft bullet liable to deform on impact. (b) is a full metal jacket, military-type bullet that should pass through soft tissue without deforming. Bullet (c) is a semi-jacketed or dum-dum design that will normally expand on impact. Similarly, bullet (d) is a hollow point design, intended to expand on impact. Bullet (e) has a steel core and is designed to pass through armour and is unlikely to deform, but the jacket may fragment.

(where the aim is to instantly take down the target and ensure that through-and-through shots do not injure passers-by) and for civilian hunting use.

Some bullets have been designed with other modifications to increase their expansion and energy transfer. For example the Winchester Supreme Expansion Technology©/Black Talon© round has six segments that peel outwards when striking the target. This effect increases the surface area presented to the tissue, causing rapid retardation and energy transfer. This increases the damage caused and makes the bullet less likely to pass through the body to potentially injure another casualty. Figure 20.6 demonstrates basic differences in bullet design.

It should be noted that even FMJ bullets not designed to deform will fragment in tissue at high velocities. This effect is observed in the standard 5.56 × 45 NATO round at speeds of over 750 ms^{-1}.

BALLISTIC PROTECTION

Attempts to protect against the effects of projectile weapons with armour have evolved with the development of the weapons themselves. Modern ballistic protection is made up of three components: mesh, plates and carriers. Carriers do not convey any protection, but position the protective armour over vital organs while causing the least limitation to the wearers' function.

BALLISTIC MESH

Ballistic mesh or soft armour is composed of a 'web' of very strong fibres, for example Kevlar® or nylon. These fibres are woven into fabric sheets, which are then overlaid to form a multi-layered material. This material absorbs and disperses the impact energy that is transmitted to the vest from the bullet, and causes the bullet to deform, or 'mushroom'. Each successive layer of material in the vest absorbs additional energy, until such time as the bullet has been stopped (11).

Because the fibres work together both in the individual layer and with other layers of material in the vest, a large area of the garment becomes involved in preventing the bullet from penetrating its target (11). Unfortunately, this means that though the bullet may not penetrate the vest, the area of tissue beneath the vest may be exposed to a large area of blunt trauma. This trauma can result in a spectrum of injury, from a simple haematoma to significant damage

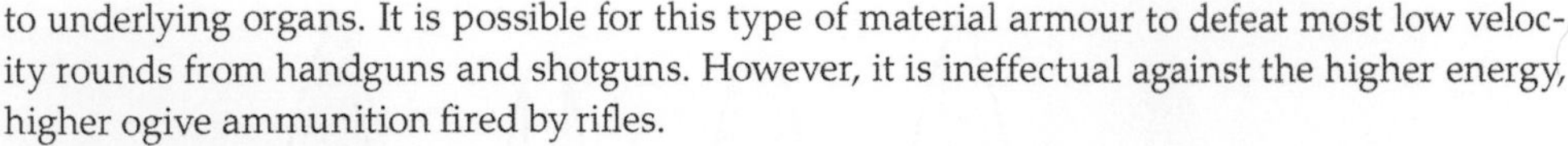
to underlying organs. It is possible for this type of material armour to defeat most low velocity rounds from handguns and shotguns. However, it is ineffectual against the higher energy, higher ogive ammunition fired by rifles.

BALLISTIC PLATES

To provide protection against high-energy ammunition, ballistic insert plates are added to ballistic mesh. Ballistic plates are traditionally manufactured from boron carbide or silicon carbide ceramic, but have also been made of steel or ultra-high molecular weight polyethylene. Ceramic plates provide the best combination of hardness, lightness and brittleness, the desirable qualities of any ballistic protection plate. The ceramic plate usually has lightweight, high-strength material similar to Kevlar attached as a backing.

The mechanism of effect of ballistic plates lies in absorbing and dissipating the projectile's kinetic energy by local shattering of the ceramic plate and blunting the bullet material on the hard ceramic. The backing then spreads the energy of the impact to a larger area and arrests the fragments, reducing the likelihood of fatal injury to the wearer.

The US National Institute of Justice (NIJ) is the internationally recognised standard for ballistic protection. In general, there are four protection levels. NIJ Levels II and IIIa require the armour to protect against handgun ammunition and tend to refer to mesh or soft armour protection systems. Most body armour issued to pre-hospital practitioners will be at this level. Levels III and IV require protection against high-velocity rifle ammunition and usually involve the use of hard armour plates. As previously mentioned, no armour will completely protect the user against injury, however, its aim is always to decrease the extent of injury the wearer experiences.

PRE-HOSPITAL ASSESSMENT AND TREATMENT

SCENE SAFETY AND COMMAND AND CONTROL

The potential dangers of attending the scene of a firearms incident are obvious. If there is any suggestion of a perpetrator at large, pre-hospital practitioners should wait in the muster area or outside the incident cordon. They should only advance to treat casualties following direct instruction from the police incident commander.

The United Kingdom has fortunately avoided significant numbers of multiple shootings such as are all too distressingly common in the United States where, in 2015, there were according to one estimate 372 mass shootings killing 475 people and wounding 1870 (12). The Dunblane incident of 1996 in which Thomas Hamilton killed 16 pupils and 1 teacher and the Whitehaven tragedy of 2011 in which Derrick Bird killed 12 and injured 11 are notable exceptions. In the event of mass shootings, the medical incident commander should consider establishing a casualty clearing station. Casualties with non-life-threatening injuries can be held there while limited resources are focused on transferring casualties with life-threatening injuries to hospital.

The majority of shootings do not therefore fit into this pattern and will simply require appropriate security cordoning of the area until the risk is eliminated and medical care when it can be provided safely. Factors which make a shooting more complex include difficulty in locating and eliminating the perpetrator, as was the case with Derek Bird or Raoul Moat, large numbers of living, or *possibly* living casualties, and major disruption to infrastructure.

ZONES AT A SHOOTING INCIDENT

The police will usually establish the following zones at an incident involving firearms.

NON-PERMISSIVE ZONE

Under no circumstances must non-specialist medical staff enter the non-permissive zone. Patients must be extracted from the non-permissive area for treatment and clinical protocols must reflect this. Police firearms teams receive standard advanced first-aid training relevant to such environments.

SEMI-PERMISSIVE ZONE

The semi-permissive zone is sometimes referred to as the *warm zone* because some risk persists but direct threat is absent. The minimal level of care necessary to save life should be provided, under instruction from the relevant commander and ideally by specially trained personnel only, such as members of a HART (hazardous area response team). Because this area is within the police cordon, an escort should be provided if clinical staff are required to enter.

PERMISSIVE ZONE

By definition, work in this area poses no risk to clinicians and all appropriate interventions are possible. However, transfer to hospital must not be delayed.

HISTORY AND ASSESSMENT

As has been previously stated, shotgun wounds are normally obvious due to their characteristic appearance. Differentiating between typically low-energy handgun GSWs and higher energy rifle GSWs can be simplified by asking casualties/bystanders if a 'long' or 'short' weapon was used. Range and direction of fire is likely to be of less relevance and is often mistaken by witnesses anyway.

It is important not to be tempted to over-interpret wounding patterns: high-energy rounds can leave small exit wounds and low-energy rounds can leave large ones as shown in Figure 20.7. Such surmise is not relevant to the initial management of the patient, and in any case is usually wrong. In the pre-hospital environment, treat the patient, not the suspected ammunition.

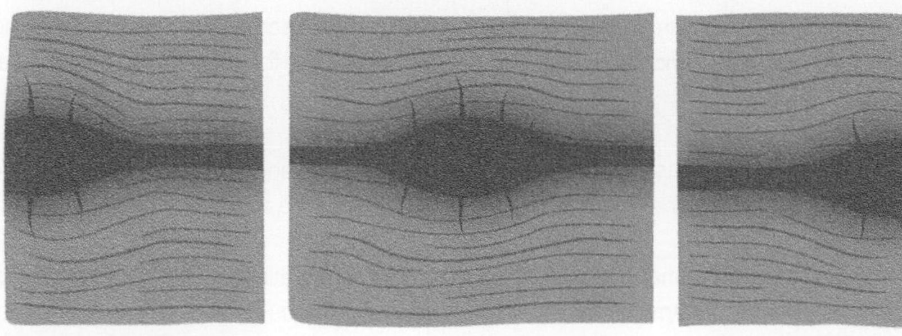

Figure 20.7 Schematic showing the variable size of entrance and exit wounds depending on bullet orientation when it strikes or leaves tissue.

Patient assessment in cases of gunshot injury follows exactly the same <C>ABCDE as in any other case of trauma. Preconceptions about the presumed severity of gunshot wounds must not influence treatment. Treatment must therefore be based on the injuries found on examination and the observed or expected physiological consequences of those injuries.

It should also be borne in mind that any predictions regarding the wound track, unreliable as these are likely to be, can only be made if the position of the victim at the *moment of impact* is known (Figure 20.8).

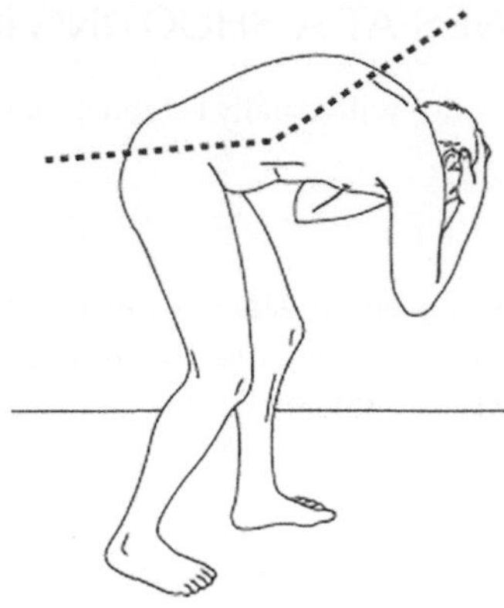

Figure 20.8 Position at impact and wound track.

PRE-HOSPITAL TREATMENT

A casualty with a GSW is no different from any other and a standard <C>ABCDE approach should be followed (Box 20.1). As previously mentioned, bullets can follow unpredictable pathways within the body, and at least some consideration should be given to spinal immobilisation particularly if the victim may have fallen as a result of being shot. Any GSW involving the torso or junctional areas has the potential to damage any structure within the thorax or abdomen and can result in rapidly fatal chest injuries. Positive pressure ventilation of a casualty with a penetrating chest injury from a GSW is a relative indication for thoracostomy.

BOX 20.1: Management of Gunshot Wounds

<C>

Massive exsanguinating external haemorrhage is unusual following a GSW but is conventionally managed by tourniquet application, pressure dressings, haemostatic dressings and fluid replacement ideally with blood products.

A

Direct trauma to the airway is likely to require intubation or a surgical airway. Loss of airway control due to loss of conscious level is managed conventionally. Facial GSWs may require the conscious patient to maintain a posture sitting up and leaning forward, and soft tissues can be held off the airway with a tongue suture.

B

Chest injuries due to GSW are managed in the same way as the same injury (tension pneumothorax, haemothorax, etc.) due to another cause. Consider thoracostomy if the patient is to be ventilated and has a chest wound.

C

The principles of hybrid resuscitation apply. Ideally resuscitation should be with blood products. The possibility of multi-cavity penetration by the round must always be considered.

D

AVPU and the Glasgow Coma Score (GCS) can be used. Penetrating injuries to the brain are usually but not invariably fatal. Treatment should therefore be active unless death is obvious on arrival.

E

Every wound must be identified by a careful all over assessment of the patient.

Haemorrhage, both compressible and non-compressible, is a common feature of GSWs and can be fatal if unchecked. A direct pressure dressing is normally sufficient to arrest extremity haemorrhage and a tourniquet should rarely be required. Bleeding from the liver or spleen, or great vessel penetration, can be rapidly fatal and suspicion of these injuries should be reported to the receiving hospital in advance of the casualty's arrival. If available, pre-hospital transfusion should be given to shocked patients, especially those with a torso GSW.

Recent military experience has clearly demonstrated that an inter- or transcranial GSW is potentially survivable; ideally transfer should be to a hospital with a neurosurgical facility and the GCS should be documented as soon as feasible and repeated en route.

SUMMARY

The management of gunshot wounds is not complex and most of the mystique and anxiety associated with shootings can be easily dispelled by a knowledge of basic ballistics. Attempts to speculate about injury patterns are unhelpful and may be dangerously misleading. A straightforward <C>ABCDE approach and an awareness that a projectile, whatever its point of entry, may have an entirely unpredictable path will ensure that critical injuries are not missed.

REFERENCES

1. Keen M. *Medieval Warfare: A History.* Oxford: Oxford University Press, 1999.
2. Crime UNOoDa. UNODC Homicide Statistics 2013. New York, 2013.
3. Office for National Statistics. Violent crime and sexual offences, 2011/12. *Statistical Bulletin*, London, 2013.
4. Maguire K, Hughes DM, Fitzpatrick MS, Dunn F, Rocke LG, Baird CJ. Injuries caused by the attenuated energy projectile: The latest less lethal option. *Emergency Medical Journal* 2007;24(2):103–105.
5. Owen-Smith MS. *High Velocity Missile Wounds.* London: Edward Arnold, 1981.
6. Fackler ML. Wound ballistics. A review of common misconceptions. *JAMA* 1988;259(18):2730–2736.
7. Harvey EN, McMillen JH. An experimental study of shock waves resulting from the impact of high velocity missiles on animal tissues. *Journal of Experimental Medicine* 1947;85(3):321–328.
8. Marshall EP, Sanow EJ. *Handgun Stopping Power: The Definitive Study.* Boulder, CO: Paladin Press, 1992.
9. Suneson A, Hansson HA, Kjellstrom BT, Lycke E, Seeman T. Pressure waves caused by high-energy missiles impair respiration of cultured dorsal root ganglion cells. *Journal of Trauma* 1990;30(4):484–488.
10. The military bullet. *British Medical Journal* 1896;2:1810.
11. DeMuth WE Jr. Bullet velocity and design as determinants of wounding capability: An experimental study. *Journal of Trauma* 1966;6(2):222–232.
12. www.shootingtracker.com/

FURTHER READING

Brooks A, Clasper J, Midwinter MJ, Hodgetts TJ, Mahoney PF. *Ryan's Ballistic Trauma.* Springer, 2011.

21 Blast injuries

OBJECTIVES

After completing this chapter the reader will

- Understand the basic science of blast injury
- Understand the patterns of injury associated with an explosion
- Be able to safely manage blast injuries in the pre-hospital environment

INTRODUCTION

The first recorded bombing in Europe occurred in Antwerp on April 4, 1585. It was a pan-European incident where the English government of Elizabeth I funded the Italian military engineer Federgio Giambelli to construct two floating bombs to destroy a bridge constructed by the Spanish who were besieging the Protestant forces in the city. Three thousand kilograms of gunpowder was used in a rudimentary shaped charge directed up at the bridge. *'A thousand soldiers were destroyed in a second of time; many of them being torn to shreds, beyond even the semblance of humanity'*. However, it was also noted that some casualties *'fell dead without a wound, killed by the concussion of the air'* (1).

An explosion is a near instantaneous oxidation of an explosive solid or fluid, converting huge amounts of chemical energy into kinetic and thermal energy. This rapid energy conversion can be immensely destructive with obviously massive potential for injury.

Explosions can occur through domestic and industrial accidents as well as deliberate actions in war or terrorist attacks. Practitioners potentially responsible for the care of casualties of explosions need to have an understanding of the unique circumstances and features of these injuries.

BLAST INJURIES IN WAR AND PEACE

Blast injuries can be considered in the military and civilian environment, however, in the modern world such distinctions are becoming increasingly blurred.

Table 21.1 Relative proportions of GSW to blast injuries

	UK, Iraq and Afghanistan	US OIF/OEF 2001–2005	Falklands	US Vietnam	US Korea
GSW	30%	19%	29%	35%	31%
Blast	70%	81%	71%	65%	69%
n	2276	1416	48	13,050	111,716

Note: OIF, Operation Iraqi Freedom (US-led invasion of Iraq 2003); OEF, Operation Enduring Freedom (US operations in Afghanistan).

BLAST INJURIES IN WAR

Contrary to popular perception, casualties from hostile action are due to explosions rather than gunshot wounds (GSWs) at a ratio of approximately 3:1. This ratio has remained remarkably consistent throughout modern high-intensity conflict as Table 21.1 shows (2–6).

Prefabricated military explosive weapons include indirect fire weapons such as mortars and artillery, rockets, mines and grenades. Non-state military forces have long favoured *improvised explosive devices (IEDs).* These are often initiated by the victim or remotely by a command wire or radio signal in order for the assailant to remain distant from their target (7). IEDs, particularly those initiated by the victim, are often concealed underground in open spaces, thus the numbers of victims are relatively limited to those directly above the blast. In order to injure large numbers of casualties, either very large devices must be employed, with associated difficulty in concealment, or multiple devices will be needed.

BLAST INCIDENTS IN THE CIVILIAN SETTING

Terrorists targeting civilians to achieve a political aim have long favoured explosive weapons due to the potential for mass casualties and terrible injuries without direct engagement of the terrorist with their target. These weapons are most effective when deployed in an enclosed, densely populated urban environment. The most significant terrorist bombings in North America and Europe are shown in Table 21.2 (8–14). These continents are amongst the least susceptible to this type of attack and similar data from other continents might reveal far more extensive casualties.

Table 21.2 Examples of terrorist bombing attacks in Europe and North America over the last 25 years

Attack	Fatalities	Injured	Suicide attack
Manchester 2017	23	139	Yes (1 bomber killed)
Boston Marathon 2013	3	264	No
Oslo bombing 2011	8	209	No
7/7 London bombing 2005	52	700	4 bombers killed
Madrid train bombing 2004	191	1,800	No
Myyrmanni bombing 2002	7	166	1 bomber killed
Omagh bombing 1998	29	220	No
Oklahoma City bombing 1995	167	592	No

The geographic range of terrorist bomb attacks on civilian targets over the last 25 years is demonstrated in Table 21.2. Sadly, the obvious conclusion is that there is a possibility of an attack of this nature almost anywhere.

COMPONENTS OF THE EXPLOSION

Explosions are complicated events that occur extremely rapidly with the release of energy and generation of large volumes of gaseous products. Their precise nature depends on the type of explosive. Professionally manufactured military- or mining-grade explosives will behave differently to home-made munitions such as fertiliser bombs which behave technically more like very rapid combustions. In general, commercial or high-grade explosives require a detonator to cause them to explode but do not require confinement. Low-grade explosives including traditional gunpowder and home-made explosives require confinement if they are to explode but do not require to be detonated.

SHOCK WAVE

The shock wave is analogous to a sound wave in that it passes through substances rather than moves them. Figure 21.1 illustrates the shock wave propagating spherically from the point of the explosion.

The shock wave travels much faster than the speed of sound (330 metres/second in air) and produces an effectively instantaneous rise in pressure for milliseconds. This rise in pressure is often referred to as the overpressure. The energy of the shock wave dissipates rapidly as it propagates away from the source explosion, proportionally to the distance, or radius (*R*) *cubed* (15). Immediately following this transient increase in pressure is a slightly longer period of negative pressure as shown in Figure 21.2.

The negative pressure component is negligible in non-experimental explosions and involves less energy but lasts longer by approximately an order of magnitude than the positive pressure component (16).

Like a sound wave, the shock wave can be reflected; therefore a casualty in a built up environment can be subjected to multiple shock waves from a single explosion as they bounce back and forth, reflected from structures near to the explosion (Figure 21.3). Similarly the shock wave can propagate around and through structures.

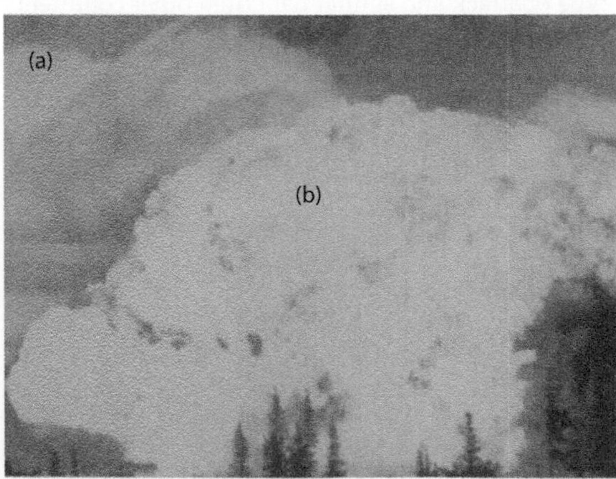

Figure 21.1 The shock wave (a) and blast wind (b).

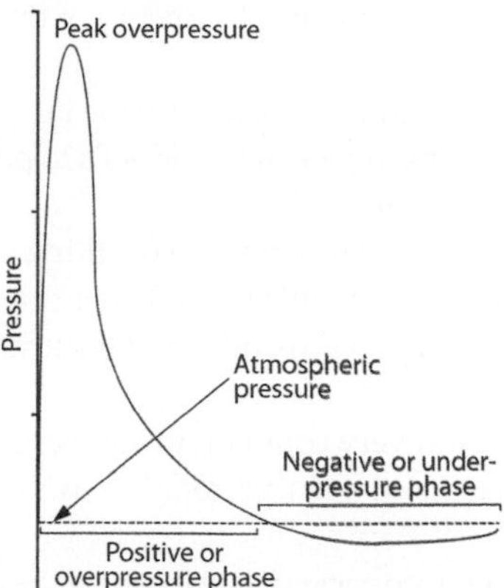

Figure 21.2 Schematic showing idealised shock wave from 'naked' explosion in an open space.

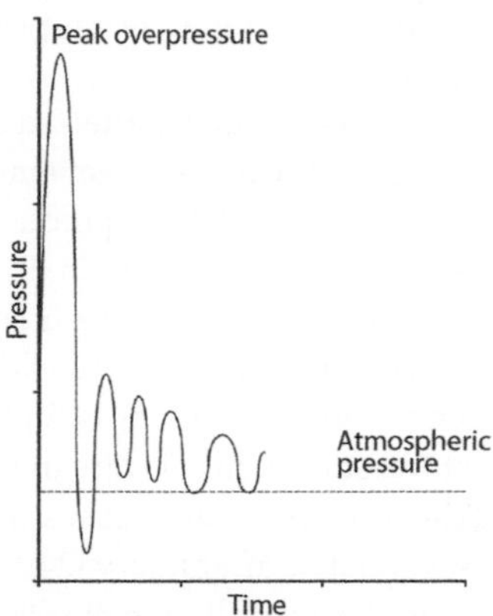

Figure 21.3 Schematic showing idealised shock wave from an explosion within a confined space showing multiple peaks of overpressure as the wave is reflected back and forth.

BLAST WIND

The gas created by the explosion expands outward at high velocity. It is this blast which carries objects such as body parts, fragments of the device and energised objects from the environment. The effect of the blast wind has a much greater range than the shock wave.

HEAT

Along with the blast wind, the combustion of explosive products continues to generate heat. This is more significant with home-made explosives and blasts in enclosed spaces. The ignition of adjacent structures can also result in propagation of the thermal effect. In some incidents a majority of casualties can be due to burns alone, although this is uncommon (17).

INJURY PATTERNS

The injury patterns produced following a blast can be predicted by the components of the explosive blast as described earlier.

PRIMARY BLAST INJURY

Clinically, in the pre-hospital environment, primary blast injuries are the least significant component of blast injury, because if a victim is close enough to a blast to be significantly affected by the effect of the blast shock wave, they are normally also severely injured by fragmentation injury and the effects of the blast wind which will be the priorities for management at scene. However, victims in buildings or vehicles may be particularly vulnerable to primary blast injury due to reflection of the blast wave.

As the shock wave moves through the casualty's body, energy is transferred into tissues particularly at interfaces between gases and tissues. This is analogous to the absorption of sound energy by the open cell foam in ear defenders: as the sound wave travels through the foam, it encounters multiple air–plastic interfaces of the foam cell and the energy of the wave is dissipated.

The organs particularly affected are those with gas–tissue interfaces, mainly the lungs, ears and bowel (18). The pressure generated by the shock wave typically must be >35 KPa to produce ear injuries and >250 KPa to produce lung or bowel injuries (19).

Blast lung injury can result in disruption at the alveolar–capillary interface resulting in lung parenchymal haemorrhage, pneumothorax and alveolar-venous fistulae (20). The incidence of blast lung in terrorist bombings varies enormously depending on proximity and enclosure but has been reported as high as 14% of casualties (21,22).

Blast intestinal injury is rare in land-based explosions but very common in submerged victims (23). The blast wave causes intramural haemorrhage and even perforation, which may occur several days after injury (24).

Ear injuries typically range from tympanic membrane to ossicle dislocation and can be a feature of up to half of blast casualties (21). It has been noted that the presence of ear injuries varies significantly depending on the position of the head relative to the blast, and even though the threshold pressure for ear damage is theoretically an order of magnitude less than that for lung injury, the absence of ear injuries is a poor surrogate for the absence of visceral injury (25).

SECONDARY BLAST INJURY

The majority of injuries are due to secondary blast effects: the impaction on the victim's body of pre-formed projectiles within the device, irregular fragments from the device, environmental debris and even tissue from other victims. These materials are accelerated by the blast wind causing widespread and often gross tissue damage and mutilation. These projectiles are accelerated radially away from the blast epicentre and follow an arced trajectory due to the effect of gravity.

Fragments and debris behave exactly like projectiles discussed in the ballistics chapter, with the caveat that they are often irregularly shaped, are subject to greater drag and therefore do not travel as far. Victims are often struck by multiple projectiles along with the tissue stripping effect of large numbers of small pieces of debris.

There have been two proposed mechanisms for the traumatic amputation of limbs. First, that the shock wave fractures the diaphysis of the long bones and then the amputation is completed by the limb being flailed by the blast wind (26). The second proposed mechanism is that the amputation occurs through the joint through a purely flail mechanism as a result of the flailing of the limb (27). In practice, it is likely that both mechanisms are involved.

TERTIARY BLAST INJURY

If a victim is thrown by the blast wind, they are at risk of sustaining blunt injury when they strike walls or objects.

BLAST INCIDENT MANAGEMENT

Each explosive incident is unique. Such incidents have the capability to cause large numbers of casualties as shown in Table 21.1; they are crime scenes with evidence which must be preserved and collected, and there is potential for injury to rescue workers.

A terrorist attack in the UK would probably be under the control of the Cabinet Office Briefing Room (COBR) as platinum command. Under the 2003 Communications Act, COBR can order the shut down of mobile phone networks and therefore communication plans should not rely on them, for example for calling in extra hospital staff. Most explosive incidents in the UK will trigger a declaration of a major incident.

SCENE CONSIDERATIONS

The scene of a blast will be under the control of the police incident commander.

Pre-hospital practitioners should be aware that terrorists are familiar with emergency service standard operating procedures and might plan a secondary device aimed at responders. This tactic was used in the 1975 Warrenpoint ambush where the secondary device killed 12 soldiers, more than the 6 killed by the primary IED (28). Triage will probably have to occur at the scene with distribution of casualties to several hospitals to avoid overwhelming a single facility's resources.

In all cases involving blast, command and control of the scene will be essential. Not only is there a potential for a large number of casualties from an explosive incident, but each one may have extremely complex poly-trauma requiring significant resources, and there is likely to be a significant level of concern over safety with the risk of building collapse or a secondary device. The horrific nature of the injuries is likely to further increase the stress on rescuers, clinicians and victims alike.

TREATMENT STRATEGIES

The aim of immediate treatment is to preserve life and to facilitate future reconstruction and rehabilitation. In practice this is focused on treating haemorrhage and preventing infection.

HAEMORRHAGE CONTROL AND RESUSCITATION

Pre-hospital management follows the <C>ABCDE process. Initially attention must be focused on extremity haemorrhage control with the use of tourniquets in the event of traumatic amputation or severe bleeding from lacerations. Multiple superficial fragment wounds do not require immediate management. Intravenous or intraosseous access (which may be particularly useful where there is limb loss) must be obtained and fluid replacement, ideally with blood products commenced. Transfer to hospital must not be delayed. The pre-hospital phase of management is part of a continuum of damage control principles (29). Treatment for primary blast injury is rarely required at scene, and careful attention to maintaining a patent airway and effective ventilation are central to management. Penetrating injury may result from high-energy fragments akin to bullet wounds, but the majority of fragment wounds will be superficial. Injuries due to translocation of the body by the blast wind are managed in the same way as conventional blunt injuries.

It is hard to exaggerate the degree of contamination in blast wounds. Explosions can drive fragments, debris, foliage, items of clothing and even tissue from other blast victims deep along tissue planes. If possible, antibiotics should therefore be administered as soon as possible in the pre-hospital setting (30).

SUMMARY

Blast injuries are often dramatic, with amputation and devastating soft tissue injuries being relatively common. It is essential that clinicians are not distracted by these injuries, but with a knowledge of how blast effects the human body, simply concentrate on the management of those injuries which are potentially life threatening. Particular attention must be paid to control of exsanguinating haemorrhage and the <C>ABCDE system followed without deviation.

REFERENCES

1. Motley JL. *The United Netherlands: History from the Death of William the Silent to the Twelve Years' Truce – 1609.* [S.l.]: John Murray, 1904.
2. Penn-Barwell JG, Bishop JRB, Roberts S, Midwinter M. Injuries and outcomes: UK military casualties from Iraq and Afghanistan 2003–2012. *Bone and Joint Journal* 2013;95B (Supp 26):1.
3. Owens BD, Kragh JF, Jr., Wenke JC, Macaitis J, Wade CE, Holcomb JB. Combat wounds in operation Iraqi Freedom and operation Enduring Freedom. *Journal of Trauma* 2008;64(2):295–299.
4. Jackson DS. Sepsis in soft tissue limbs wounds in soldiers injured during the Falklands Campaign 1982. *Journal of the Royal Army Medical Corps* 1984;130(2):97–99.
5. Hardaway RM 3rd. Viet Nam wound analysis. *Journal of Trauma* 1978;18(9):635–643.
6. Reister FA. *Battle Casualties and Medical Statistics: U.S. Army Experience in the Korean War.* Washington, DC: Surgeon General, 1973.
7. Ramasamy A, Hill AM, Clasper JC. Improvised explosive devices: Pathophysiology, injury profiles and current medical management. *Journal of the Royal Army Medical Corps* 2009;155(4):265–272.
8. Biddinger PD, Baggish A, Harrington L, d'Hemecourt P, Hooley J, Jones J, Kue R, Troyanos C, Dyer KS. Be prepared—The Boston Marathon and mass-casualty events. *New England Journal of Medicine* 2013;368(21):1958–1960.
9. Sollid SJ, Rimstad R, Rehn M, Nakstad AR, Tomlinson AE, Strand T, Heimdal HJ, Nilsen JE, Sandberg M. Oslo government district bombing and Utoya island shooting July 22, 2011: The immediate prehospital emergency medical service response. *Scandinavian Journal of Trauma, Resuscitation and Emergency Medicine* 2012;20(1):3.
10. Aylwin CJ, Konig TC, Brennan NW, Shirley PJ, Davies G, Walsh MS, Brohi K. Reduction in critical mortality in urban mass casualty incidents: Analysis of triage, surge, and resource use after the London bombings on July 7, 2005. *Lancet* 2006;368(9554):2219–2225.
11. Turegano-Fuentes F, Caba-Doussoux P, Jover-Navalon JM, Martin-Perez E, Fernandez-Luengas D, Diez-Valladares L, Perez-Diaz D et al. Injury patterns from major urban terrorist bombings in trains: The Madrid experience. *World Journal of Surgery* 2008;32(6):1168–1175.
12. Torkki M, Koljonen V, Sillanpaa K, Tukianinen E, Pyorala S, Kemppainen E, Kalske J, Arajarvi E, Keranen U. Triage in a bomb disaster with 166 casualties. *European Journal of Trauma* 2006;32(4):374–380.
13. Potter SJ, Carter GE. The Omagh bombing—A medical perspective. *Journal of the Royal Army Medical Corps* 2000;146(1):18–21.
14. Mallonee S, Shariat S, Stennies G, Waxweiler R, Hogan D, Jordan F. Physical injuries and fatalities resulting from the Oklahoma City bombing. *JAMA* 1996;276(5):382–387.
15. Taylor G. The formation of a blast wave by a very intense explosion I. Theoretical discussion. *Proceedings of the Royal Society of London A: Mathematical and Physical Sciences* 1950;201(1065):159–174.

16. Owen-Smith MS. *High Velocity Missile Wounds.* London: Edward Arnold, 1981.
17. Chapman CW. Burns and plastic surgery in the South Atlantic campaign 1982. *Journal of the Royal Naval Medical Service* 1983;69(2):71–79.
18. Guy RJ, Kirkman E, Watkins PE, Cooper GJ. Physiologic responses to primary blast. *Journal of Trauma* 1998;45(6):983–987.
19. Ritenour AE, Baskin TW. Primary blast injury: Update on diagnosis and treatment. *Critical Care Medicine* 2008;36(7 Suppl):S311–S317.
20. Guy RJ, Glover MA, Cripps NP. The pathophysiology of primary blast injury and its implications for treatment. Part I: The thorax. *Journal of the Royal Naval Medical Service* 1998;84(2):79–86.
21. Mellor SG, Cooper GJ. Analysis of 828 servicemen killed or injured by explosion in Northern Ireland 1970–84: The Hostile Action Casualty System. *British Journal of Surgery* 1989;76(10):1006–1010.
22. Ritenour AE, Blackbourne LH, Kelly JF, McLaughlin DF, Pearse LA, Holcomb JB, Wade CE. Incidence of primary blast injury in US military overseas contingency operations: A retrospective study. *Annals of Surgery* 2010;251(6):1140–1144.
23. Huller T, Bazini Y. Blast injuries of the chest and abdomen. *Archives of Surgery* 1970;100(1):24–30.
24. Mellor SG. The pathogenesis of blast injury and its management. *British Journal of Hospital Medicine* 1988;39(6):536–539.
25. Hill JF. Blast injury with particular reference to recent terrorist bombing incidents. *Annals of the Royal College of Surgeons of England* 1979;61(1):4–11.
26. Hull JB, Cooper GJ. Pattern and mechanism of traumatic amputation by explosive blast. *Journal of Trauma* 1996;40(3 Suppl):S198–S205.
27. Singleton JAG, Gibb IE, Bull AMJ, Clasper JC. Blast-mediated traumatic amputation: Evidence suggesting a new injury mechanism. *Bone and Joint Journal* 2014;96B(Suppl 9):1.
28. Edwards A. *The Northern Ireland Troubles: Operation Banner, 1969–2007.* Oxford: Osprey, 2011.
29. Midwinter MJ. Damage control surgery in the era of damage control resuscitation. *Journal of the Royal Army Medical Corps* 2009;155(4):323–326.
30. Penn-Barwell JG, Murray CK, Wenke JC. Early antibiotics and debridement independently reduce infection in an open fracture model. *Journal of Bone and Joint Surgery British Volume* 2012;94(1):107–112.

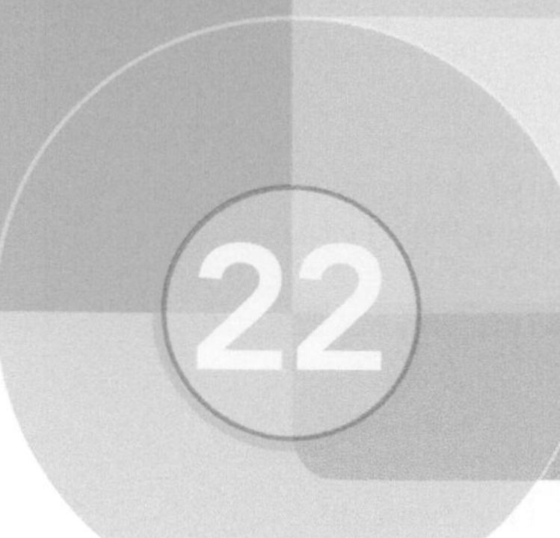

22 Trauma management in the austere pre-hospital environment

OBJECTIVES

After completing this chapter the reader will

- Understand the concept of austerity as applied to trauma management
- Be aware of the constraints an austere environment places on the management of the trauma victim
- Be able to plan a trauma response appropriate to an austere operating environment

INTRODUCTION

In the United Kingdom and developed world, we are increasingly comforted by the protection of a robust pre-hospital care system. An ambulance, fully equipped and staffed by highly trained paramedics, is never far away, more often than not backed up by a helicopter-borne critical care service. Unfortunately, timely, excellent care for the ill and injured is not ubiquitous. Many states lack the finances or infrastructure to provide medical services even in key urban areas, and in remote parts there may be no professional help coming. Other areas are so remote that even with the full support and funding of government, the pre-hospital phase can be prolonged: even in the direst emergency and under perfect conditions, a patient from the British Antarctic Survey base at Halley (located 75°35′S, 26°39′W) is 12 hours from an operating theatre (1).

Trauma, on the other hand, is universal. Road deaths account for 1.24 million people a year worldwide (91% occurring in low- or middle-income countries) and as many as 50 million people are injured (2). Trauma is the ninth leading cause of death worldwide and a greater cause of mortality than malaria. Thus there is a pressing need for those working in austere environments to understand how to deliver the best trauma care with the resources available.

WHAT IS AUSTERITY IN THE MEDICAL CONTEXT?

Austerity conjures images of hostile climates and scarce population, but in medical terms it simply means that resources are limited. *Resource-constrained* is an equivalent term. Austere environments can include:

- Remote expedition environments such as a jungle, mountain or desert.
- Conflict environments such as Syria and Afghanistan.
- Rural communities with difficult access routes and vehicle availability in developing countries such as Sierra Leone, Sudan and Central African Republic.
- Rural communities with difficult access in developed countries such as the Scottish Highlands.
- The humanitarian disaster environment where there has been disruption to normal healthcare infrastructure and personnel.
- Any environment with a lack of skilled healthcare workers and resources.

The implication is that in these environments access to one or more key resources will be limited. In terms of pre-hospital trauma care, these constraints tend to fall into three broad domains: *capability, capacity* and *access*. These domains may be chronically limited – for example in a less economically developed country (LEDC) where total spending on healthcare and infrastructure is a small proportion of a tiny gross domestic product and there have been decades of underfunding or degradation from conflict. Alternatively, resources may be acutely reduced after natural disasters such as earthquake and flooding, or because of a sudden increase in population at risk, for example in the case of a large refugee population moving into the area, fleeing a conflict elsewhere. Expeditions may be limited by what personnel can carry, use and purchase whilst in the field.

CAPABILITY

The capability of medical services is dependent on several factors, any or all of which may be limited in an austere environment. Components include equipment (including drugs and consumables with potential for resupply), personnel and their level of training, and the secondary care capability in the area.

EQUIPMENT

Medical equipment is expensive and in resource-poor areas there may be significant constraints on both what can be afforded and what is available for purchase even if there are funds. There is often lack of funding available to maintain equipment, purchase replacement parts or develop the skills to implement repairs. Once broken, equipment may remain unserviceable, permanently reducing capacity or even capability.

Equipment must be transported and so the scaling that can be taken to the patient depends on whether it needs to be man-portable or is vehicle delivered. The latter will also depend on the availability and capability of the transport platform.

There is no generic list of equipment that should be available for trauma management in the pre-hospital environment, although recommendations and minimum standards are suggested for trauma care in general (3).

Ideally, infection control measures mandate single-use items, but in resource-poor environments these may not be practical, as the number needed along with the space taken up by individual packaging may be prohibitive. Reusable equipment is often more robustly designed which also suits the environment, though this often also means heavier and bulkier. Resupply needs to be considered – turnaround time is longer if there is no simple off-the-shelf replacement or a period of sterilisation is required.

Disposal of single-use equipment, packaging and waste or sharps is also important. Many areas will not have dedicated facilities for processing these by-products. Adequate sharps bins and clinical waste bags must be built into the stock carried and resupply options.

Locally sourced drugs may vary considerably in availability, quality and cost. Imported supplies are likely to be much more expensive and resupply opportunities less frequent. Medical gases may be available in canisters, but the weight and bulk soon becomes an issue without good transport. Oxygen concentrators are becoming smaller and cheaper but suffer from similar constraints, as well as the need for a reliable power supply. Single-use chemical oxygen generators are also becoming more widely available.

TRAINED PERSONNEL

Medical personnel are often in critically limited supply, both in terms of their absolute numbers, and in terms of their specialist training. In Sierra Leone in 2010 there were 0.03 physicians per 1000 population, compared to 2.7 in the UK (3 per capita) (4) – as a result in 2008 there were only five anaesthetists in total across ten government hospitals. Where resources are stretched so thin, generalism is a valued commodity – any surgeon will be expected to be able to perform basic general, obstetric and orthopaedic procedures. Conversely there will be very limited access to specialist surgeons and so to more complex definitive procedures. The same Sierra Leone study found that at that time a chest drain could be placed at 60% of the hospitals, an open fracture managed at 80% and a laparotomy performed at only 20% (5).

SECONDARY CARE

The capability of the secondary care network is critical to understanding the level of pre-hospital care that should be provided. The pre-hospital delivery of trauma care is rarely definitive; it is a bridge, preventing or minimising deterioration of the patient's condition until they can be transported to a higher echelon. A severe head injury, retrieved within 30 minutes, intubated, resuscitated and with ongoing sedation requirements cannot be managed in a local hospital that has neither surgeons, a CT scanner, nor an intensive therapy unit (ITU). Without adequate secondary care support, pre-hospital care becomes futile at best; a distraction and waste of scarce resources at worst (6,7). Any attempt to provide pre-hospital care in a remote or austere environment needs to be planned carefully in the light of these constraints. The level of care that can be provided is rarely limited in these environments by the skill set of the practitioner; far more common it is the logistical issues surrounding the availability and transport of equipment, or the duration of travel to a higher level of care that limits what can reasonably be done.

PRACTICE POINT

The level of pre-hospital care must be congruent with the available secondary care receiving facilities.

Constraining factors other than resources include cultural and political issues. The care that is delivered must be culturally acceptable and the practitioner should be mindful of the complexities around, for example, the treatment of an unaccompanied woman by a Western male team in Afghanistan.

CAPACITY

Even where the capability exists, the capacity of the system may be critically inadequate. Occasionally this can occur even in developed urban settings (for example during epidemics or a major incident) but is usually limited in duration and rarely has a major impact on the delivery of care. In resource-poor areas, such capacity issues may be chronic and severe, as evidenced by the fact that the only 3.5% of surgical procedures occur in the poorest third of the world (8). In some areas of South Africa, residents describe ambulances as almost non-existent or arriving hours after patients have died (7).

These chronic problems may be dramatically worsened when many patients present with a similar illness or mechanism of injury, for example large numbers of crush injuries after large earthquakes or fragmentation wounds after a large explosion. Because these patients are all competing for the same limited resources, pinch points in the system such as operating theatres become critical.

Where problems affect the wider populace (such as the cholera outbreak in Haiti or people fleeing a village during a conflict), the intrinsic medical infrastructure (probably already weakened by the situation) will struggle to cope with the increased demand across all specialties; the simple numbers of beds, staff and basic drugs become the issue. Finally there will be conflicting demands on non-medical assets and infrastructure (communications and transport assets in particular), which may exacerbate pre-existing shortages.

In the context of medical support to expeditions or military operations, the capacity should be clearly defined before setting off. Sadly, because of poor planning – particularly on expeditions – the limited capacity for a given treatment is often not discovered until the drugs start to run low.

ACCESS

DISTANCE

The nearest medical resource, be it first responder, ambulance or medical facility, may be some distance away. In the United States the average distance to hospital for an urban resident is only 5.5 miles, rising to 35.9 miles for people in rural areas (9). In a Kenyan study, 66% of accident victims reached a hospital within an hour (10). In Sierra Leone distances between hospitals can be in excess of 200 km; while the majority of surgical patients there have to travel less than 80 km to get to a hospital, the state of the roads means that in some cases even this journey can take days (5).

INFRASTRUCTURE AND TRANSPORT PLATFORMS

The patient's location and ease of access to that location will determine the required level of transport capability for a particular situation. While in the UK this is usually a smooth road easily covered by a standard ambulance; in other areas it may need to be a modified 4 × 4 vehicle, helicopter or even boat. Even if a platform is available, limited fuel supply, maintenance and parts may restrict its use.

Communications infrastructure is also critical. A delayed call will inevitably result in delayed arrival of medical assistance. In developing countries where the onus is usually on the patient's family or good Samaritans to transport them, pre-hospital times for fractured femurs in one study in four low-income countries averaged 6 days (10,11).

ENVIRONMENTAL

Access to remote areas when weather is poor (for example during the monsoon) may be especially difficult. Air support is often equally limited. In extreme examples, areas may become completely inaccessible, preventing any access to additional healthcare facilities. Evacuation from the British Antarctic Survey base at Halley is impossible for over 5 months of the year (1).

SECURITY AND CONFLICT

Health workers and patients are particularly vulnerable in areas of conflict or where security is limited or absent. Recent examples include hospitals being targeted in Syria, and polio immunisation teams executed in Pakistan (12,13). The International Committee of the Red Cross (ICRC) specifically recognises the risk to healthcare workers in such regions (14).

Purposeful deprivation of health resources has been seen as a strategy in various conflicts, and while internationally condemned, is difficult to overcome politically (12,15). Even if facilities and staff are not overtly targeted, healthcare provision can be made harder through a variety of administrative means (restricted access to visas, control of movement through checkpoints, etc.). Thus the freedom to provide pre-hospital care is intricately linked to the cultural and political situation on the ground.

STRATEGIES FOR DELIVERY OF GOOD PRE-HOSPITAL CARE IN AUSTERE ENVIRONMENTS

PLANNING

In order to effectively plan a pre-hospital function in an austere environment, the mission needs to be clearly defined. Whether an enduring service, expecting to manage many casualties over a period of time, or a 'one-shot' capability such as to provide cover for a brief expedition, the problem can be broken down into several parts (see Box 22.1).

BOX 22.1: Key Planning Questions

- What is the population at risk?
- What spectrum of conditions will be managed and for how long? How will resupply take place?
- Where is the next level of care, and what is the ceiling of care that can be provided there? How far away is it?
- What platform will transport the team and casualty, and how long does it take to get to the next level of care?
- How much treatment can be done in one episode before resupply?
- How will the response be activated?
- How do I guarantee the safety of the team?
- Do I need additional non-medical facilitators?

WHAT IS THE REMIT OF MY SERVICE?

Will the service be supporting a specified group (for example an expedition) or will it be available to all comers? Will the service or facility be working alone (expedition) or at the request of the host nation as a small part of the multi-national response to a disaster? These questions are fundamental to understanding the mission and need to be answered in as much detail as possible. They impact every aspect of the planning process, from the visas and paperwork allowing entry to the country through to the list of drugs carried, and the communications network and command and control structure that co-ordinate pre-hospital care.

PRACTICE POINT

Clarity regarding eligibility for care, and hence the scope of the service to be provided, is absolutely essential.

WHAT SPECTRUM OF CONDITIONS WILL BE MANAGED AND FOR HOW LONG? HOW WILL RESUPPLY TAKE PLACE?

It is unusual to be asked to provide a service for trauma victims alone, even if, for example after an earthquake, this appears to be the thrust of the intervention. It is essential therefore that clinicians and organisers are aware of the other likely presenting problems and be prepared and able to manage them. Effective plans must be in place to replace drugs and consumables.

WHERE IS THE NEXT LEVEL OF CARE, AND WHAT IS THE CEILING OF CARE THAT CAN BE PROVIDED THERE? HOW FAR AWAY IS IT?

There is no point delivering a level of care that exceeds the capability of the next echelon – intubation of a head-injured patient before delivery to a hospital that has no CT scanner, neurosurgical capability or ITU is futile. Where pre-hospital critical care interventions are feasible because they are appropriate to the local secondary care facilities, then the resources needed to support them must be calculated. Oxygen, power for ventilators and drugs to maintain sedation in particular become limiting factors in the prolonged transfer of such patients.

WHAT PLATFORM WILL TRANSPORT THE TEAM AND CASUALTY, AND HOW LONG DOES IT TAKE TO GET TO THE NEXT LEVEL OF CARE?

As already noted this determines the amount of equipment that can be transported, how far and how quickly. This in turn constrains what interventions can be undertaken and the amount of consumables needed to perform them.

HOW MUCH TREATMENT CAN BE DONE IN ONE EPISODE BEFORE RESUPPLY?

In particular, this limits the flexibility of the system to respond to multiple casualties or to attend consecutive incidents without returning to base. This is largely a logistical issue in terms of the quantity of consumables carried.

HOW WILL THE RESPONSE BE ACTIVATED?

The method of activation will impact on time to dispatch, and will also impact on workload and effectiveness. If calls come from multiple sources without a reliable screening mechanism ('intelligent tasking') then there is little control over whether the resource is deployed appropriately (16). High-level pre-hospital care interventions are only of benefit if they are given to the small percentage of trauma patients that actually need them.

HOW DO I GUARANTEE THE SAFETY OF THE TEAM?

Given that medical care will be harder to provide in an austere environment, it is essential that all reasonable precautions are taken to look after all members of the team. This personal preparation – from fitness, control of ongoing medical conditions and vaccinations before deployment, through to hydration, rest and safe food during the deployment – is critical. The wider political and social context also impacts on the ability of personnel to move safely around the area.

DO I NEED ADDITIONAL NON-MEDICAL FACILITATORS?

Drivers, guides and translators also provide local and cultural knowledge, security and situational awareness that may be essential to the safe and effective provision of care. In some cases these roles may be fulfilled by a single person; in others when operating as part of a wider network there may be larger numbers of locals involved in a variety of roles.

UNDERSTANDING THE PATIENT JOURNEY

When the transfer time is prolonged and resources are limited, care must be taken to deliver care efficiently. A good example of this is in the use of analgesia. In order to make the patient as comfortable as possible, and yet also conserve resources, careful mapping of the anticipated analgesic needs against the journey to the next echelon of care is critical. For the purposes of planning, the journey can be broken down by how permissive the situation is – a military concept regarding enemy activity, which can be extended to imply whether the environment is amenable to safe intervention or whether it is less than ideal (semi-permissive) or overtly dangerous (non-permissive). Periods of high or low medical activity – assessment or intervention (such as analgesic demands) – can then be laid over this environmental timeline. This allows the practitioner to plan ahead and modify either the sequence of tasks or the method chosen to best complete them in order to best suit the needs of the patient and the situation.

To demonstrate these principles we will return to the Halley Antarctic scenario and an overturned vehicle. Initially the patient is inaccessible (wedged upside down inside a vehicle) but in a warm, sheltered environment. It is semi-permissive at best – intervention is difficult but the patient is in no immediate danger from the environment. Once the patient is removed from the vehicle, the rescuers have 360-degree access making interventions easier, but the temperature is –10°C and an immediate risk to both casualty and rescuer; a non-permissive environment. If a tent could be erected as work to extricate the patient progressed, then they could be moved to a warm, sheltered environment with 360-degree access; in other words, a more permissive environment. However, once the patient has been stabilised, they face a 2-hour journey in the back of a cramped vehicle with poor light; again, semi-permissive at best. When they reach a warm, well-lit base, then the environment becomes permissive again, until transfer to the plane to fly out.

Now overlay the periods of demand. The extrication from a semi-permissive environment may require fast-acting analgesia or sedation. If the patient is relatively easy to access, then intravenous access is ideal. If only the upper torso can be reached, then an intraosseous needle (sternal or humeral) might be the only accessible option. If no part of the patient can be easily reached and pain control is a priority, then intranasal (e.g. fentanyl) or inhaled agents (entonox, methoxyflurane) might be ideal initial options. Intravenously, fentanyl or ketamine might be preferred agents because of their rapid onset and relative cardiovascular stability. All of these options allow almost immediate progression to extrication.

Once the patient has been extricated to the tent, then there is time for a longer acting analgesic to be administered (such as IV morphine) as additional access is secured. While a tent is not an ideal situation to perform many medical procedures, those that need to be done within the next 2 hours should be done now. It will be impossible to do anything more than the most basic care during the next stage of the trip. The philosophy of *treat then transfer* is appropriate when *treat during transfer* is impossible. Primary survey interventions and resuscitation should be followed by reduction and splintage of the limbs if needed and thorough precautions against hypothermia. If the patient needs to micturate, now is the time! Top-up analgesia will be possible later but not easy, so oral analgesics should be given for their long duration of action, and additional IV analgesia drawn-up and labelled ready to give. The same is true for IV fluids. If appropriate forethought has taken place, then the 2-hour trip to base should now be comfortable, warm and require minimal additional intervention.

INDIVIDUAL COMPONENTS OF CARE

In this section we consider some adaptations to standard techniques, equipment or drugs that may be more suitable in some austere environments.

ANAESTHESIA AND AIRWAY MAINTENANCE

Pre-hospital emergency anaesthesia requires a specialist skill set and ideally an array of equipment to cover a range of eventualities. Rendering a breathing patient apnoeic in the pre-hospital arena is dangerous, especially if environmental conditions are difficult (cold, dark, cramped, noisy). It should be performed with a trained assistant, oxygen saturations, waveform $ETCO_2$ monitoring, non-invasive blood pressure and ECG (17). The necessary drugs (especially muscle relaxants) degrade and so an effective cold chain and resupply mechanism is critical to maintaining their efficacy. In very austere environments the risks and logistical constraints of pre-hospital emergency anaesthesia will often outweigh the benefits of a spontaneously breathing patient without a secured airway; simpler options such as a nasopharyngeal airway and left lateral positioning may be preferred, and a clear and consistent policy should be in place.

Where pre-hospital emergency anaesthesia is necessary and appropriate, every effort should be made to ensure success at the first attempt and so adequate pre-oxygenation, use of a bougie, careful positioning and effective teamwork with the assistant are essential.

Failed intubation drills are likely to be simple, for example a supraglottic airway or even direct progression to cricothyroidotomy, as stocking a wide range of additional difficult airway equipment is simply not feasible.

Cricothyroidotomy can be done awake, without paralysis, and by a lone practitioner and has the highest success rate when performed using an open technique (18). These surgical airways may even prove a valuable first line in carefully selected patients in austere environments where there are not the skills, equipment or ability to maintain an anaesthetic. Those with significant facial injuries/burns and airway compromise could potentially be managed spontaneously by ventilating with local anaesthetic, a scalpel and a cuffed tube.

BREATHING

Oxygen delivery is difficult and relies on either cylinder supply (large and heavy), concentrators (electrically driven, bulky and low flow) or manufacture units (costly chemical process, single use such as the O2Pak™). As a result, it is usually in short supply. Thus high-flow oxygen will be used much more sparingly in an austere environment than would be the UK norm. What little there is can be made to go further with specialist low-resistance reservoir bag systems which maximise inspired oxygen for a given flow rate (for example Topox™), but these are considerably more expensive than standard systems.

Mechanical ventilation will rely on either relatively unrestricted gas supply or electricity, and ventilators are usually bulky. There have been attempts to manufacture ventilators that resolve these issues and some companies now provide lightweight, multiple-use non-electrical ventilators. The Sure-vent 2™, for example, is a disposable plastic ventilator allowing multiple uses of the same device with different patients and with no need for electrical power.

If a ventilator is not feasible, then manual ventilation via bag–valve–mask (BVM) may need to continue for long periods. While such use of manpower is intensive, it is sometimes advantageous in the difficult pre-hospital environment; there is immediate tactile feedback – disconnection results in immediate loss of resistance and increasing pressures can also be felt easily. On the back of a dark, vibrating, noisy moving platform, these cues will be far more easily detected than alarms on a mechanical ventilator.

Other breathing interventions remain largely as normal in UK practice. In areas of conflict where rates of penetrating chest injury are high it is prudent to also carry commercial chest seals (Russell™, Bolin™) for open pneumothoraces rather than having to improvise one on scene.

CIRCULATION – ACCESS

Intravenous access remains the gold standard for the delivery of fluids and drugs pre-hospital no matter how challenging the environment. Emergency access can be achieved easily and quickly by less skilled personnel with the use of intraosseous access. However these systems are usually heavier and bulkier than simple cannulae (powered units in particular tend to be larger) and are only licensed for use for up to 24 hours. Whatever technique is used, it must still be performed in as aseptic a manner as possible (or if placed in an emergency, exchanged as early as practical for an aseptically placed means of access) and extremely well secured.

RESUSCITATION FLUIDS AND STRATEGIES

In the context of non-compressible truncal trauma in particular, UK practice has moved towards a model of limited pre-hospital fluid administration. There is considerable evidence that early normotensive resuscitation with crystalloids in these patients is harmful (19,20). However these approaches have been shown to be time-limited options, harmful if maintained for long periods, leading to the concept of novel hybrid resuscitation (21). Permissive hypotension for the first hour after injury is beneficial – only giving boluses of fluids to maintain a degree of hypotension (for example to a radial pulse). This strategy is not acceptable in all patient groups – being inappropriate in head injuries and paediatric trauma in particular.

Furthermore it has been proven harmful if a more normal blood pressure is not re-established within 2 hours (21). So after this first hour fluids will have to be given to maintain end organ perfusion (indicated for example by adequate urine output) accepting that bleeding is still not definitively controlled and that some additional coagulaopathy may result.

One intervention that has been shown to be of clear value in this setting is tranexamic acid, which is cheap and easy to carry and should be administered to all patients considered at risk of significant bleeding or shock (22). Freeze-dried blood products such as lyophilised plasma (e.g. Lyoplas™) are increasingly available, and may have a role in some specific circumstances.

Combining strategies like hybrid resuscitation with newer fluid options could provide a novel solution to an endemically challenging problem, particularly in LEDCs, where resuscitation timelines are longer and access to gold standard products is constrained by cost.

DISABILITY

Cervical spine immobilisation has become a staple of pre-hospital care in the Western world over the last 30 years. More recently, concerns have been mounting around the number of patients who are immobilised unnecessarily for the benefit of the very few who have significant spinal injuries (23). Some patients may also come to harm as a result of spinal immobilisation. There can be no doubt that immobilisation can be very uncomfortable if prolonged and once the decision has been taken to apply it, practitioners may be reluctant to remove it. Conscious co-operative patients without major distracting injuries can be encouraged to self-extricate and settle themselves down for further evaluation. Then rules such as the NEXUS or Canadian C-Spine Rules can be applied before taking the decision to apply formal immobilisation. Even if these non-specific decision rules are positive, in the truly austere or isolated environment, the increased difficulty in managing and transporting the patient may outweigh the very small risk of an unsecured spine and large studies in the past have shown no evidence of harm from such a strategy (24).

ENVIRONMENTAL

In an attempt to reduce the impact of fixed constraints from the environment, those that can be modified need to be aggressively managed. One of these is temperature. There are many single-use warming systems available for field use, which have been proven to be effective in military settings (such as HPMK™ and Blizzard™). Techniques such as splintage and transfer by stretcher are low-tech and largely independent of the level of resource in the area. Particularly with prolonged evacuation times, great care must be taken to ensure that the patient is comfortable, well padded at all contact or pressure points, and kept warm during transfer. This has a huge impact on analgesic requirements but also minimises further bleeding and injury.

ANALGESIA

Well-described concepts such as the *analgesic ladder* are just as effective in austere environments, but consideration should also be given to onset time, duration and route. Combining these concepts (as previously illustrated) will maximise patient comfort, particularly during challenging phases such as extrication and transport. All routes of administration may have a role, but intranasal, inhalational, intraosseous and rectal are probably neglected, with the focus on oral and intravenous administration seen in UK practice.

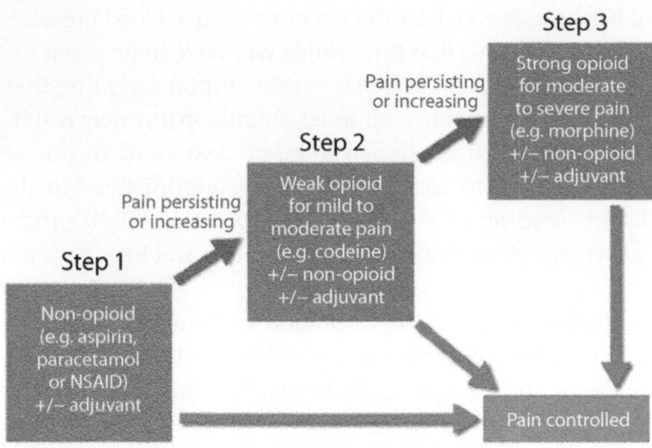

Figure 22.1 The analgesic ladder.

Agents should be selected to maximise the options in terms of analgesic strategies, so that fast-acting, high-efficacy agents as well as longer-acting agents need to be carried, covering the spectra of duration and potency. Local anaesthesia may also have a role in prolonged evacuation from, for example, remote expeditions, and the impact that adequate pain relief has on mobility should never be underestimated. A well-placed haematoma block after a fall while mountaineering has allowed climbers with splinted fractures to the upper limb to climb/ski themselves off the hill – averting an otherwise challenging rescue attempt (Figure 22.1).

PROLONGED FIELD CARE

As evacuation times become longer, more and more patient needs will become evident beyond normal trauma and critical care management. There are many ways to think of these, but a basic strategy is called HITMAN (25) (Box 22.2).

BOX 22.2: HITMAN

H **Hydration** – IV or oral fluids.
Hygiene – Plan for the patients' need to micturate and defaecate. Consider how best to keep the patient clean.

I **Infection** – Antibiotics, wound cleaning and dressing (including changes). Check cannulation sites regularly for signs of erythema.
Monitor contact areas, and exclude compartment syndrome.

T **Tubes** – Ensure they are secured and protected, but also whether they are necessary given the fact that they are a high septic focus risk. Consider urethral catheterisation.
Temperature control – Both monitoring for fever and avoiding hypothermia.

M **Medication** – Beyond simply analgesics and antibiotics. Does the patient need antiemetics or their own regular medicines (for example antimalarials)?

A **Analgesia**

N **Nutrition** – Ensure adequate nutrition if they are able to eat.
Notes – Document thoroughly.

THE DISASTER ENVIRONMENT

There is increasing interest in the standards of medical care provided following a disaster, such as the Haiti earthquake or Typhoon Haiyan. Any community affected by a disaster should receive a minimum standard of health provision even in the event of extensive infrastructural, human and logistical damage. Pre-hospital teams from the wider international community may comprise part of any effort to assist with meeting these basic healthcare needs.

Although very much environmental and location dependent, the healthcare systems of many affected countries are significantly degraded immediately following a sudden onset disaster. There is not only structural damage to health facilities, but also disruption to water, power, logistics and access – all of which will influence the functioning integrity of an individual health facility and the national health system. This will often also be compounded by a reduction in available healthcare workers, either directly through injury and deaths, or loss of relatives, housing and other personal affects which limit their ability to continue in their work. If the disaster hits an already resource-constrained environment, such as Haiti, then the impact on community health provision is even more significant. Injury patterns and health needs will vary after different disasters and over time following the disaster. Common immediate health needs after an earthquake or typhoon include traumatic injuries (in particular wounds and limb injuries), which require triage, resuscitation, surgery and postoperative care. Days and weeks after the disaster, health needs change; communicable diseases and vector-borne diseases increase, and malnutrition and exacerbation of chronic disease become more prevalent.

Medical care during a disaster is likely to be delivered by both local and international providers. Collaboration between the two is fundamental. In these circumstances, the most effective method of healthcare delivery by far is local clinicians within local health systems, strengthened as needed by external resources. Where international medical teams are needed (and invited), they must work with the local health authorities and integrate within the health cluster to target those needs identified by the disaster-affected country.

These teams must be self-sufficient in order not to draw on the already stretched resources of the affected country. Ideally this means that they should come complete with logistical support including vehicle(s) and fuel; they should bring their own habitat, medical equipment and resupply. They should be able to manage their own water and sanitation needs. Alongside their equipment, they clearly must have the skills both to deliver the relevant medical capability and to look after themselves. Ideally this should involve specific training in humanitarian principles, team-focused training and foreign medical team standards. Finally, they must have adequate experience and information to facilitate effective decision-making in the context of the local community and culture, and the resources available. An ideal starting point for the development of such experience is the *UK International Emergency Trauma Register (UKIETR)*, which seeks to identify interested professionals and direct them to appropriate training (26).

SUMMARY

Austere environments provide unique challenges for pre-hospital trauma care. By their very nature these settings limit some or all of the resources available to the practitioners and so require imagination and flexibility to make the most of what is available. Planning and forethought become essential tools. To achieve the greatest effect, the individual or team requires a deep understanding of the environment, the people, the geography and the society in which they will operate, as well as the non-clinical skills to ensure they can function in that environment safely, comfortably and effectively.

REFERENCES

1. Marquis P, British Antarctic Survey Medical Unit Manager, Personal communication, December 2013.
2. World Health Organisation. Media centre factsheets. July 2013. http://www.who.int/mediacentre/factsheets/fs310/en/.
3. World Health Organization. Guidelines for essential trauma care. 2004. http://www.who.int/violence_injury_prevention/publications/services/guidelines_traumacare/en/.
4. The World Bank. World Development Indicators databank, Physicians per 1000 population. http://databank.worldbank.org/data/views/reports/tableview.aspx.
5. Kingham TP, Kamara T, Cherian M, Gosselin RA, Simkins M, Meissner C, Foray-Rahall L, Daoh KS, Kabia SA, Kushner AL. Quantifying surgical capacity in Sierra Leone. *Archives of Surgery* 2009;144(2):122–127.
6. Eisenburg MF, Christie M, Mathew P. Battlefield neurosurgical care in the current conflict in southern Afghanistan. *Neurosurgical Focus* 2010;28(5):E7.
7. Sun JH, Shing R, Twomey M, Wallis LA. A strategy to implement and support pre-hospital emergency medical systems in developing, resource-constrained areas of South Africa. *Injury* 2014;45:31–38.
8. Bickler SW, Spiegel DA. Global surgery – Defining a research agenda. *Lancet* 2008;372: 90–92.
9. Nallamothu BK, Bates ER, Wang Y. Driving times and distances to hospitals with percutaneous coronary intervention in the United States. *Circulation* 2006;113:1189–1195.
10. Macharia WM, Njeru EK, Muli-Musiime F, Nantulya V. Severe road traffic injuries in Kenya, quality of care and access. *African Health Science* 2009;9(2):118–124.
11. Matityahu A, Elliott I, Marmor, M. Time intervals in the treatment of fractured femurs as indicators of the quality of trauma systems. *Bulletin of the World Health Organization* 2014;92(1):40–50.
12. Amnesty International. Climate of fear in Syria's hospitals as patients and medics targeted. October 25, 2011. http://www.amnesty.org/en/news-and-updates/report/climate-fear-syrias-hospitals-patients-and-medics-targeted-2011-10-25.
13. BBC News. Pakistan polio team hit by deadly attack. March 1, 2014. http://www.bbc.co.uk/news/world-asia-26397602.
14. International Committee of the Red Cross. The healthcare in danger project. http://www.icrc.org/eng/what-we-do/safeguarding-health-care/solution/2013-04-26-hcid-health-care-in-danger-project.htm.
15. United Nations News Centre. February 24, 2009. http://www.un.org/apps/news/story.asp/story.asp?NewsID=30005&Cr=sri+lanka&Cr1=#.UyQ_stzA7Hg.
16. Thurgood A, Boylan M. Activation and deployment. In *ABC of Prehospital Care*, T Nutbeam, M Boylan (eds.). Oxford: Wiley-Blackwell, 2013.
17. Association of Anaesthetists of Great Britain and Ireland (AABGI) Standard for pre-hospital RSI. http://www.aagbi.org/sites/default/files/prehospital_glossy09.pdf.

18. Hubble M, Wilfong D, Brown L, Hertelendy A, Benner RW. A meta-analysis of pre-hospital airway control techniques part 2: Alternative airway devices and surgical cricothyroidotomy success rates. *Prehospital Emergency Care* 2010;14:515–530.
19. Bickell WH, Wall MJ, Pepe PE, Martin RR, Ginger VF, Allen MK, Mattox KL. Immediate versus delayed fluid resuscitation for hypotensive patients with penetrating torso injuries. *New England Journal of Medicine* 1994;331:1105–1109.
20. Kasotakis G, Sideris A, Yang Y, de Moya M, Alam H, King DR, Tompkins R, Velmahos G. Aggressive early crystalloid resuscitation adversely affects outcomes in adult blunt trauma patients: An analysis of the Glue Grant database. *Journal of Trauma and Acute Care Surgery* 2013;74(5):1215–1221.
21. Midwinter M, Woolley T. Resuscitation and coagulation in the severely injured trauma patient. *Philosophical Transactions of the Royal Society B: Biological Sciences* 2011;366(1562):192–203.
22. CRASH2 Collaborators. The importance of early treatment with tranexamic acid in bleeding trauma patients: An exploratory analysis of the CRASH-2 randomised controlled trial. *Lancet* 2011;377(9771):1096–1101.
23. Connor D, Greaves I, Porter K, Bloch M. Pre-hospital spinal immobilization: An initial consensus statement. *Emergency Medical Journal* 2013;30(12):1067–1069.
24. Hauswald M, Ong G, Tandberg D, Omar Z. Out-of-hospital spinal immobilization: Its effect on neurological outcome. *Academic Emergency Medicine* 1998;5(3):214–219.
25. Corey G, Lafayette T. Preparing for operations in a resource-depleted and/or extended evacuation environment. *Journal of Special Operations Medicine* 2013;13(3):74–80.
26. UK International Emergency Trauma Register. http://www.uk-med.org/trauma.html.

23 Mass casualty situations

OBJECTIVES

After completing this chapter the reader will

- Understand the underlying principles of major incident management
- Understand the principles of prioritisation (triage) of trauma victims
- Be aware of the generic structure of a major incident response

INTRODUCTION

The UK National Health Service Emergency Preparedness Framework (2013) defines a significant incident or emergency as 'one that cannot be managed within routine service arrangements'. The response will require special procedures, involve more than one emergency service, the wider National Health Service (NHS) and even the local authority (1). This is a very broad definition designed to capture the traditional *major incident* but also to accommodate extreme health system pressures such as an infectious disease outbreak, perhaps a flu epidemic in winter, or a logistics challenge such as a fuel tanker driver strike.

A mass casualty situation is defined by the World Health Organization as simply one where an event generates 'more patients at one time than locally available resources can manage using routine procedures' (2).

In considering such broad terms, for the pre-hospital responder in a rural area with limited facilities, a simple road traffic collision with a handful of casualties may meet this definition, whereas in an urban area with more resources the event would be readily manageable within available resources and without special arrangements. The ability to manage a situation can be considered under the term *surge capacity* where the ability to manage depends upon 'staff, stuff and structure' (3), that is having sufficient staff with the equipment they need following a plan defined by a command system. In essence, they need a *major incident response*.

In terms of numbers, specific terms are applied (Table 23.1) (4). Likewise, in terms of type, there is recognised terminology (Table 23.2) (1).

Table 23.1 Terminology

NHS level	Numbers
Major	10s
Mass	100s
Catastrophic	1000s

Table 23.2 Incident descriptors

Nature of incident	Definition
Big bang	Transport incident, explosion, series of smaller events
Rising tide	Developing infectious disease epidemic, evolving staffing crisis/industrial action
Cloud on the horizon	A threat such as chemical or radiation release elsewhere where there is time to prepare
Headline news	Public or media alarm about a pending issue
Internal incident	Loss of utilities, fire, or breakdown of core equipment such as IT failure
CBRN	Deliberate release of chemical, biological or radiological material
HAZMAT	Incident involving hazardous material

The scope to be covered in the chapter relates to the pre-hospital phase of managing a mass casualty incident. Planning for such events is constantly evolving using the emergency planning cycle (Figure 23.1) (5).

The intentions are that guidance and future responses are sensitive to the perceived risks or threats, and also to learn from exercises and critical analysis of actual events. The science behind emergency preparedness and response is dynamic; the literature is replete with case studies and narratives of major incidents, but the formal academic study and developing science of emergency preparedness, resilience and response is evolving rapidly. It is not possible to carry out formal studies; development and evolution arise from post-hoc incident investigation and from expert consensus (6).

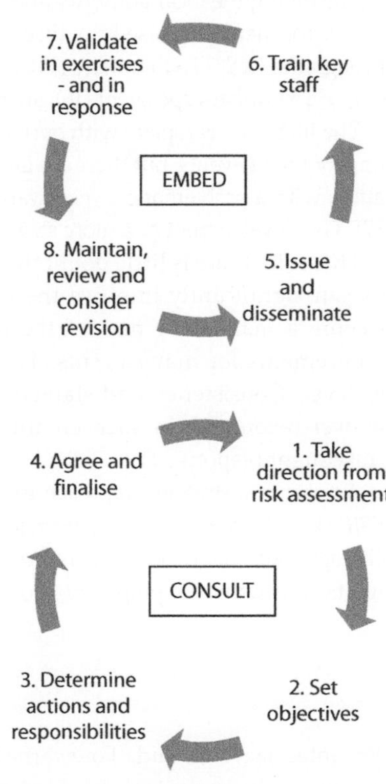

Figure 23.1 The emergency planning cycle. (From Civil Contingencies Act Enhancement Programme, Chapter 5 (Emergency planning): Revision to emergency preparedness, 2011, https://www.gov.uk/government/uploads/system/uploads/attachment_data/file/61028/Emergency_Preparedness_chapter5_amends_21112011.pdf.)

RESILIENCE AND PREPARATION

Disaster management consists of four distinct components:

- Mitigation
- Preparedness
- Response
- Recovery

The first two of these involve recognising the hazards that exist and taking steps to reduce their potential impact.

Hazards can be anticipated. Natural challenges such as a town that is built in a flood zone or technological ones such as a large airport or an industrial chemical plant raise specific threats that can be proactively addressed and the risk reduced through preparation.

Often underestimated, mass gathering medicine has evolved to consider the challenge simply of large numbers of people gathered together (7). Predictive tools have been developed that consider the nature of the challenge and describe the level and type of resources that should be put in place to manage this. Perhaps the world's greatest recurring challenge is the annual Hajj to Mecca (8), but even such relatively regular events as UK Premier League football matches carry a risk that should be mitigated and prepared for (9). In the UK there is official guidance in this regard for sports stadia and other crowd events, the *Green Guide* and *Purple Guide* (10,11). Through careful preparation and risk assessment, the potential consequences can be reduced; there are examples of where this has been well managed (12) and equally of where disaster has followed (13).

In terms of specific natural or technological hazards, local communities will typically have a risk register and plan for those hazards that figure most highly. Flooding has been a recurrent challenge in parts of the UK and the potential impact is far wider than simply the immediate emergency service local response (14). An optimal system response is complex and wide ranging, involving the local authority and government agencies over months. The current UK political environment has raised the threat of terrorism to a significant level and general preparation through the *CONTEST* strategy (15), and specific threats such as a *marauding terrorist firearms incident*, or a Mumbai-type event (16), are now regular features of the mass casualty exercise schedule.

The literature is replete with narrative descriptions of exercise reports and public health planning for major events, but there are far fewer that honestly critique the effectiveness of that preparation, with a problematic level of variance in the reporting and identification of learning points (17). The development of a more structured academic approach is necessary but slow to evolve.

This said, there is little doubt that education and training of emergency service responders can significantly improve the incident response and involvement in such events has become a mandatory part of the responding personnel training cycle and of licencing requirements for many events. This apparent effectiveness is not without its challenges however. Consistency and standardisation are a challenge (18) and sometimes there can be over-resourcing in such environments that undermines the value of training for the subsequent response (19).

As part of a strategic approach to this challenge, the UK Emergency Services introduced the *JESIP* (*Joint Emergency Services Interoperability Programme*) (20) that is now established training for all responders, applying the core principles of cooperation and communication has evolved and significantly improved preparation for a response and so increased system resilience.

THE ALL HAZARDS APPROACH

Cervantes Saavedra said, 'Forewarned is forearmed, to be prepared is half the victory'. When a disaster occurs current expert opinion is that the strategic emergency response should be based upon a common and practised multi-agency standard framework which can be adapted for the specific needs of the event, an *All Hazards* approach (21).

This leads to the JESIP doctrine which is the principles-based philosophy capturing this approach that defines the tactical and operational command (20). The themes are co-location, communication, co-ordination and shared situational analysis, the intention being that there is a connected situational awareness that allows for intelligent flexibility in the response.

There will always be unexpected challenges and adaptation is key to mounting an effective and efficient response. The challenges of adverse weather, darkness and remoteness all compound an effective response to a mass casualty incident.

A model health response to a mass casualty incident will involve the entire health economy, from the emergency first responders to the community services for the area. Civil contingencies documents from the 1990s approach major incidents in a very limited response-oriented way (22), but the breadth of the necessary response and the need to integrate all responders into a coordinated whole for the duration of the response, including the recovery period, has become more evident and the command system now captures all parties from the blue-light emergency services to category 2 responders defined by the Civil Contingencies Act 2004 (23) to include utility and water companies and even the Environment Agency.

Being aware of the complexity of the wider mass casualty response, the core principles of mounting a response, particularly as it relates to the pre-hospital environment, can best perhaps be considered using the principles taught in the entry qualification programme, Major Incident Medical Management and Support, or MIMMS® (24). This is essential knowledge for anyone who responds to trauma in the pre-hospital environment.

MIMMS PRINCIPLES: METHANE AND CSCATTT

Over the last two decades, basic training in the management of a significant incident was taught through the MIMMS philosophy (24). To facilitate recall of the different components of this structured approach the mnemonic CSCATTT is used (Box 23.1).

BOX 23.1: MIMMS CSCATTT mnemonic

Command and control
Safety
Communication
Assessment
Triage
Treatment
Transport

The first step in any mass casualty or major incident is to recognise it as such. The first lesson taught in the programme is DECLARE IT! There are a variety of anecdotal tales of delays and missed opportunities to manage an incident arising from failure to recognise the magnitude of the challenge and mobilise the necessary resources. During basic training, significant emphasis is placed on the need for those first responding to an incident to have a relatively low threshold for activating the response, with the reassurance that it can always be stood down later. The emergency services would rather begin to escalate their response and then stand it down as more information becomes available than have an unnecessary period of delay 'to be absolutely sure'. It is now accepted that this should be done using the METHANE mnemonic (Box 23.2) (6).

BOX 23.2: MIMMS METHANE mnemonic

M	Major incident *declared* or *stand by*
E	Exact location
T	Type of incident
H	Hazards present and potential
A	Access, the direction of approach
N	Numbers of casualties, with nature and type
E	Emergency services present and required

For the responding pre-hospital personnel from the health system, the structure of the response is perhaps best considered using the CSCATTT.

It is generally recognised that the early phase of the response is often based upon incomplete information and it is necessary that each aspect is considered and planned for during this period. Failing to consider each will cause difficulty as the response builds. The initial responders are unlikely to form the command element for the full incident, but their early decisions will build the foundation upon which the subsequent response is built. There is clearly a huge pressure to begin moving patients to hospital, but it is unlikely that patients will be moved from scene during the first 30 minutes; addressing the CSCATTT components is fundamental to a robust response.

COMMAND AND CONTROL

In describing the oversight function at a mass casualty event, it is usual to consider it in the context of a *big bang*-type event. The structure and principles can then be adapted to more protracted events as required.

Ideally, the first ambulance crew on scene should recognise the incident as a major one and activate the cascade. They should take a command function and begin to structure the response until relieved by more senior personnel with specific training to take on the role of *ambulance incident commander* (*AIC*) and other core command roles.

By the very nature of such an incident, there is typically confusion during the first phase and the responding emergency services need to function almost on *autopilot*. This is helped by the inclusion of action cards, giving step-by-step instructions, in emergency plans. A detailed understanding is not required; the responder adopts an identified role and follows the list of instructions in sequence. It is only later that adaptation and modification might be required and the trained commanders are typically in the leadership functions at this point.

Command is a vertical transmission of authority and instruction. Whilst this is a clear concept to the police and fire services, it is not natural in the health service where clinicians are accountable for their actions on a patient-by-patient basis. In the environment of a major incident, a command hierarchy is essential.

The current and established command system in the UK operates a 'medallion' approach with *gold* (*strategic*) command remote from the scene but coordinating the wider health service response and ensuring business continuity, *silver* (*tactical*) at scene leading the direct response and, as required, *bronze* (*operational*) commanders moving forward and taking charge of specific functions such as patient triage or scene rescue (Figure 23.2) (4).

STRATEGIC COMMAND

Strategic command involves senior officers, typically chief officers or executives, who have responsibility for providing the resources to support the incident response and is usually remote from the scene of the incident. Whilst ensuring that there is sufficient support deployed, they are also responsible for maintaining the function of the wider health system during the time of strain and thinking about continuity going forward. This may require calling on mutual aid from adjacent areas and appraising senior government infrastructure of events. The response

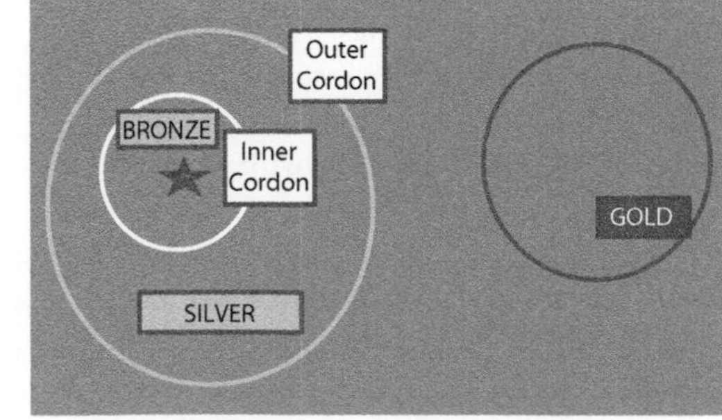

Figure 23.2 Command circles at an explosion.

may require the involvement and coordination of a much wider range of organisations beyond the emergency services, potentially including the local authority, environment agency and even utility companies.

The gold commanders from the lead responding agencies can be brought together as a *strategic coordinating group* (SCG), typically chaired by the police, to mount a joint response. In events of sufficient magnitude there may be a number of SCGs that are brought together through a regional committee before communicating vertically to the Major Incident Coordination Centre (MICC) at the Department of Health and, through them, to the Cabinet Office Briefing Room (COBR) and the Civil Contingencies Committee (CCC) (4).

TACTICAL COMMAND

Tactical command is the level that leads the response at the scene of the incident, taking charge as the *ambulance incident commander* (AIC), overseeing and responsible for delivering a proportionate response. They will usually be supported by a *medical incident advisor* (MIA) and a number of additional specialist staff. The tactical commanders from each of the attending emergency services should cooperate as a *command team* with shared understanding of the situation and agreed assessment of the risks and challenges (Figure 23.3) (20).

During the early stages of the response there is a need to agree the flow in and out of the incident area for responding vehicles, the evacuation plan and the treatment and management thresholds for casualties. Whilst the specific details will be defined by local geography, such as the availability of buildings and the nature of the road network, the structure is fairly clear (Figure 23.4).

The nature of the incident and the range and type of casualties will determine the evacuation plan. The ambulance incident commander should determine the destination hospitals and the rate of patient flow to each based upon the nature of the injuries. Strategic command should be aware of this and facilitate capacity in those receiving facilities by providing support as necessary.

OPERATIONAL COMMAND

The AIC and MIA roles are ideally hands-off positions. There are a number of different functions at the incident scene and oversight of these is typically delegated. Examples might include sectoring of a large incident scene, management of the casualty clearing station, vehicle parking and loading, and perhaps oversight of patient decontamination. Each of these operational functions is overseen by a command element that feeds back to the AIC.

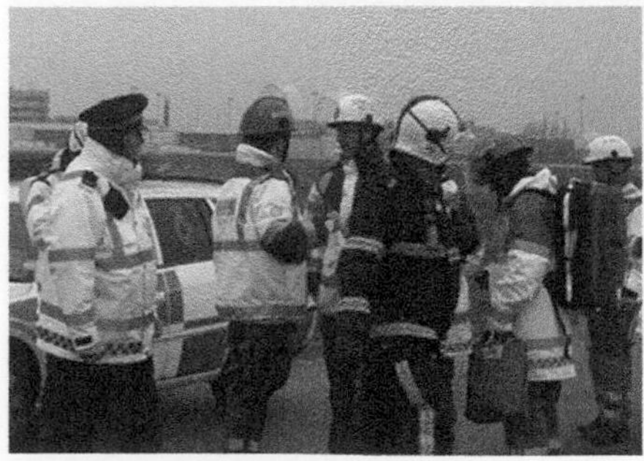

Figure 23.3 Scene command team.

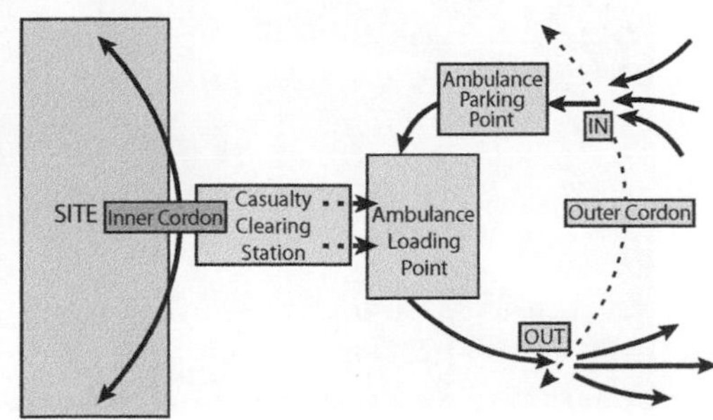

Figure 23.4 Patient flow at a mass casualty incident.

With a specific remit for patient care, at the casualty clearing station there should be an operational commander overseeing the ongoing triage and also delivery of clinical care to the injured whilst awaiting evacuation. This is likely to be the base for the majority of the medical assets working at scene, and often an operational medical incident advisor is required to support this and ensure that only appropriate clinical interventions are provided.

SAFETY

The scene of a major incident will be an environment with inherent hazards that pose a risk to rescuers. Responsibility for mitigating and managing these risks rests with the strategic command team and should be managed through *DORA* (*Dynamic Operation Risk Assessment*). The challenges are constantly changing and must be continually reassessed. Basic pre-hospital emergency medicine principles apply; the Safety 1-2-3. Personal safety of the rescuers must be considered, then that of the scene before finally addressing the safety of the survivors, both casualties and the involved but not injured.

PERSONAL SAFETY

Employers have an absolute duty under health and safety legislation to minimise the risk to their staff in the pursuance of their duties. The effect of this can be seen through the evolution of PPE, the personal protective equipment worn by staff entering an environment over the last few years (Figure 23.5).

A reflective jacket was all that was considered necessary 30 years ago; now a responder would not be allowed to enter an emergency scene without full personal protection. Whilst the necessary level of protection is subject to the dynamic risk assessment, judgement about the level of personal protection can be applied; the responder should have the full level of protection

(a)

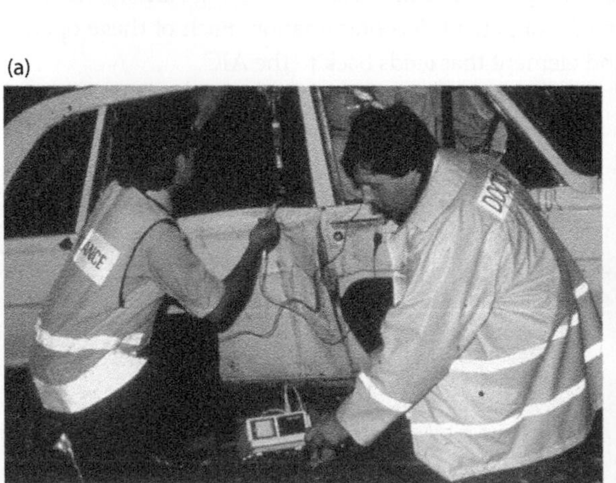

(b)

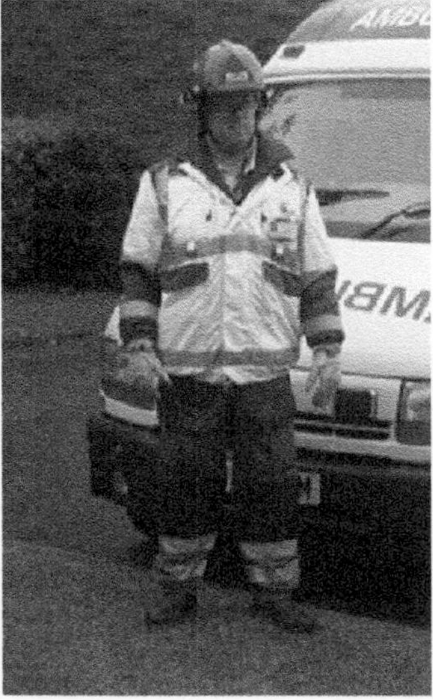

Figure 23.5 Evolving PPE (a) old and (b) new.

necessary. Where a hazard, such as a toxic environment, potentially exists, the basic training is to withdraw to a safe position and call for a higher level of protection. The 'Stay Out, Get Out, Call HART' principle, where HART is the hazardous area response team, is the norm (25).

SCENE SAFETY

As part of the command assessment of the scene and the planning for management by the scene command team, a security (Silver) cordon and a safety (Bronze) cordon are defined, and entry to each should be controlled. If there is a fire, chemical or radiation hazard, the inner cordon will be secured by the fire service; in a terrorist or firearms incident the police may control this cordon.

Once it has been deemed safe to enter an incident scene, the rescuers can begin to attend to those involved. This assumes that the scene can be contained. In a terrorist explosion, for example, those involved and still able to walk will self-evacuate and 'starburst' in all directions. It is unlikely that a cordon to contain a large number of people could be drawn in sufficient time to control the dispersal.

CASUALTY SAFETY

Those involved in a major incident may be affected by a number of unknowns. There have been many examples of chemical contamination affecting both casualties and rescuers. Bio-hazards, either from body fluids from those injured or deceased and spread by an explosive force, including for example the contents of toilets on trains or aircraft, are a theoretical risk to all. To date there has not been a significant issue with radiation contamination, but it is regarded as only a matter of time before this occurs and decontamination of all involved may become necessary. In a terrorist event there is always a potential danger from a terrorist masquerading as an injured person.

There are other risks to rescuers such as MMMF (man-made material fibre) and toxic fumes from burning components that may be relatively concealed and must be guarded against (26). They should be recognised in the DORA from the scene command team, but may come through direct contact with patient clothing after evacuation or through 'off-gassing'.

COMMUNICATION

Communication both at the scene between the different levels of command and the emergency services and also from the scene to the remote command chain is vital to the smooth running of even the most straightforward response to a mass casualty incident. This also includes communication from the scene to the identified receiving hospitals.

There have been many examples of communication systems failing at the scene of a major incident. Radio systems have often been overwhelmed by the volume of traffic or lack of area coverage. The encrypted digital TETRA (Terrestrial Trunked Radio) radio network, known as Airwave, is now the standard for the emergency services in the UK. Whilst not invulnerable, it has multiple layers of redundancy and so allows relatively smooth interservice communication.

Following the London experience with the terrorist events of 2005, well-known communication black spots, such as tunnels and the London Underground, have now been TETRA enabled. There are still some remote areas that remain inaccessible, but coverage is now almost universal.

The emergency services have become increasingly dependent upon the use of mobile phone cellular technology. Dependency on mobile telephones has become an area of vulnerability; there are a limited number of users permitted in each 'cell' and capacity can readily be exceeded. The danger of this dependency has been shown serially through communication difficulties at mass events. The amount of traffic to be carried overwhelms the network and the mobile phones become ineffective.

A system was developed, termed *ACCOLC* (*Access Overload Control*), where specified mobile phone cell areas could be closed to all but those pre-registered and so priority mobile phone traffic. This option was managed centrally and was never shown to work effectively in practice. The system was changed to *MTPAS* (*Mobile Telecommunications Privileged Access System*) where there is more local control of the priority SIM cards for the 'entitled organisations', Category 1 responders to a major incident (27).

In any event, technological solutions can always fail and the old style 'runner' system may need to be instituted. To avoid the 'Chinese whispers' phenomenon, messages should ideally be written.

THE MEDIA

The 24-hour news organisations have become extremely effective at communicating details of an evolving emergency situation. It is quite possible that news reporting, particularly live video from the scene, may give vital information to the more remote commanders and to the wider health response before the normal communication channels can generate a properly informed report. The capacity to view this information flow is a key part of an emergency control centre infrastructure.

There should be strict adherence to policy regarding media communication by all involved in responding to an incident. Only official communications, typically though the command hierarchy and managed by the police, should be made. Any statements or information given out must to be checked for accuracy, avoid speculation and be approved in advance.

Clear guidance is given that the media should be proactively managed by the command elements; transmission of public safety information and reassurance can be disseminated if this aspect of the response is properly addressed. Uncontrolled, the media can cause increased public distress and mislead. Syndication of sources and active engagement can help manage the insatiable demand from the news media. Awareness of news deadlines and regular updates from command officers can be very helpful.

PRACTICE POINT

Use the media proactively to inform and advise the public and prevent panic.

SOCIAL MEDIA

Social media is a relatively new phenomenon, often providing Twitter feeds and video from within the emergency scene by those involved in the incident or witnessing it unfold (Figure 23.6). Termed *backchannel communication*, this modality cannot be easily managed or controlled but should certainly be watched by the responding emergency services; there may be useful information contained within it (28). It is increasingly common for the gold

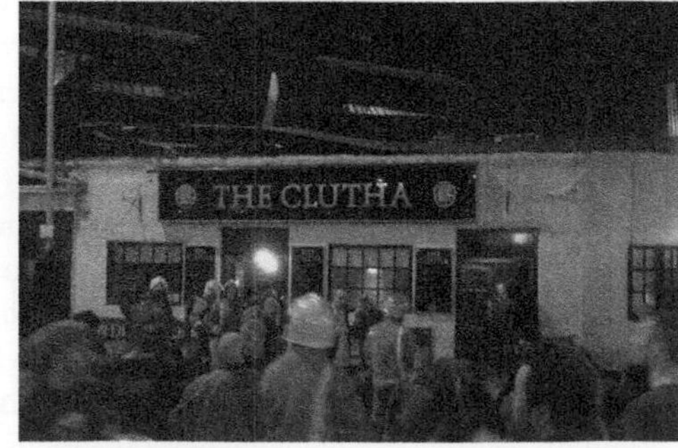

Figure 23.6 Real-time images and video via social media within minutes of an incident.

command to ensure that the ambulance service communications team is monitoring the feed and putting out statements of its own into the domain to inform the public and deflect any potential misleading information.

ASSESSMENT

The first step in managing a major incident is to recognise it and declare it. The initial report should use the framework of the METHANE mnemonic.

The most important aspect of using the acronym is that it is comprehensive and both the sender and recipient of the message understand the structure of the report. Sending all of this information in a first report will allow the system to construct an appropriate and proportionate response.

REPORT REFINEMENT AND CASCADE

As the response begins and more information becomes available about the scale and full nature of the incident, and more experienced and trained commanders arrive at the incident scene, a more detailed needs analysis of the situation will be constructed.

The level of resources to be brought to the scene will depend on the nature of the event and the numbers involved. The AIC and MIA will need to decide how the injured are going to be managed and to where they are to be evacuated: intelligent dispersal rather than simply evacuation to the nearest hospital. Appropriate hospitals will be notified and information sought on the numbers of injured that can be received. Preparation and exercising can help with planning in this area but real-time information will be necessary. Local knowledge by the commanders of the capability and specialist skills of the hospitals will be important in determining how far the activation process radiates from the scene. For example, in an incident involving multiple patients with significant major burns, the cascade may need to go as far as the National Burn Bed Bureau, beginning the search for dedicated burn bed capacity around the UK. A similar process may be necessary if there are significant numbers of critically injured children through the Children's Intensive Care networks.

TRIAGE

A mass casualty incident is one where there are typically more people injured than there are resources *immediately* available to provide the necessary care. In this situation there is a need to determine priority for both treatment and evacuation from the scene; it is a resource-constrained environment. The prioritisation of casualties must be objective and reproducible, ideally based on evidence. The process must be dynamic; patients can deteriorate or improve after contact with the responding personnel, and it must be flexible to accommodate the capacity available to manage the load. The process should occur serially; at the incident scene, at entry to the casualty clearing station (CSS; *front triage*), at departure from the CCS (*rear triage*) and again on arrival at hospital.

The terms *sieve* and *sort* have become the terminology used, arising from the MIMMS programme. An initial screen is applied at the point of first contact and then further more detailed reviews are performed at subsequent stages (24). This has become the UK standard.

TRIAGE SIEVE

To be acceptable for this environment, the system must be quick, reliable and reproducible. A number of systems have been described. The current first look, primary triage or sieve is based upon *START* (*Simple Triage and Rapid Treatment*) (29) (Figure 23.7).

This approach is based on each patient being reviewed in under 30 seconds, rapid assessment for the number and severity of the injured to be determined, and providing the incident command team with information to begin to make decisions about the resources required and plan for the evacuation. Priorities for treatment are identified and then the limited resources can be directed to those in most urgent clinical need.

There is a range of documentation systems for labelling the casualties and a danger of the process losing sight of its purpose in discussion about the best way to do this. Examples of these include the use of coloured clothes pegs or slap bands, the *SMART tag* and the *Cambridge Cruciform System* (Figure 23.8). Each has an increasing level of complexity, but the principle is the same: clear and quick to apply but adjustable if there is a need to upscale or downgrade the category.

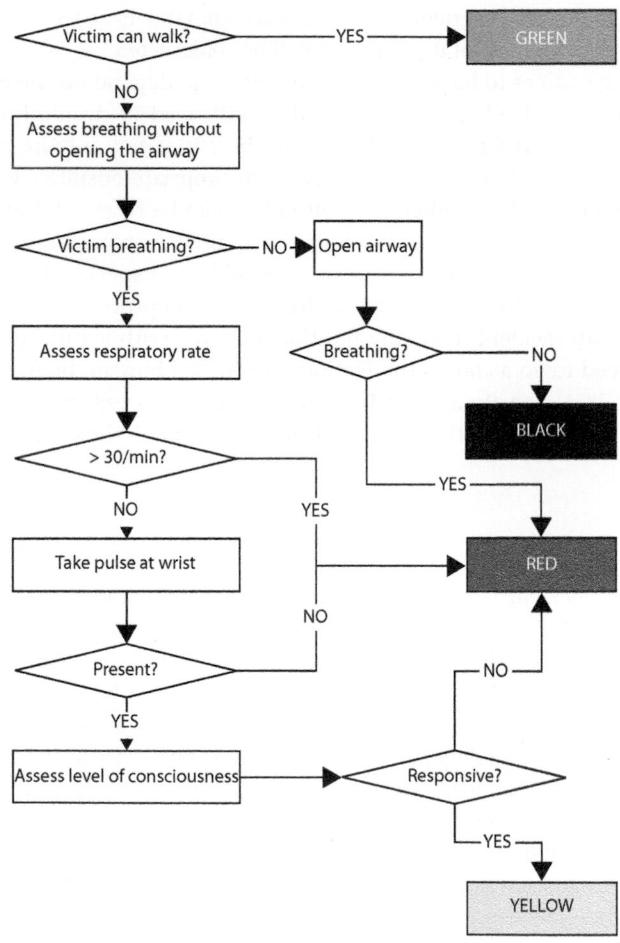

Figure 23.7 The triage sieve based on START.

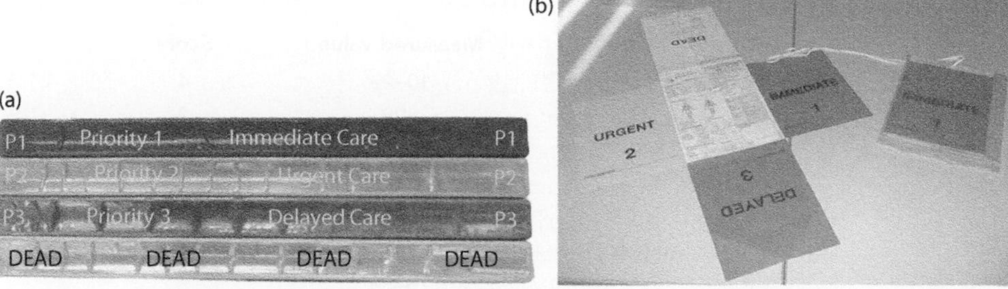

Figure 23.8 Triage (a) slap bands and (b) Cambridge Cruciform triage label.

CHILDREN AND TRIAGE

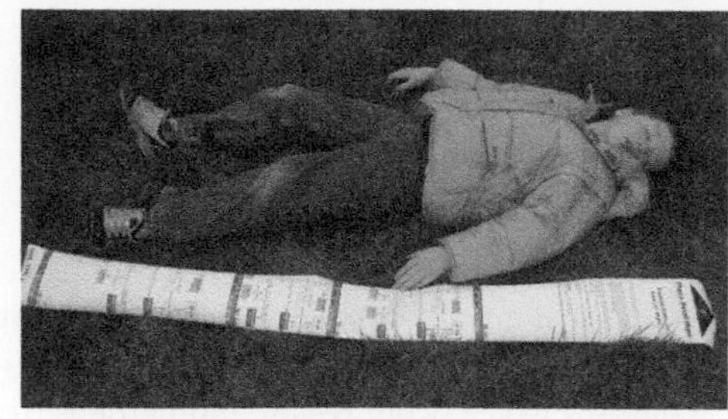

Figure 23.9 Paediatric sizing tape.

Children have different physiology to adults and there is therefore a need to accommodate the child's weight or size in determining the normal range of their physiology. This is difficult to do both in a hurry and from recall. The generally accepted approach is to use the standard START algorithm but with a sizing 'tape', such as the Broselaw tape, with different physiological parameters for respiratory rate and pulse rate for different sizes of children marked on it (30) (Figure 23.9).

T1 HOLD

An additional category of *immediate but no intervention* has been described (31). In principle, this is used for circumstances when there are too many critically injured casualties for the system to manage and the *immediate* category needs to be subdivided. Essentially, this category is *too sick to receive treatment at the current time* and these casualties are put to one side of the evacuation chain. This is contrary to the current principles of clinical practice and, whilst the concept is a useful one when under huge pressure, any decision to introduce this category would need to come from the most senior command level at the incident. The decision to implement this protocol is not one for the operational personnel within the scene.

TRIAGE SORT

Once the casualties have been sieved and the number and severity of the injured has been determined, there needs to be recognition that the first process is 'rough and ready'. The 'sort' is a more detailed and clinically informed process but requires a higher level of clinical skill and may not be appropriate in the early stages of the response to an incident.

Determining the severity of injury is often a retrospective process once the details of the injuries are known. The Injury Severity Score (ISS) is an anatomical injury-based system but can only be applied retrospectively. It is more appropriate to use the patient's physiological

Table 23.3 Triage Revised Trauma Score

Physiological variable	Measured value	Score
Respiratory rate	10–29	4
	>29	3
	6–9	2
	1–5	1
	0	0
Systolic blood pressure	>90	4
	76–89	3
	50–75	2
	1–49	1
	0	0
Glasgow Coma Scale	13–15	4
	9–12	3
	6–8	2
	4–5	1
	3	0

status using simple readily measured parameters: the pulse rate, systolic blood pressure, Glasgow Coma Score (GCS) and perhaps oxygen saturation through pulse oximetry. Each variable has a different predictive value and there are a variety of systems that weight these factors to produce a categorical triage score. In the UK the most common system is the Triage Revised Trauma Score (TRTS) (32) which is the basis for the triage sort (Table 23.3).

Table 23.4 Triage categories and scores

Priority	TRTS
T1	1–10
T2	11
T3	12
Dead	0

This system can then be used to assign a more refined triage category to each casualty (Table 23.4).

Triage to this detail is a time-consuming process when clinicians are busy providing care, but it more accurately determines which patients are in need of intervention more urgently. The use of such an objective tool helps make the decision on which patient should be treated next in a very difficult situation.

TRIAGE ACCURACY

Triage is intended to be an objective and reproducible process, but the reality is that in an emotional environment responders find it difficult to apply rigorously. Likewise, any simple system is relatively crude and has an error rate. Over the 25 years that the described triage principles have been established, there have been few occasions where the system has been consistently and reliably applied. In the 1990s, responders rarely used the system at all, but more recently it has been shown to be capable of being used effectively and influencing evacuation decisions (33).

Analysis has shown that there is consistent *over-triage*: responders put the injured in a more urgent category than warranted, particularly when children are triaged. Over-triage will clog the system and delay essential treatment for others in need. At the same time, there are some

Table 23.5 2 × 2 triage table

	Critically injured	Non-critically injured
Higher priority	Correct high triage	Incorrect high triage (over-triage)
Lower priority	Incorrect low priority (under-triage)	Correct low triage

patients for whom the triage process fails to recognise the urgency of their situation and unnecessary delay is incurred, that is 'under-triage' (Table 23.5).

Inaccurate triage potentially means that resources are not distributed in an optimal manner and, further down the evacuation chain, people are evacuated to hospital in an order that may not benefit the most severely injured. Analysis of incidents shows how significant field triage decisions can be in a potentially resource constrained environment. An over-triage rate of 64% occurred in some locations of the London bombings in 2005, and this would potentially cause significant issues for patients if hospital resources were being overwhelmed (33).

Emergency responders understand the principles of triage but often allow other factors to influence their decision process, undermining its efficacy. Less injured casualties will often not be willing to comply with evacuation decisions, preferring to stay with their friends and relatives who might be more severely injured. It cannot be reasonable to expect a parent to leave their severely injured child to comply with the evacuation chain. This requires the system to rigorously apply the triage decisions but allow for some flexibility in terms of the nature and timing of the evacuation of some patients in some categories.

TREATMENT

The capacity to provide care at the scene of a mass casualty incident is, by the nature the incident, relatively limited. There are a range of tiers of potential care:

- Bystander first aid
- Treatment at the scene
- Casualty clearing station interventions
- Discharge from the scene
- Diagnosis of death

BYSTANDER CARE

Many members of the public caught up in a mass casualty incident have first aid training and often healthcare providers are involved but not injured. Members of both groups will want to provide immediate assistance to the injured. Simple treatments such as opening an airway in an unconscious casualty or applying a pressure dressing to a bleeding wound in the first few minutes can be life-saving. Following the London bombings, *NHS major incident dressing packs* have been forward deployed to transport hubs to facilitate this good Samaritan casualty care (34).

TREATMENT AT THE SCENE

Medical assistance to the emergency services involved in extricating casualties from a complex environment will often be required, and safe provision of analgesia can significantly improve the speed and efficiency of the process. The presence of an experienced doctor who can work with the paramedics and other rescue personnel to risk assess the interventions being proposed and, with the rescuers, determine the process of extrication can create a significant momentum.

Within the Medical Emergency Response Incident Team (MERIT) there will be people who are limited to being able to work in the *casualty clearing station* (CCS) and others who are sufficiently experienced to move forward into the scene. The need for this support will be determined by the tactical command team.

CASUALTY CLEARING STATION INTERVENTIONS

The management of the injured in a mass casualty response involves the creation of a CCS, a focal point through which all casualties pass for assessment and from where they will be evacuated to an appropriate hospital for their injuries. With any resource-constrained environment there is the potential for a queue, or delay, before evacuation. The environment may be one where the more detailed triage sort is applied and prioritisation more accurately determined.

There are also potential opportunities to provide clinical interventions that can reduce the urgency or triage category of some casualties. Traction splint application to fractured long bones or chest drain insertion for a significant chest injury such as a tension pneumothorax can decrease the time pressure for onward movement. This activity can facilitate more intelligent sieving, allowing for example the more urgent evacuation from the field of those for whom nothing beyond fluid resuscitation can be done in the CCS such as intra-abdominal bleeding.

The level of intervention in the CCS depends on the clinical skill and competence of those staffing it. Historically this capability was provided by *mobile medical teams* drawn from the local hospitals. Now this should be done by the personnel on the *MERIT*, with a consequent significant increase in the range of interventions that can be competently performed.

The MERIT should provide the medical staff to support the ambulance service in this environment, and its members should both understand the clinical expectations and have practised them. They should also be familiar with the demands of intelligent evacuation and the role of senior clinical input in assisting with evacuation priority decisions.

DISCHARGE FROM SCENE

Often a significant number of people at the scene of a major incident will have sustained no or only very minor injuries. Depending upon the nature of the incident, many may not require hospital treatment. The use of experienced health personnel to assess the triage category *green* casualties, including those involved but not injured, and discharge them from the scene to the care of the police, can significantly reduce the burden for transport for the ambulance service and allow focused use of resources.

DIAGNOSIS OF DEATH

The diagnosis of death is an important legal step in the management of an incident scene. Whilst a lower priority than the care of the injured, at some point this procedure will be required from the responding clinicians.

The initial triage sieve will already have identified those who are deceased. The labelling process leaves the body in situ and since the location of a deceased person is important to the incident investigation and possibly also identification of the dead, there are only two reasons to move a body:

- To gain access to a living person who is trapped within the incident
- To prevent destruction of the deceased person's body such as in the event of a fire

The police will manage the remains under their regulations on behalf of HM Coroner once the living have been evacuated from the scene.

EVACUATED POPULATIONS

In some major incidents, particularly of the *rising tide* and *cloud on the horizon* types, there can be a significant displacement of the population. Examples might include a river flooding an urban area or an industrial incident with the potential for a toxic gas cloud spreading over a residential district. If such an evacuation takes place, most people will be able to self-evacuate but residential facilities such as nursing homes and schools will need assistance. Resilience planning for primary care trusts requires them to maintain a record of all those who are potentially vulnerable within their community so that they can be identified and support provided during the evacuation.

Local authorities have a responsibility to establish care facilities for their population, should they be displaced, frequently involving the use of public buildings such as sports facilities and schools. Many of those moved will not have brought their regular medications with them, and a primary care treatment facility, together with a pharmacy, may be necessary to accommodate the essential medication re-provision needs. Whilst most able-bodied people can sleep on a camp bed and live in a communal resource for a brief period of time, the more highly care-dependent, often elderly, people will require more specialised support.

TRANSPORT

In a *big bang* or *conventional* incident, the evacuation of the injured from the scene to hospital is the final stage in the clinical response.

EVACUATION

There have been occasions where those involved have largely self-evacuated to hospital and there has been little emergency service control of this flow; in the Manchester terrorist bombing in 1996 many of the injured took themselves to the local hospitals. There have been other examples where, without any real coordination or planning, the emergency services have evacuated the injured to local hospitals (termed the *Vietnam concept* or *scoop and run*), but caused significant confusion in doing so. A good exemplar of this was the response to the Ramstein Air Show disaster in Germany in 1988 which resulted in the relatively uncontrolled evacuation of the injured to over 50 health facilities across northern Europe (35).

In planning terms for evacuation to hospitals, the science behind emergency preparedness has adapted the concept of surge capacity and this now equates to the number of injured persons and the severity of their injuries that can be accommodated in each facility per unit time.

Allowing for the time delay between a hospital receiving notification of the declaration of a mass casualty incident and the transport of the first injured by ambulance, there is an expectation that a hospital should be able to empty its emergency department (ED), creating an initial surge capacity equivalent to the number of resuscitation bays for red/immediate casualties and the number of major/trolley bays for the number of T2/urgent casualties. As an example, for a large ED, this might equate to 6 reds and 16 yellows in the first instance; for a smaller department, this may only be 2 reds and 6 yellows.

After this initial influx, there will be a smaller but continuing capacity as the first casualties are managed and moved onwards into the hospital. This continuing capacity is expected to be of the order of half the initial wave per hour for up to 4 hours. The exact flow rate will depend upon the nature of the injuries but this might equate to 18 reds and 48 yellows for a large receiving hospital and 6 reds and 18 yellows for a smaller hospital. This would certainly stretch the services that are available but should not exceed their capacity and lead to a degradation in the standard of care.

The role of the AIC/MIA health command is to try to manage the flow and ensure that no location is completely overwhelmed. This will require communication between the hospitals and the control team, often achieved by dispatching an ambulance liaison officer to each destination hospital.

As an additional complexity, if there are injuries requiring specialist treatment, ideally the patients should be moved directly to a facility with those specialist services available on site, reducing the need for onward secondary transport. Examples of such injuries might be neurosurgical injury or significant burns of a complex orthoplastic injury. However, the presence of associated injuries which could not be appropriately managed at a specialist facility might make this course of action unsafe, and in many cases casualties will be secondarily transferred to specialist facilities after a more general assessment and resuscitation.

Fundamental to an effective dispersal plan, effective and sufficiently clinically senior 'rear triage' is key. Experienced clinical judgement with a knowledge of the facilities of the surrounding hospitals, properly informed by the physiological triage sort and with clinical assessment of the injuries can allow intelligent disperal.

MODE OF TRANSPORT

Evacuation is carried out by ambulance. Old style vehicles used to be able to carry two stretchers, one being the normal transport trolley and a second a series of sideways facing seats that could be used as a stretcher if necessary. Ambulance safety and design issues have now eliminated this option and each ambulance is only able to transport a single stretcher patient.

The management of the rear of the casualty clearing station requires careful planning. There needs to be a free flow for vehicles in and out of the 'pinch point' and active management of potential congestion through a parking and queuing system (Figure 23.10).

Around the scene of a major incident, the traffic network will often become gridlocked as a result of road closures and traffic diversions. The police will aim to create *blue light* routes through the congestion to allow more free movement to the designated hospitals.

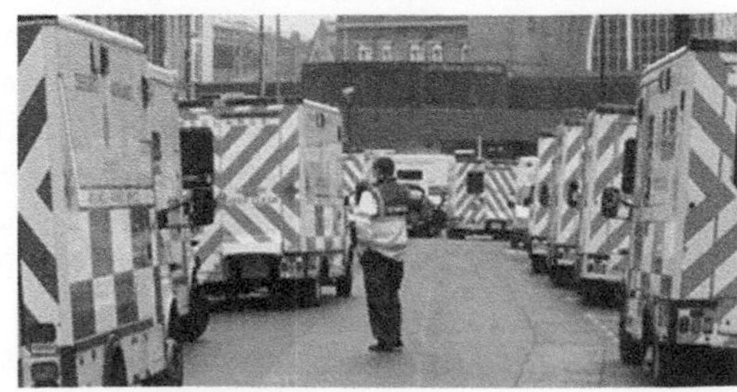

Figure 23.10 Ambulance parking.

In many incidents, a significant number of the casualties may have only minor injuries and other management options may be available. In some incidents, public transport such as buses might be commandeered to transport these individuals to a hospital some distance from the scene, protecting the nearer hospitals for the more significantly injured. There may also be alternative treatment locations such as walk-in centres which can provide simple dressings and basic treatments.

If there is sufficient capacity, it may be possible to screen and discharge those with no or minimal injuries from scene, removing the need to transport to hospital. These people will need to be processed by the police for investigation and documentation purposes but can be discharged by the health system.

HELICOPTERS

Over the last few years, a network of charitable UK air ambulances has developed with the capacity collectively to significantly impact on the care provided at an incident scene (Figure 23.11). In the first instance, they can carry both personnel and specialist equipment to the incident to support the MERIT function and then also provide for the evacuation of patients to specialist centres. This is increasingly pertinent with the establishment of major trauma networks but also applies for such injuries as large burns.

There is such potential to call on this resource, particularly in more remote locations, that some ambulance service emergency plans now have a specialist air movement officer as well as an ambulance parking officer to help manage the air traffic.

MERIT: MEDICAL EMERGENCY RESPONSE INCIDENT TEAM

Traditionally, mobile medical teams might have been brought to scene from the local emergency departments, but with the development of pre-hospital emergency medicine as a sub-specialty, this provision has evolved and current emergency preparedness guidance recommends that there is a dedicated medical asset administered by the ambulance service. Termed a *MERIT*, and drawn from across the region rather than from a specific location, it should be mobilised to the scene to provide additional medical support to the scene.

New Ideas

Medical provision at the scene of a major incident is provided by members of MERITs (see text) trained and equipped to work in challenging pre-hospital environments.

Part of the person specification for the role is that these medical staff should be familiar with the pre-hospital environment, have trained for it, and come both equipped and prepared for the environment of the casualty clearing station and forward into the scene of the incident as deemed necessary by the tactical commanders, the AIC and MIA.

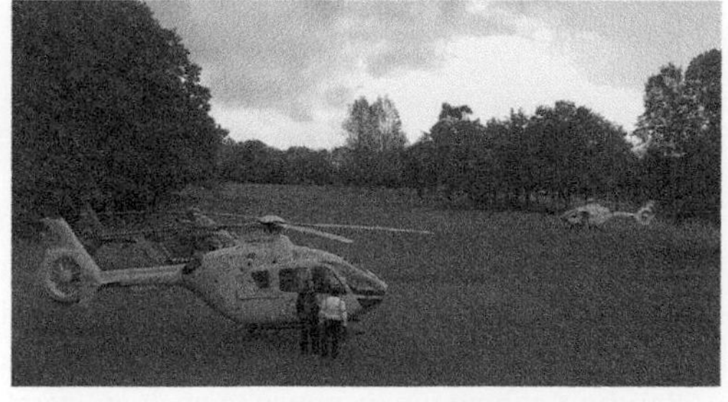

Figure 23.11 Charitable air ambulances.

The number and type of MERIT response will depend upon the size and nature of the incident. There is a range of potential roles, including:

- Work at the casualty clearing station – Assisting and supporting ambulance crews with the delivery of care in a relatively controlled environment.
- Work *forwards* at the scene (bronze) in support of paramedics in the scene wreckage managing and extricating the injured.
- '*Clearing the scene*' – Not all those involved are physically injured and some may not need transfer to hospital. Clinical review and discharge of those with no physical injuries from the scene to the care of the police may be an appropriate disposition.
- Diagnosing death – It may be necessary for a doctor to be assigned to work with a police officer and to officially 'diagnose death' on those who have perished in the incident, ensuring that the time of determination and location are properly recorded.

The National Burn Plan calls for specialist skills in the form of a *BAT* (*burns assessment team*) to be made available to manage a significant burn injury incident, a sub-group of the MERIT (36). This team of specialist practitioners is most likely to be best deployed to the designated receiving hospitals, but there may be circumstances where their deployment to support the medical staff in the CCS may be beneficial, allowing for the direct transfer of seriously burned patients to burn units around the country.

RECOVERY

Major incident scenes have typically managed to evacuate their injured casualties within 4 hours of the incident. There is usually a period of intense activity, beginning with considerable confusion which then becomes more organised and can function very effectively. All mass casualty events are likely to be followed by a detailed investigation of the circumstances of the event, but also of the actions of those who responded to provide assistance.

A detailed log of the decision-making and actions taken in response to the information available at the time is invaluable when any formal investigation is carried out. Many NHS emergency plans have a specific 'loggist' role, a person who accompanies the command element to document the activities and time stamp the decisions. 'If it wasn't written down, it never happened'.

PRACTICE POINT

For major incidents as for the care of a single patient: 'If it wasn't written down, it never happened'.

SUMMARY

Every clinician who is involved in the management of trauma victims in the pre-hospital environment is likely, sooner or later, to be involved in a major incident, whether it is a road traffic collision involving multiple vehicles, a crash involving a bus full of schoolchildren or more rarely a terrorist incident. It is essential therefore that every clinician has at least a basic understanding of how the response to such an event is organised, hence the inclusion of major incident management in this manual.

REFERENCES

1. National Health Service. Emergency Preparedness Framework. 2013. Accessed January 5, 2015. http://www.england.nhs.uk/wp-content/uploads/2013/03/eprr-framework.pdf.
2. World Health Organization. Mass Casualty Management Systems. 2007. Accessed January 5, 2015. http://www.who.int/hac/techguidance/MCM_guidelines_inside_final.pdf.
3. Kaji A, Koenig KL, Bey T. Surge capacity for healthcare systems: A conceptual framework. *Academic Emergency Medicine* 2006;13(11):1157–1159.
4. Department of Health. Mass casualties incidents: A framework for planning. 2005. Accessed January 5, 2015. http://webarchive.nationalarchives.gov.uk/20130107105354/http://www.dh.gov.uk/prod_consum_dh/groups/dh_digitalassets/@dh/@en/documents/digitalasset/dh_063393.pdf.
5. Civil Contingencies Act Enhancement Programme. Chapter 5 (Emergency planning): Revision to emergency preparedness. 2011. Accessed January 5, 2015. https://www.gov.uk/government/uploads/system/uploads/attachment_data/file/61028/Emergency_Preparedness_chapter5_amends_21112011.pdf.
6. Radestad M, Jirwe M, Castrén M, Svensson L, Gryth D, Ruter A. Essential key indicators for disaster medical response suggested to be included in a national uniform protocol for documentation of major incidents: A Delphi study. *Scandinavian Journal of Trauma and Resuscitation Emergency Medicine* 2013;21(1):68.
7. Arbon P, Bridgewater FH, Smith C. Mass gathering medicine: A predictive model for patient presentation and transport rates. *Prehospital and Disaster Medicine* 2001;16(3):150–158.
8. Memish ZA, Stephens GM, Steffen R, Ahmed QA. Emergence of medicine for mass gatherings: Lessons from the Hajj. *The Lancet Infectious Diseases* 2012;12(1):56–65.
9. Leary A, Greenwood P, Hedley B, Agnew J, Thompson D, Punshon G. An analysis of use of crowd medical services at an English football league club. *International Emergency Nursing* 2008;16(3):193–199.
10. Department of Culture, Media and Sport (CMS). *Green Guide – Sports Grounds Safety Authority 2007.* Accessed June 28, 2015. www.safetyatsportsgrounds.org.uk/publications/green-guide.
11. Health and Safety Executive. The event safety guide: A guide to health, safety and welfare at music and similar events. 1999. Accessed June 28, 2015. www.thepurpleguide.co.uk/.
12. Mahoney EJ, Harrington DT, Biffl WL, Metzger J, Oka T, Cioffi WG. Lessons learned from a nightclub fire: Institutional disaster preparedness. *Journal of Trauma and Acute Care Surgery* 2005;58(3):487–491.
13. Elliott D, Smith D. Football stadia disasters in the United Kingdom: Learning from tragedy? *Organization & Environment* 1993;7(3):205–229.
14. Carroll B, Balogh R, Morbey H, Araoz G. Health and social impacts of a flood disaster: Responding to needs and implications for practice. *Disasters* 2010;34(4):1045–1063.
15. Home Office. CONTEST: The United Kingdom's strategy for countering terrorism. The Stationery Office, 2011.
16. Shankar D, Agrawal M, Rao HR. Emergency response to Mumbai terror attacks: An activity theory analysis. *Cyber Security, Cyber Crime and Cyber Forensics: Applications and Perspectives* 2010:46–58.
17. Ranse J, Hutton A. Minimum data set for mass-gathering health research and evaluation: A discussion paper. *Prehospital and Disaster Medicine* 2012;27(6):543–550.

18. Ingrassia PL, Prato F, Geddo A, Colombo D, Tengattini M, Calligaro S, La Mura F, Franc JM, Della Corte F. Evaluation of medical management during a mass casualty incident exercise: An objective assessment tool to enhance direct observation. *Journal of Emergency Medicine* 2010;39(5):629–636.
19. Romundstad L, Sundnes KO, Pillgram-Larsen J, Røste GK, Gilbert M. Challenges of major incident management when excess resources are allocated: Experiences from a mass casualty incident after roof collapse of a military command center. *Prehospital and Disaster Medicine* 2004;19(2):179–184.
20. JESIP. Joint Emergency Services Interoperability Programme. 2015. Accessed June 28, 2015. http://www.jesip.org.uk/.
21. Cabinet Office. Emergency response and recovery. 2013. Accessed June 28, 2015. https://www.gov.uk/government/publications/emergency-response-and-recovery.
22. Cabinet Office. Dealing with disaster. 2001.
23. Office C. Civil Contingencies Act 2004. Accessed June 28, 2015. http://www.legislation.gov.uk/ukpga/2004/36/contents.
24. Carley S, Mackway-Jones K. *Major Incident Medical Management and Support.* Oxford: Blackwell, 2005.
25. NARU. Hazardous Areas Response Team 2015. Accessed July 16, 2015. http://naru.org.uk/naru-work-activities/naru-work-activities-capability-deliverables-hart-programme/.
26. CFRA. Fire and Rescue Service Operational Guidance GRA 4.1 Incidents involving transport systems - Road 2009. Accessed July 15, 2015. https://www.gov.uk/government/uploads/system/uploads/attachment_data/file/14907/gra-4-1.pdf.
27. Government U. Public safety and emergencies – guidance Resilient communications 2014. Accessed July 12, 2015. https://www.gov.uk/resilient-communications.
28. Sutton J, Palen L, Shklovski I (eds.). Backchannels on the front lines: Emergent uses of social media in the 2007 southern California wildfires. Proceedings of the 5th International ISCRAM Conference, Washington, DC, 2008.
29. Gebhart ME, Pence R. START triage: Does it work? *Disaster Management and Response* 2007;5(3):68–73.
30. So T-Y, Farrington E, Absher RK. Evaluation of the accuracy of different methods used to estimate weights in the pediatric population. *Pediatrics* 2009;123(6):e1045–e1051.
31. Buma AH, Henny W. *Triage: Ballistic Trauma*. Springer, 2005, pp. 527–534.
32. Moore L, Lavoie A, Abdous B, Le Sage N, Liberman M, Bergeron E et al. Unification of the revised trauma score. *Journal of Trauma and Acute Care Surgery* 2006;61(3):718–722.
33. Challen K, Walter D. Major incident triage: Comparative validation using data from 7th July bombings. *Injury* 2013;44(5):629–633.
34. Government U. Coroner's Inquests into the London bombings of 7 July 2005: Review of progress 2012. Accessed July 15, 2015. https://www.gov.uk/government/uploads/system/uploads/attachment_data/file/97988/inquest-7-7-progress-report.pdf.
35. Martin T. The Ramstein airshow disaster. *Journal of the Royal Army Medical Corps* 1990;136(1):19–26.
36. Department of Health. NHS Emergency Planning Guidance. Planning for the management of burn-injured patients in the event of a major incident: Interim strategic national guidance 2011. Accessed July 15, 2015. https://www.gov.uk/government/uploads/system/uploads/attachment_data/file/215643/dh_125842.pdf.

24

Retrieval and transport

OBJECTIVES

After completing this chapter the reader will

- Have knowledge of the criteria used in deciding the most appropriate transport method
- Understand the constraints, duration and limitations of air transfer
- Understand the need for organisational systems for patient retrieval

INTRODUCTION

Following patient assessment and stabilisation, transport to definitive care is a critical part of the injured patient's journey. Retrieval and transport can be divided into four types as shown in Table 24.1.

It is widely recognised and clearly supported by the evidence that the retrieval phase of patient care carries significant risks to both the patient (1–3) and to pre-hospital clinicians (4–7). A well-planned and well-governed approach to patient retrieval is therefore essential as part of any organisation providing pre-hospital care. The use of dedicated teams to undertake retrieval may improve patient outcomes (8–9).

The following principles must be applied to all trauma patients:

- Transport from scene should be directly to definitive care whenever possible.
- Patients must be stabilised as much as is possible before transport, especially by air.
- When helicopter transport is available the clinician must make an informed decision as to whether this is the fastest and safest mode of transport.
- For prolonged transfers redundancy is required for equipment, consumables and power.
- Accurate and timely communication with the receiving centre is essential.

PRE-TRANSFER MANAGEMENT AND TRIAGE

A thorough primary and rapid secondary survey at scene should be used to determine the potential hospital capabilities required for each patient. Pre-hospital trauma scoring and triage tools should be employed where possible (10–12). The choice of receiving hospital should be

Table 24.1 Retrieval classification

Primary retrieval	Retrieval from the scene of an incident to hospital
Secondary retrieval	Retrieval from a healthcare facility with basic facilities on site
Tertiary retrieval	Retrieval from a secondary care facility to definitive tertiary care
Quaternary retrieval	International repatriation

based on this assessment, ensuring where possible that all relevant surgical and critical care facilities which the patient may need are available on the one site. This prevents unnecessary secondary and tertiary retrievals, which add delay and risk (13,14).

When direct retrieval to definitive care will be prolonged, the decision to bypass nearer hospitals must take into account the clinical condition of the patient and the skills of the clinical personnel on scene. For example the ability to provide pre-hospital anaesthesia, ventilation and blood transfusion may make a prolonged journey safe to undertake which would not be possible if only basic airway, breathing and circulation management techniques were available. Within each trauma network, guidelines should be available describing how and when the decision to bypass facilities should be made.

When there is debate about appropriateness of triage, telephone or telemedicine advice from a senior doctor experienced in pre-hospital care can be of significant benefit. Longer transfer times and transport by air should lower the clinician's threshold for pre-transfer intubation and ventilation. This reduces the risk of patient deterioration during the retrieval phase.

Pre-alerting the receiving hospital improves the initial care provided for seriously injured patients (15). In particular requesting a hospital trauma team response or the immediate availability of blood and blood products or radiological imaging are important.

In cases where transport to a nearby hospital is required for stabilisation before secondary transfer to definitive care, alerting the local secondary retrieval service as early as possible is beneficial.

The decision regarding the most appropriate destination for a retrieval may, thus, be complex, involving consideration of evacuation times, geographical location of health service assets, clinical capability of crew (and thus the level of intervention they might perform), and the nature and likely progression of the patient's injuries. For air retrieval other factors will include weather and the time of day. Thus the 30-year-old unconscious patient with an apparently isolated head injury as a result of a fall will probably be best transferred to a regional trauma centre with neurosurgery on site 30 km away. If, however, there are airway problems or his physiology is significantly abnormal, then transfer to the nearest hospital is most likely to be the correct decision. If a pre-hospital critical care team is on scene, they may be able to optimise the patient sufficiently to allow safe transfer directly to the major trauma centre.

DECIDING ON MOST APPROPRIATE TRANSPORT METHOD

Two main transport modalities are generally available for primary retrievals: land ambulance and helicopter ambulance. For retrievals between hospital facilities, fixed-wing aircraft may also be used.

It is clinically safer to transfer a patient by land than air. Patient assessment in terms of examination and auscultation is easier due to lower noise levels. Equipment alarms are audible in road vehicles but not in rotary aircraft where helmets and headphones are routinely worn. In the event of patient deterioration it is usually straightforward to stop the ambulance allowing re-assessment and correction of the problem with adequate space to work. The same is not possible in a helicopter. Physical space within an air ambulance is often restricted and crew members' physical movement and communication abilities may be restricted by safety equipment such as harnesses, helmets, life jackets and immersion suits.

Therefore the benefits of air transfer in terms of speed over prolonged distance must be balanced against the more limited ability to assess and treat the patient during transfer.

Road ambulances allow direct transfer in one vehicle from the scene to the emergency department. With some helicopter transfers and all fixed-wing journeys, an ambulance journey is required to initially reach the aircraft and for transportation from the aircraft to the hospital at the receiving end. Each patient movement risks dislodging equipment and takes considerably more time than one would anticipate.

If the road transfer time is less than 45 minutes it may be faster to go by road ambulance (16). When driving times exceed 45 minutes, then helicopter retrieval should be considered. In general, fixed-wing retrieval is only appropriate for journeys exceeding 100 miles.

PRACTICE POINT

If the road transfer time is less than 45 minutes, it will normally be faster and clinically safer to go by road ambulance.

Although a 30-minute transfer by road ambulance to a major trauma centre may appear slower than a helicopter flying time of 7 minutes, the time taken for a more detailed pre-flight patient assessment, helicopter loading and unloading times (as well as time for the airframe to be called and arrive if it was not the primary response) mean that the land transfer will be quicker, as well as safer and allowing better patient observation and monitoring. Conversely, aeromedical evacuation is likely to be more comfortable for the patient.

PATIENT PACKAGING FOR RETRIEVAL

Patients should be carefully packaged before transfer. Good packaging aims to achieve patient comfort, spinal immobilisation and thermal insulation. Effective equipment management also ensures that invasive lines and other equipment are adequately secured.

The gold standard device to use for trauma patient packaging is a vacuum mattress. This forms a rigid but conforming stretcher for the patient to lie on and, for short distances, to be carried with. Pressure areas risks are minimised, reducing the danger of skin ischaemia. For short primary retrievals to hospital a scoop stretcher is an acceptable method of patient support. The scoop has the advantage of being applied and removed with minimal patient movement thus maintaining clots which have formed and minimising discomfort for injured casualties. Rescue boards (long spine boards) are for extrication only and should not be used to transport patients.

PRACTICE POINT

Rescue boards (long spine boards) are for extrication only and should not be used to transport patients.

For all retrievals, especially prolonged transfers in cold weather conditions, patients should be insulated against heat loss. Vacuum mattresses act as effective insulators, supplemented with blankets over the patient and head insulation. Patients on scoop stretchers require additional thermal protection. Insulation kits comprising of bubble wrap-type material are commercially available, as are warming blankets such as the Blizzard® blanket, which incorporate chemically based heating elements.

NEW IDEAS

Active warming blankets consisting of insulated blankets and several chemically based warming blocks are an effective way of treating and preventing hypothermia amongst trauma victims and have been extensively used by the military in Afghanistan.

When packaging patients for transport it is good practice to ensure that access to intravenous cannulae, thoracostomies, chest drains and arterial lines is possible. This can, however, be challenging. Cognisance should be paid to which side of the vehicle the stretcher is mounted against. In such cases only one side of the patient will be easily accessible during transport.

It is good practice to provide patients with ear protection during air transfer. This includes ventilated patients who are liable to the same hearing damage risks. Anaesthetised patients should have eye protection in place.

With head-injured patients there are a number of techniques which can be employed to reduce intracranial pressure. These include placing the patient in a 10 degrees head up position (17), loosening or removing cervical collars (18) when head blocks are in place, and using adhesive tape to secure endotracheal tubes rather than circumferential tube ties.

EQUIPMENT FOR TRANSFER

Pre-hospital care providers should ensure that they have sufficient equipment and consumables for the duration of the journey. This means that it is advisable to have at least twice the amount estimated to be required to allow for unseen delays: this includes drugs, fluids, oxygen and battery power for electrical devices.

Time should ideally be taken to optimise equipment alarm parameters according to individual patient physiology. During movement, clinicians may lose the ability to effectively observe the patient and so become more reliant on monitor and ventilator alarms. Inappropriately adjusted alarms which display frequently may reduce their impact and the clinician's response when a true emergency occurs.

Equipment display brightness should be adjusted to optimise the information on the screens. Dull screens can be difficult to see in daylight, and in noisy aircraft, clinicians are more reliant on visual alarm messages than audible ones.

Equipment must be procured with pre-hospital care and retrieval requirements in mind. It should also be noted that there are complex regulations regarding carriage of equipment in airframes to which all operators are subject. The following characteristics must be considered:

- Weight and bulk; the smaller and lighter the better
- Durability when dropped

- Weather proofing
- Battery duration
- Battery power monitoring

It is advisable to carry backup equipment to deal with equipment failure. A monitor can be replaced by a pulse oximeter and a portable capnometer device such as the EMMA™ (Figure 24.1). These two small pieces of equipment can provide measurements of heart rate, oxygen saturation, respiratory rate and end tidal CO_2. A bag valve mask can replace the work of a non-functioning ventilator.

Considerable risk is associated with unsecured equipment during transfer. Equipment items become projectiles during sudden changes in vehicle speed and direction and during collisions. Equipment can be secured in bespoke retainers, on equipment bridges or in specially designed transfer trolleys.

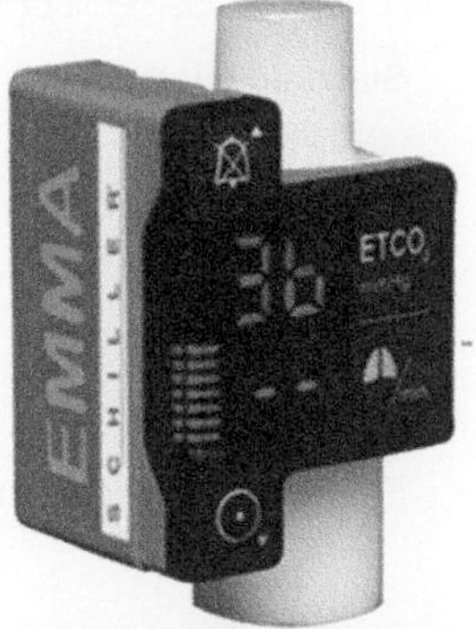

Figure 24.1 The EMMA™ capnometer.

CLINICAL GOVERNANCE AND SAFE TRANSPORT SYSTEMS

Patient retrieval is widely regarded as being a hazardous activity. Limited equipment and personnel combined with environmental challenges place patients and personnel at risk. Robust clinical governance systems are therefore necessary to maximise safety (19). Components of a retrieval clinical governance system are described in Table 24.2.

National standards and guidelines exist around the provision of care for transport of critically ill and injured adults (20,21) and all those involved in critical care transport should audit themselves against these standards.

ROTARY WING PATIENT TRANSFER

Helicopter transfer is ideal for patients when the road transfer time exceeds 45 minutes. Time to load and unload patients must be taken into account, as should time for land ambulance transfers to and from the aircraft. Helicopter operations are restricted during periods of poor weather and reduced visibility.

Clinicians working with helicopters should be suitably trained as medical passengers (22). Training should include the use of in-flight communications equipment, personal protective equipment (Table 24.3), emergency exit use, cabin security and moving around the aircraft. Personnel operating regularly on rotary aircraft over water should complete helicopter underwater escape training.

Helicopters used for patient transport vary considerably in size and capability. The smallest helicopter ambulances can carry three people – the pilot, patient and a medical attendant. Larger helicopters, especially those used for search and rescue operations, may have two pilots and a navigator.

Some helicopters are fitted with hydraulic winches to allow rescuers and clinical personnel to be deployed to patient locations which are not suitable for landing. Following stabilisation, patients can be winched in stretchers onto the aircraft. The size of the airframe determines what may be achieved in flight. Smaller airframes will inevitably result in limited access to the patient,

Table 24.2 Elements of retrieval system governance

Standard operating procedures	Service specific SOPs dealing with clinical conditions, equipment and transport logistics which must be regularly updated in light of experience and incidents.
Checklists	Two person 'check and response' checklists are advisable including: pre-mission checklist, emergency anaesthesia, procedural sedation and leaving scene.
Equipment management	Daily check system, post-mission two-person checks, regular full equipment pack checks.
Significant event management system	Low threshold for event reporting within the team. Facilitated by paper, app based or online reporting. Effective investigation, communication and system change framework in place.
Audit	Continual audit of clinical and operational effectiveness.
Training and simulation	Regular scheduled and job planned training and simulation.
Emergency action cards	Pre-planned action cards for emergencies such as equipment failure, accidental extubation and unexpected patient deterioration.
Debriefs	Mandatory, structured post-retrieval team debriefs.
Clinical governance meetings	Regular clinical governance meetings to discuss cases and events.
Transfer standards	Applying standards applicable to critical care transfer as described by the Intensive Care Society and the Association of Anaesthetists of Great Britain and Ireland.

Table 24.3 Personal protective equipment for helicopter medical personnel

At all times:
- Helicopter helmet with visor and communication system
- Toe protector boots
- Flame-retardant flight suit
- High-visibility jacket

Dependent on conditions and training:
- Immersion survival suit
- Life jacket
- Short-term air supply
- Personal locator beacon

and so a 'treat-then-transfer' policy should be adopted. Larger airframes, such as the Eurocopter 145 and military support helicopters, may be large enough for procedures to be carried out in flight, allowing a 'treat-during-transfer' policy, which will reduce pre-hospital time for the patient. The largest airframes of all, such as the CH-47 Chinook, enable a full suite of interventions to be carried out in flight, bringing the emergency department to the patient. Motion sickness is common amongst crew members and patients alike. Awake patients should be given an anti-emetic.

It is hazardous to approach helicopters while the rotor blades are turning, especially when they are shutting down or starting up as they can be rotating below head height. If the helicopter has landed on sloping ground, the blades will be closer to ground level on the side higher up the slope. If at all possible the helicopter should shut down before personnel and patients move

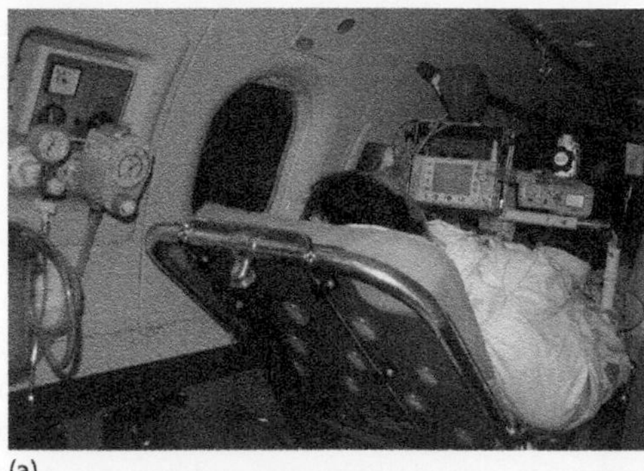
(a)

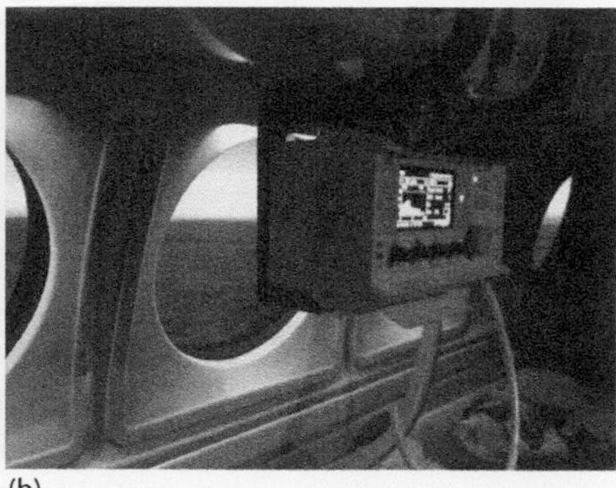
(b)

Figure 24.2 (a) Equipment secured to bridge attached to stretcher. (b) Ventilator secured on retainer attached to aircraft.

around the aircraft. If this is not possible, then the crew should listen to the directions of the pilot before leaving the aircraft.

On level ground, the aircraft should be approached from the front in the 10 to 2 o'clock arc. Movement around the tail rotor should be avoided completely. It is imperative that the pilot knows that people are moving near the aircraft and must give permission for them to enter or leave the rotor disc.

Medical equipment should be secured using a medical bridge or equipment retaining brackets (Figure 24.2). Equipment should ideally be flight tested by an avionics engineer before it is certified for use in flight. Defibrillation and external pacing are possible in flight, but it is essential to inform the pilot before it is activated.

FIXED WING PATIENT TRANSFER

As with helicopters, the size and capabilities of fixed-wing aircraft are very variable. Generally there is more room to move around and less need for constant harness use by the crew. Fixed-wing aircraft also tend to be less noisy, allowing more effective communication and patient assessment when it is needed. Again, it is essential that equipment is secured appropriately according to aviation regulations. The potential clinical effects of the reduction in atmospheric pressure due to altitude must be considered. Air-filled spaces will expand. These include:

- Endotracheal tube cuffs
- Gas in the pleural space
- Pneumocranium

Changes in air pressure may necessitate replacement of air with saline in endotracheal tube cuffs (23). In some fixed-wing aircraft, it may be possible to increase cabin pressurisation to sea level during the flight. In rare instances maintaining a low flight altitude may be necessary, however, risks to flight safety must be fully discussed with the aircraft captain.

Rapid acceleration during takeoff may lower the patient's blood pressure due to reduced venous return. This is usually transient and causes no harm. In haemodynamically unstable patients and those with increased intracerebral pressure, decreases in venous return may be more detrimental, and hence adequate and appropriate filling of the vascular compartment, ideally with blood products, is advised.

Land ambulance transfers at the referring site and the receiving centre airfield are essential when using aeroplanes. Time for these transfers needs to be factored in to the transport time estimate.

SUMMARY

Appropriate and careful selection of the method of transfer of a patient from the scene of an accident are essential in achieving optimum outcomes. Where possible, patients should be transferred directly to definitive care, but the factors influencing this decision, like those influencing mode of transport, are complex, and good decision-making requires experience. Careful pre-transfer stabilisation is essential before transfer, especially by air, and patients must be carefully packaged and equipment well secured before transfer.

Transfer by air limits the ability to assess the patient, detect deterioration and carry out interventions. Although it may seem rapid, time for transport to and from the aircraft and loading and unloading the patient may mean that road transfer from the scene is a faster method for the patient to reach definitive care. It must not be forgotten that patient retrieval is clinically and physically hazardous and that robust, safe organisational systems are therefore a necessity.

REFERENCES

1. Flabouris A, Runciman WB, Levings B. Incidents during out-of-hospital patient transportation. *Anaesthesia and Intensive Care* 2006;34(2):228–236.
2. Uosaro A, Parvianen I, Takala J, Ruokonen E. Safe long-distance interhospital ground transfer of critically ill patients with acute severe unstable respiratory and circulatory failure. *Intensive Care Medicine* 2002;28:1122–1125.
3. Maccartney I, Nightingale P. Transfer of the critically ill adult patient. *British Journal of Anaesthesia CEPD Reviews* 2001;1:12–15.
4. Holland J, Cooksley DG. Safety of helicopter aeromedical transport in Australia: A retrospective study. *Medical Journal of Australia* 2005;182:17–19.
5. Lutman D, Montgomery M, Ramnarayan P, Petros A. Ambulance and aeromedical accident rates during emergency retrieval in Great Britain. *Emergency Medicine Journal* 2008;25:301–302.
6. Kahn CA, Pirrallo RG, Kuhn EM. Characteristics of fatal ambulance crashes in the United States: An 11-year retrospective analysis. *Prehosp Emergency Care* 2001;5:261–269.
7. Hinkelbein J, Dambier M, Viergutz T, Genzwuerker HV. A six-year analysis of German emergency medical services helicopter crashes. *Journal of Trauma* 2008;64:204–210.
8. Gilligan JE, Griggs WM, Jelly MT, Morris DJ, Haslam RR, Matthews NT, Everest ER, Bryce RL, Marshall PB, Peisach RA. Mobile intensive care services in rural South Australia. *Medical Journal of Australia* 1999;171:617–620.
9. Britto J, Nadel S, Maconochie I, Levin M, Habibi P. Morbidity and severity of illness during interhospital transfer: Impact of a specialised paediatric retrieval team. *BMJ* 1995;311:836–839.
10. Bruijns SR, Guly HR, Bouamra O, Lecky F, Lee WA. The value of traditional vital signs, shock index, and age-based markers in predicting trauma mortality. *Journal of Trauma and Acute Care Surgery* 2013;74(6):1432–1437.

11. Raum MR, Nijsten MW, Vogelzang M, Schuring F, Lefering R, Bouillon B, Rixen D, Neugebauer EA, Ten Duis HJ; Polytrauma Study Group of the German Trauma Society. Emergency trauma score: An instrument for early estimation of trauma severity. *Critical Care Medicine* 2009;37(6):1972–1977.
12. Hasler RM, Kehl C, Exadaktylos AK, Albrecht R, Dubler S, Greif R, Urwyler N. Accuracy of prehospital diagnosis and triage of a Swiss helicopter emergency medical service. *Journal of Trauma and Acute Care Surgery* 2012;73(3):709–715.
13. Atkins ML, Pinder AJ, Murphy PG. Quality of care during the transfer of the critically ill neurosurgical patients in West Yorkshire: A comparison with national guidelines. *Journal of Neurosurgical Anaesthesiology* 1998;10:293.
14. Vyvyan HAL, Kee S, Bristow A. A survey of secondary transfers of head injured patients in the south of England. *Anaesthesia* 1991;4:728–731.
15. Porter JM, Ursic C. Trauma attending in the resuscitation room: Does it affect outcome? *American Surgeon* 2001;67(7):611–614.
16. Black JJM, Ward EM, Lockey DJ. Appropriate use of helicopters to transport trauma patients from incident scene to hospital in the United Kingdom: An algorithm. *Emergency Medicine Journal* 2004;21:355–361.
17. Ng I, Lim J, Wong HB. Effects of head posture on cerebral hemodynamics: Its influences on intracranial pressure, cerebral perfusion pressure, and cerebral oxygenation. *Neurosurgery* 2004;54(3):593–597.
18. Davies G, Deakin C, Wilson A. The effect of a rigid collar on intracranial pressure. *Injury* 1996;27(9):647–649.
19. Hearns S, Shirley PJ. Retrieval medicine: A review and guide for UK practitioners. Part 2: Safety in patient retrieval systems. *Emergency Medicine Journal* 2006;23:943–947.
20. Whiteley S, Mccartney I, Mark J, Barratt J, Binks R. Guidelines for the transport of the critically ill adult (3rd edtion). London: Intensive Care Society, 2011. http://www.ics.ac.uk /professional/guidance_transport_3_3_.
21. Safe Transfer of Patients with Brain Injury. The Association of Anaesthetists of Great Britain & Ireland, 2006. http://www.aagbi.org/sites/default/files/braininjury.pdf.
22. JAR-OPS 3. Commercial air transportation (helicopters). Joint Aviation Authorities, 2007, page 1-B-11. http://www.jaa.nl/publications/jars/606970.pdfpage.
23. Shirley P. Transportation of the critically ill and injured patient. *Update in Anaesthesia* 2004;18.

25 Handover and documentation

OBJECTIVES

After completing this chapter the reader will

- Understand the importance of optimal handover and good documentation
- Be able to provide a structured pre-alert message
- Understand the legal and regulatory obligations relating to patient health care records

INTRODUCTION

Knowledge of the events prior to hospital admission may help facilitate appropriate patient care. Elements of information are passed verbally at handover, but a written (often electronic) report must be prepared that is left at the hospital for reference and does not omit any important details (1). Unfortunately, there is a well-recognised tendency for emergency department staff to rely on the verbal handover with up to 50% of clinicians failing to refer to pre-hospital documentation despite its usefulness (2). This may be exacerbated by the use of electronic recording systems by ambulance trusts. Thus initial decision-making in the emergency department is often based on a combination of the handover provided by the pre-hospital practitioner and the rapid evaluation of the patient. Despite its importance, there is usually only one opportunity to provide a handover, and receiving clinicians are often focused on commencement of patient assessment which distracts them from listening carefully.

PRACTICE POINT

The aim of an effective clinical handover is to pass information, professional responsibility and accountability seamlessly between the pre-hospital team and hospital clinicians (3).

Unfortunately, it is well recognised that the handover of patients in hospital between health care professionals is a particularly hazardous time (4). This is due to the potential for misinterpretation, dilution or total loss of information (5). There is likely to be no difference when pre-hospital practitioners hand over to emergency department staff on arrival at hospital. Indeed, it may be of greater importance, as any lost information may not easily be retrieved or be available from any other source.

Information conveyed to the hospital trauma team is highly variable. Whilst some studies have found that on average 70% of transmitted information is received and documented, others have found this to be as low as 36% (2,6,7). Stiell et al. used the term *information gaps* to describe the information that an emergency department clinician requires to manage a patient optimally but which is found to be missing (8). As a result, emergency department stays were found to be delayed by up to 60 minutes. A failure of high-quality pre-hospital handover of information is likely to increase these information gaps resulting in increased length of stay, delayed treatment and poorer patient outcomes (6). This is perhaps not surprising as few pre-hospital care practitioners have had any formal training in handover provision (9,10).

PRE-ALERT

Communication with the receiving hospital must begin at scene. The establishment of regional trauma, cardiac and stroke networks in the United Kingdom has resulted in pre-hospital staff bypassing local hospitals in favour of specialised facilities located further away. Information on patient condition, intervention and expected time of arrival at the health care facility is essential in preparing the hospital to receive the patient. This may include the alerting and mobilisation of specialised medical staff such as a trauma team, the preparation and allocation of a resuscitation bay, activation of massive transfusion protocols, and the alerting of ancillary services such as imaging and laboratory personnel. Where a pre-alert is passed, evidence suggests that definitive treatment is instituted faster than when it is not (11). Pre-alert information for seriously ill or injured paediatric patients is particularly useful to the receiving team, as details of the child's demographics and physiology allows appropriate equipment to be prepared and accurate calculation of drug dosages prior to their arrival (12).

Pre-alert information may be passed directly from scene or via a central control room to the hospital. Studies have suggested that pre-alerting is generally done poorly, with the majority of patients with an Injury Severity Score (ISS) greater than 15 not being pre-alerted (13). Furthermore, up to 75% of patients with traumatic injury who were alerted by the ambulance service fell outside of the inclusion criteria for major trauma, as defined by the Trauma Audit Research Network (14). In the UK, criteria have been developed to identify those who would benefit most from direct transfer to a major trauma centre (MTC). This mandates the need for a pre-alert message.

The majority of pre-hospital care information is transmitted via ambulance control rooms to the hospital (15). This method prevents direct two-way communication between pre-hospital staff at scene and hospital clinicians and risks information being diluted or altered, particularly if personnel passing the message to the receiving hospital are non-clinical. Ideally, communication between pre-hospital staff at scene, ambulance control and the receiving hospital should be made via a conference call. This allows direct transmission of information between scene and hospital and permits a recording to be made for accurate documentation, whilst ensuring a continuous flow of information through ambulance control.

HOSPITAL HANDOVER

The delivery of key information during a pre-alert message and at patient handover to the receiving hospital team is vital in maintaining continuity of care and ensuring patient safety (16).

All communication, whether passed by radio, mobile phone or face to face, at patient handover should be done with accuracy, clarity and brevity.

An effective handover is most likely to be delivered when the pre-hospital practitioner is experienced, confident and succinct. A noisy environment, inattention by receiving hospital staff and constant interruptions during handover have been cited as key reasons why information may be lost or become distorted during handover (7,9,10). Information conveyed to the receiving team at handover may have important implications for the patient's ongoing management and ideally all receiving clinical hospital staff should be apprised of this information. On the patient's arrival at hospital the emergency department team leader should confirm that there are no life-threatening conditions that may require immediate intervention, for example cardiac arrest or catastrophic haemorrhage. In such a case handover may instead be directed towards the individual team leader or scribe (9). If the patient is stable, however, handover may be undertaken before transfer of the patient onto the hospital bed (10). This prevents the natural tendency for medical staff to commence patient treatment before or during handover from the pre-hospital care personnel (17). The performance of a *'five second check'* for immediately life-threatening issues such apnoea or life-threatening haemorrhage before the handover will ensure that critical issues are not missed.

ATMIST

Structured templates have been developed for pre-hospital use in order to convey information in a systematic manner. This allows a handover and pre-alert to be provided in a rapid, standardised manner. Their usage is now commonplace, with the ATMIST handover being seen by many UK ambulance services as the standard of care and in the military setting as a pre-hospital key performance indicator (18). This mnemonic has largely superseded ASHICE (see Box 25.1). The aim should be to complete handover in 45 seconds. It is sometimes difficult to convey a perception of the patient in the pre-hospital setting in a way that receiving staff have a full appreciation of it (10). Photography taken at scene or of an injury prior to application of a dressing can often improve this understanding.

BOX 25.1: ATMIST and ASHICE

Age and sex
Time of injury and hospital arrival
Mechanism of injury
Injuries sustained
Signs and symptoms
Treatment administered

Age
Sex
History
Injuries sustained
Condition of patient
Estimated time of arrival

DIGITAL TECHNOLOGY

Despite the wide availability of digital photography, evidence suggests that fewer than 10% of pre-hospital responders routinely provide photographic images, although 75% of hospital clinicians believe such images to be beneficial (15). Like written documentation it must be remembered that any stored photographic material remains part of the patient record and as such patient confidentiality must be maintained. Digital material may also be subject to data protection laws and may be requested by law enforcement agencies in the event of an inquiry or prosecution.

Increasingly, technological innovations such as telemedicine are playing an integral role in the transmission of information between scene and hospital. One non-trauma example of this is the transmission of electrocardiograms to centres offering percutaneous coronary intervention. This allows the rapid identification of patients who may benefit from such procedures and allows the receiving centre time to prepare or mobilise the appropriate staff.

In addition, advice and support can now be provided to emergency services at the scene of an incident with the help of digital media. Specialist paramedics such as those in the *hazardous area response team* (*HART*) carry live-feed cameras, permitting recordings of the environment in which the individual is working. This data can then be transmitted back from the scene to a control centre where information regarding the patient's condition, injury and environment can be disseminated to the relevant personnel.

PATIENT DOCUMENTATION

Documentation of pre-hospital events is a critical element in patient care, ensuring that the patient continues to receive optimal management. It may also be relied upon to facilitate an appropriate response in the event of a complaint, legal proceedings or coroner's inquest.

PRACTICE POINT

Good records, good defence; poor records, poor defence; no record, no defence.

If a vital sign has been observed or a drug has been administered, but neither have been recorded, the assumption will be made that such actions have not been performed, the consequences of which may be disastrous. In one study pre-hospital documentation was only found to be adequate, when compared to a set of emergency care standards, two-thirds of the time (19). Good clinical records contain sufficient information to allow another health care professional to reconstruct a patient encounter without relying on memory or assumption. In general, clinical records that contain adequate information to permit continuity of care will also be satisfactory for other purposes (20).

There are many different forms of pre-hospital documentation that will ultimately form part of the patient's health care record. These are listed in Box 25.2.

PATIENT REPORT FORMS

In the main, most UK ambulance services use a patient report form (PRF) with a standardised *check box*, *circle* or *fill-in-the-box* format or alternatively an ePRF system. This form details key demographic patient information, dates, times and incident numbers. Space is allocated for details of drug administration and specific interventions such as insertion of an airway adjunct. Many pre-hospital organisations have a list of common approved abbreviations or codes that may be used. Space may also be provided for freehand text to describe the

BOX 25.2: Types of Pre-Hospital Documentation

- Patient report form (PRF) (paper or electronic)
- Text messages
- Printouts from monitoring equipment
- Electrocardiograms (ECGs)
- Video or audio recordings
- Digital photography
- Ultrasonography scans (USS)
- Written correspondence between health care professionals

mechanism of injury, clinical findings and management of the patient. The PRF then becomes a part of the patient's medical record. Its main role is to allow sufficient documentation of the patient's condition to allow other health care professionals to continue optimal patient management. It may also be used as a reference document for legal purposes, for example if the patient wishes to proceed with a claim of alleged assault or in the event of legal proceedings for clinical negligence (21).

BOX 25.3: Uses of Pre-Hospital Clinical Material

Clinical audit
Publication
Research
Education
NHS administration
Managerial requirements
Charity presentations

Whilst the main purpose of the PRF is to provide an accurate record to facilitate continuity of care, pre-hospital data may have a wide variety of other uses subject to the necessary caveats regarding confidentiality (Box 25.3).

CONTENT

Good documentation must include the following:

- Incident number
- Patient details and demographics
- Patient's history or mechanism of injury
- Relevant clinical findings on examination
- Time stamps
- Drugs administered
- Patient observations
- Decisions made, actions taken and who is making the decisions
- Any information given to the patient
- Follow-up arrangements
- Any information surrounding patient refusal of examination, treatment or hospital admission
- Signature and date

The guidelines for doctors in Good Medical Practice (GMC 2013; Box 25.4) provide useful guidance for all clinicians.

All patients have a right to expect a timely response when requesting the attendance of an emergency service. The time of call is often taken as the closest reliable marker of injury onset time and may have important implications for further management of the patient. As an example, it is important to ascertain the time of burn injury, as this influences fluid administration, whilst the time to defibrillation for a patient in cardiac arrest has important implications for patient outcome. In the United Kingdom response time targets for the ambulance service have been set by the government, making the documentation of response times essential.

As a minimum the following response times should be recorded by all pre-hospital practitioners attending an incident (22).

- Time of call
- Time of response
- Time of arrival at scene and/or patient
- Time leaving scene
- Time of arrival at hospital (if appropriate)

BOX 25.4: Good Medical Practice Guidelines for Doctors

Record your work clearly, accurately and legibly

- Documents (including clinical records) must be clear, accurate and legible. Wherever possible records should be made at the same time as the events recorded or as soon as possible afterwards.
- Records that contain personal information about patients, colleagues or others must be kept securely, and in line with any data protection requirements.
- Clinical records should include:
  - relevant clinical findings
  - the decisions made and actions agreed, and who is making the decisions and agreeing the actions
  - the information given to patients
  - any drugs prescribed or other investigation or treatment
  - who is making the record and when

It may also be appropriate to document any delays in patient treatment or transportation, such as those due to adverse weather conditions or patient location.

As well as recording positive findings, it is also advisable to document important negatives. For example, following comprehensive assessment of a patient, it may be deemed that immobilisation of the cervical spine is unnecessary. If the patient subsequently wishes to make a complaint or institute legal proceedings, any documentation will be relied upon to provide a robust defence of the decisions made at the time of the incident. It must be remembered that this may not occur until years after the original event.

As patients have a right to access their own medical records under the *Data Protection Act 1988*, it is imperative that documentation is professional and in keeping with that expected by colleagues and regulatory bodies. The use of abbreviations should be avoided where possible, as this will prevent ambiguity when read by other medical personnel and avoid distress to patients and their relatives, especially if misinterpreted. The Health and Care Professions Council states that paramedics must *'understand the need to use only acceptable terminology'* in making records, whilst the Nursing and Midwifery Council recommends *'that records should be factual and not include unnecessary abbreviations, jargon, meaningless phrases or irrelevant speculation'* (23,24).

REFUSAL OF CARE OR NON-HOSPITAL ATTENDANCE

Patients who request the attendance of pre hospital personnel but subsequently refuse assessment or attendance at hospital represent 50%–90% of litigation cases in some studies (25,26). Patients under the influence of alcohol or illicit drugs and those with central nervous system impairment or mental illness represent the most difficult to fully evaluate. It is therefore imperative that particular care is taken to document findings, advice given and patient disposition in these groups of patients (27).

Meticulous documentation is also essential in the event that the clinical condition does not mandate the patient travelling to hospital or if the patient refuses admission. A thorough assessment must be undertaken with adequate documentation explaining any treatment administered, any self-care instructions and any red flag warning signs that the patient or carer should look out for in case of subsequent deterioration. It is also recommended that under these circumstances a record is made of the patient's capacity to consent or refuse treatment along with a note of any witnesses present at the time of patient discharge. This is particularly important if the patient is left with their next of kin or parent who may be involved in the provision of ongoing care or supervision. In some cases discussion may have taken place with other health care providers, for example the patient's general practitioner, a hospital specialist, or incident commander, in the event of a major incident and these discussions must be fully documented. Whilst it is appreciated that critical interventions play an essential role in determining patient outcome, so too does an understanding of the decision-making process resulting in a management plan.

PRESENTATION

All handwritten notes should be made in indelible black ink such that is clear to the reader and allows legible copies of the original notes to be made by photocopier or scanning if necessary. In some cases copies are made at the time of documentation on to carbon paper. All notes made must be legible. Indeed, some advocate the use of printing words rather than cursive handwriting (22).

Poorly recorded information may be just as hazardous to a patient as missing information. Poorly presented documentation which is unclear, inaccurate or difficult to follow may result in errors and misinterpretation. The features of good documentation are listed in Box 25.5.

BOX 25.5: Features of Good Documentation

- Specific with accurate records of events and the mechanism of injury
- Contemporaneous
- Concise; providing sufficient, clear information
- Objective; avoiding assumptions, for example 'alleged assault' rather than 'assault'
- Objective; stating the facts and avoiding subjective comments
- Accurate
- Legible if handwritten

ALTERATIONS, ADDITIONS OR AMENDMENTS

If information needs to be amended or added to a patient record, it must be ensured that any entry is signed or initialled and the date and time of the amendment recorded. This will help to prevent accusations of deception and claims that the new entry is being passed off as part of the original record (20). If an error is made, this should be struck through with a single line so that the original entry can still be read, and initialled, timed and dated.

Under the Data Protection Act 1988, patients also have the right to amend any factual inaccuracies in their medical records or, if appropriate, to have them permanently removed. Patients do not, however, have the right to ask for entries expressing a professional opinion to be changed. Where there is dispute over a professional entry, the patient's view should be documented alongside any further advice sought from regulatory and indemnity organisations (21).

CONTEMPORANEOUS NOTES

In theory notes should be written contemporaneously. However, in the critically injured patient, treatment may need to be provided en route to hospital and it may not be possible to make a record during this time. It is also recognised that in the pre-hospital environment the majority of documentation is prepared in sub-optimal conditions, for example in a moving vehicle or whilst administering patient treatment. In addition, the pre-hospital practitioner may only have a short period of time to construct a verbal handover and document all the necessary patient details and findings before arriving at their destination. Where it is not possible to complete a comprehensive record of patient care before arrival at hospital, this should be completed at the earliest opportunity thereafter, usually following verbal patient handover. This will allow proficient recall of events and prevent important omissions of information that other members of the health care team would otherwise rely upon to make treatment and prognostic decisions regarding ongoing patient care.

COPIES

It is often necessary to record notes in a manner that permits multiple copies to be made. This allows an original copy to be kept by the organisation or individual who made the record, whilst permitting subsequent copies to be distributed elsewhere, such as being left with the patient who does not travel to hospital. In the event that the patient is later admitted to hospital, copies can also be given to the receiving health care facility, ideally with a duplicate forwarded onto the patient's usual doctor or general practitioner.

ELECTRONIC RECORDING

The use of electronic media to record, process and store data is an essential part of modern life. Collection and storage of all recorded data, allowing legible presentation either on screen or in the form of printouts, is particularly desirable. Further benefits could also be achieved if collated data was then shared with other health care systems in primary and secondary care.

Many automated devices currently store a wealth of useful data, for example defibrillators accurately record the time of defibrillation, presenting cardiac rhythm and duration of monitoring, whilst monitoring equipment records the exact time of the vital sign values. Ideally this information would be immediately integrated into the patient's health care record; however, this requires a standardised interface for all medical devices which is not currently available. Nevertheless, data storage cards within the aforementioned devices do permit recording of information and knowledge of how to access this may be useful in particular circumstances (27).

ELECTRONIC PATIENT REPORT FORM (ePRF)

A growing number of pre-hospital providers are moving away from paper-based patient documentation to electronic devices, as these devices help to improve the accuracy and legibility of recorded data. They also allow comprehensive data collection that can then be used to audit the quality and consistency of care provided, whilst avoiding the need for costly storage. A range of devices and software platforms are available from rugged laptops to smaller tablets and personal pocket computers with a varying ability to interface with other health care provider IT systems. Such devices allow immediate access to clinical decision support tools such as National Poisons Databases, drug formularies and national guidelines. They are also able to provide information on previous patient attendances, allowing comparison of clinical material such as electrocardiograms.

Some systems have been integrated with the IT of local emergency departments allowing immediate sharing of information from the time of input, prior to patient arrival. Not only does this help to minimise administrative delays at hospital by preventing duplication of workload but it also optimises patient handover, enabling immediate continuity of patient treatment. In addition the patient's hospital notes and previous admissions may be easily made available prior to the patient's arrival.

In the UK there is a national strategy to develop the ePRF as part of the NHS National Programme for IT, resulting in a transition from hard copy patient report forms to an electronic system. The NHS Information Standards Board has produced national guidance on the minimum clinical information that emergency NHS ambulance personnel in England are required to record. Its purpose is to improve the comparability of recorded data recorded on the form across all ambulance services and other health care providers (28). This guidance states that the following items of data that must be included on the ePRF:

- Details of the patient
- Details of the incident
- Details of the ambulance crew
- Details of the presenting complaint
- Details of patient assessment
- Details of patient treatment or interventions made
- Details of drug administration
- Patient past medical history
- Patient pain score
- Destination hospital or details of discharge at scene if applicable

Whilst some fields on the ePRF may be autopopulated by data collected by the ambulance call centre, such as time of call to the emergency services or time of arrival of the first responder, the remainder must be inputted manually by the pre hospital-practitioner. The majority of input fields are mandatory thus minimising the risk of incomplete data collection. Some data fields may only apply if a particular condition is met, for example trauma. In addition, ambulance trusts are able to add additional fields that are considered appropriate for regional service delivery, such as clinical performance indicators (28).

In the future, sychronisation of pre-hospital electronic patient data with the records of other health care facilities such as general practices or community hospitals may allow the sharing of important information such as allergies, chronic diseases or prescribed medications. This knowledge would help to assist the practitioner in their management of the patient and improve patient safety, particularly where the patient or relative was unable or unwilling to provide this information themselves (27).

AUDIOVISUAL RECORDING

The *General Medical Council* (GMC) has issued comprehensive guidance on the creation and use of audiovisual material, such as video recordings or photographic material. This includes a wide range of recording devices including digital cameras, video cameras and mobile phones. Specific guidance on the use of these devices is provided with reference to both adult and paediatric patients and those who lack capacity to consent to usage of such material. Most pre-hospital organisations provide guidance as to how any material taken should be used or stored, but the principles remain the same.

The essential principles of audiovisual recording (29) include maintaining the patient's privacy and dignity; ensuring, when possible, that consent has been obtained before making any recordings; and stopping recording and/or deleting images following any patient request to do so. If the images are to be used for any purpose, the patient's consent must be obtained and recordings must be stored in an appropriately secure place. However *'if you judge an adult to lack capacity and where treatment must be provided immediately, recordings may still be made where they form part of an investigation or treatment that you are providing in accordance with common law'* (29).

Visual recordings made of the scene or injuries sustained may enhance teaching, training and assessments of health care professionals and students. If such material is to be used for any purpose other than for *direct* patient benefit, then further consent must be obtained from the patient. Where possible the recording should be anonymised or coded (29). It is important to bear in mind that even insignificant details may still make the patient identifiable.

LEGAL REQUIREMENTS

Strict rules govern the recording and storage of patient information. This includes all written and digital documentation, clinical or non-clinical data. In the United Kingdom, a named individual, usually a senior member of the organisation (Caldicott Guardian), must take responsibility for protecting patient confidentiality and enabling appropriate information sharing. Most pre-hospital organisations will have guidelines detailing how, what and when patient information should be recorded and how this should be stored. Good information governance should not be underestimated and heavy fines have been imposed on health care organisations in the UK which have failed in their responsibility to keep patient information confidential and secure (30).

CONFIDENTIALITY AND ACCESS TO MEDICAL DOCUMENTATION

Maintaining patient confidentiality is not only central to maintaining a therapeutic patient relationship but is also a legal principle which must be maintained even following the death of the patient. It is also a condition of registration with the *GMC, Nursing and Midwifery Council,* and the *Health and Care Professions Council.*

The principle of confidentiality extends beyond that of divulging confidential patient information to ensuring that any written documentation is securely stored (31). Medical records should not be left in a position where unauthorised access may easily occur.

Despite the need to keep all patient data confidential there are occasions when such information may be disclosed. This is discussed next.

DISCLOSURE WITH CONSENT

Health care records may be disclosed to other parties if the patient gives their consent. Requests from insurance companies or individuals involved in legal proceedings (for example personal injury claims) are common and information may only be disclosed with written agreement from the patient. It is important to ensure that any information provided only extends to that agreed in the written authority the patient provides.

DISCLOSURE WITHOUT PATIENT CONSENT

Disclosure without patient consent may only occur if the disclosure is required by law, for example by court order or is judged by the practitioner to be in the public interest. In determining whether there is a public interest justification to breach confidentiality, it is necessary to weigh the harm that is likely to arise from non-disclosure of information against the possible harm to the patient of disclosure. The police may also request disclosure of information in certain defined situations when the information is required for the prosecution of a criminal case or in the interests of public safety. There are clearly established regulations regarding the disclosure by clinicians of information to the police. Information *must* without exception be disclosed if the clinician is ordered to do so by a court.

DISCLOSURE TO CLINICAL TEAM MEMBERS

Most patients understand that personal information will be shared with other health care professionals in order to facilitate their ongoing care. The sharing of information should be on a need-to-know basis only, and patients have the right to request that particular information remain confidential. Where this occurs, the patient's request should be respected unless the withholding of information from other health care team members would put the patient or others at risk of serious harm or death.

RELATIVES

Patient's relatives are often present at the scene of the incident or may arrive before the patient is transported to hospital. If the patient is conscious with capacity to consent, the easiest method is to ask the patient themselves if they will give permission to discuss their condition and treatment with their relatives and if so, the degree of detail. Where a patient is not able to provide consent to this disclosure, it is still possible to discuss personal information with a patient's relatives. The GMC states *'you may need to share personal information with a patient's relatives, friends or carer to enable you to assess the patient's best interests'*. Deciding how much detail to disclose is a matter of individual judgment when determining what is in the patient's best interests. It is important to ensure that only relevant information pertaining to the particular condition is discussed.

THE POLICE

In general the police have no more right of access to medical records than anybody else, except in the following circumstances:

- Under the Road Traffic Act where the police may require the name and address of someone suspected of some form of traffic offence
- When the patient consents to disclosure
- To comply with a court order
- When public interest in disclosure outweighs the public interest in preserving patient confidentiality

When victims of violence refuse police assistance, disclosure may still be justified if others remain at risk, such as domestic violence where children may be at risk, or when the assault involved the use of weapons. The GMC states that where a patient has received gunshot or knife wounds, doctors have a duty to inform the police immediately (32). In general this extends only to the release of the patient's personal details such as name and address. However, it may also be appropriate to disclose confidential health care information of the patient. The police have a duty to consider whether there is a likelihood of further attacks.

CHILD PROTECTION

In any case where there is concern over a child's welfare, the child's best interests must be made paramount. This may require disclosure of confidential information to social services or the police, and wherever possible the parents' consent to disclosure should be obtained. This may not always be required however, if doing so would put the child at increased risk of injury.

SPECIAL CIRCUMSTANCES

In the event of a mass casualty scenario, modifications may need to be made to documentation. Triage cards often provide a useful place to document patient details, injuries and destination. This can be supplemented later on by more comprehensive medical notes or by the completion of a PRF.

There are many other forms of documentation that pre-hospital care practitioners may have to complete in line with their routine duties, for example critical incident report forms, inoculation injury forms, administration forms or police statements. The same diligence in completing these forms must be shown as when completing any other patient documentation.

SUMMARY

Handover and documentation are skills that are rarely taught but are as essential as any other in the provision of good quality pre-hospital care. A failure of either can lead to duplication of effort, loss of information and patient harm. It is essential that when a pre-alert is passed to hospital all key elements that may allow a hospital to prepare for patient arrival are passed. Using a standardised format such as ATMIST allows this to be achieved with relative ease. The primary role of good documentation is to assist with continued patient care. It also acts as reference to hospital clinicians of the events pre-hospital, for research and audit, and in case of complaint or legal proceedings. As such, meticulous documentation must occur with every patient contact. As well as moral and regulatory body obligations, the *Data Protection Act 1988* places specific duties upon each individual and organisation handling patient data. These duties are reinforced by the Caldicott principles (33). The format of data can vary from written records to electronic patient report forms through to audiovisual recordings and digital images. The pre-hospital practitioner must stay aware of the guidance available to them and the constraints these may pose. It is likely that electronic documentation will play an increasingly significant role. The introduction of the electronic patient report form (ePRF) and its integration with other NHS IT systems is likely to improve safety and efficiency of pre-hospital care medicine.

In general, only individual patients themselves may consent for what, how and when records can be made and shared about them (34). Most patients recognise that documentation will be made and shared with others within the health care team in order to continue to manage their health care. However, separate consent is required if this information is to be used for any other purpose (e.g. publication). Despite this, there are occasions when it may be possible to disclose information without the patient's consent. Such situations are uncommon, and pre-hospital practitioners are encouraged to seek guidance from their regulatory, employing or medico-legal organisation where they feel this is appropriate.

REFERENCES

1. Murray SL, Crouch R, Ainsworth-Smith M. Quality of the handover of patient care: A comparison of pre-hospital and emergency department notes. *Int Emerg Nurs.* 2012; 20(1):24–7.
2. Yong G, Dent AW, Weiland TJ. Handover from paramedics: Observations and emergency department clinician perceptions. *Emerg Med Australas.* 2008;20(2):149–55.
3. Jeffcott SA, Evans SM, Cameron PA, Chin GS, Ibrahim JE. Improving measurement in clinical handover. *Qual Saf Health Care.* 2009;18(4):272–7.
4. Safe handover: safe patients. British Medical Association Junior Doctors Committee 2004.
5. Evans SM, Murray A, Patrick I, Fitzgerald M, Smith S, Cameron P. Clinical handover in the trauma setting: A qualitative study of paramedics and trauma team members. *Qual Saf Health Care.* 2010;19(6):e57.
6. Carter AJ, Davis KA, Evans LV, Cone DC. Information loss in emergency medical services handover of trauma patients. *Prehosp Emerg Care.* 2009;13(3):280–5.
7. Evans SM, Murray A, Patrick I, Fitzgerald M, Smith S, Andrianopoulos N, Cameron P. Assessing clinical handover between paramedics and the trauma team. *Injury.* 2010;41(5):460–4.
8. Stiell A, Forster AJ, Stiell IG et al. Prevalence of information gaps in the emergency department and the effect on patient outcomes. *CMAJ.* 2003;169(10):1023–8.
9. Thakore S, Morrison W. A survey of the perceived quality of patient handover by ambulance staff in the resuscitation room. *Emerg Med J.* 2001;18(4):293–6.
10. Owen C, Hemmings L, Brown T. Lost in translation: Maximizing handover effectiveness between paramedics and receiving staff in the emergency department. *Emerg Med Australas.* 2009;21(2):102–7.
11. Learmonth SR, Ireland A, McKiernan CJ, Burton P. Does initiation of an ambulance pre-alert call reduce the door to needle time in acute myocardial infarct? *Emerg Med J.* 2006;23(1):79–81.
12. McInerney JJ, Ward CT, Hussan TB. Strategies to improve communication at the pre-hospital/accident and emergency interface. *Prehospital Immediate Care.* 2000:176–9.
13. Brown E, Bleetman A. Ambulance alerting to hospital: The need for clearer guidance. *Emerg Med J.* 2006;23(10):811–14.
14. Crystal R, Bleetman A, Steyn R. Ambulance crew assessment of trauma severity and alerting practice for trauma patients brought to a general hospital. *Resuscitation.* 2004;60:279–82.
15. Budd H, Almond L, Porter K. A survey of trauma alert criteria and handover practice in England and Wales. *Emerg Med J.* 2007;24:302–4.
16. Bruce K, Suserud BO. The handover process and triage of ambulance-borne patients: The experiences of emergency nurses. *Nurs Crit Care.* 2005;10(4):201–9.
17. Talbot R, Bleetman A. Retention of information by emergency department staff at ambulance handover: Do standardised approaches work? *Emerg Med J.* 2007;24(8):539–42.

18. Stannard A, Tai N, Bowley D et al. Key performance indicators in British military trauma. *World J Surg.* 2008;32:1870–3.
19. Selden BS, Schnitzer PG, Nolan FX. Medicolegal documentation of prehospital triage. *Ann Emerg Med.* 1990;19(5):547–51.
20. MPS factsheet, Access to Health Records. www.medical protection.org/uk/factsheets
21. MPS booklet, MPS Guide to Medical Records. www.medical protection.org/uk/booklet
22. Harkins S. Documentation: Why is it so important? *Emerg Med Serv.* 2002;31(10):89–90, 93–4.
23. HPC, Standards of proficiency – Paramedics. http://www.hpc-uk.org/assets/documents/1000051CStandards_of_Proficiency_Paramedics.pdf (accessed 25 May 2013).
24. NMC, Record keeping – Guidance for nurses and midwives. http://www.nmc-uk.org/Documents/NMC-Publications/NMC-Record-Keeping-Guidance.pdf (accessed 25 May 2013).
25. Soler JM, Montes MF, Egol EB et al. The ten year malpractice experience of a large urban EMS system. *Ann Emerg Med.* 1985;14:982–5.
26. Ayres JR. Jr: The law and You: Causes of lawsuits: Emergency Medical Update (video-cassette series). Winslow, Washington, Ellen Lockert and Assoc, Inc., 1988 Vol1 P4.
27. Felleiter P, Helm M, Lampl L, Bock KH. Data processing in prehospital emergency medicine. *Int J Clin Monit Comput.* 1995;12(1):37–41.
28. Ambulance Electronic Patient Report: Standard specification Information Standards Board for Health and Social Care 2011. www.isb.nhs.uk/documents/isb-1516/amd-48-2010/1516482010spec.pdf
29. GMC, Making and Using Visual and Audio Recordings of Patients – Guidance for Doctors (2011). www.gmc-uk.org/recordings
30. NHS Trust fined £325,000 following data breach affecting thousands of patients and staff. Information Commissioners Office Press Release. http://www.ico.org.uk/news/latest_news/2012/nhs-trust-fined-325000-following-data-breach-affecting-thousands-of-patients-and-staff-01062012 (accessed 25 May 2013).
31. GMC, Confidentiality – Guidance for Doctors (2009). www.gmc-uk.org/recordings
32. GMC Confidentiality: Reporting Gunshot and Knife Wounds (2009).
33. The Caldicott Guardian Manual 2010 Department of Health UK.
34. Information Commissioners Office: Principles of data protection. http://www.ico.org.uk/for_organisations/data_protection/the_guide/the_principles (accessed 2 June 2013).

FURTHER READING

Borst N, Crilly J, Wallis M, Paaterson E, Chaboyer W. Clinical handover of patients arriving by ambulance to the emergency department – A literature review. *International Emergency Nursing* 2010;18:210–20.

Chapleau W, Pons P. *Emergency Medical Technician: Making the Difference.* Elsevier, 2006.

General Medical Council. Consent – Patients and doctors making decision together. Guidance for Doctors 2008. www.gmc-uk.org/recordings.

The Information Commissioners Office. http://ico.org.uk.

Data Protection Act 1988. http://www.legislation.gov.uk/ukpga/1998/29/contents.

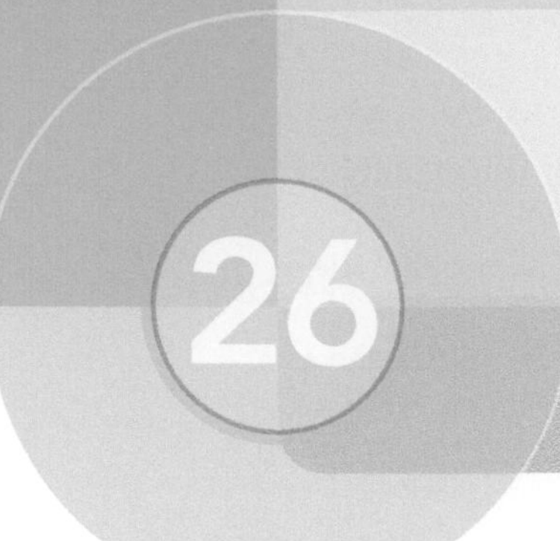

Law and ethics in pre-hospital care

OBJECTIVES

After completing this chapter the reader will

- Understand the important legal principles relevant to the practice of pre-hospital care
- Be aware of some of the ethical challenges of pre-hospital practice
- Be more able to practise in the pre-hospital environment safely and within the law

INTRODUCTION

Central to the issues of lawful and ethical practice in pre-hospital trauma care is the concept of accountability. Whilst clinicians and leaders have a considerable degree of freedom and autonomy in making clinical and policy decisions, they are accountable for their actions and for the decisions they make. Oxford Dictionaries regard those who are accountable as being 'required or expected to justify actions or decisions' (1). The ability to justify one's decisions or actions is important, but it is equally important to know who it is that can call us to account for our decisions or actions. That professionals engaged in the provision and delivery of any aspect of healthcare are accountable to their patients is obvious. However, there are also official bodies charged with the responsibility of protecting the interests of service users, acting on their behalf and calling clinicians and leaders to account. In particular, clinicians and leaders are subject to the accountability requirements of their professional regulator and in law. They are also expected, partly as a matter of professional regulation but also as a matter of personal integrity, to operative within an ethical framework.

This chapter will address some of the issues faced by those involved in pre-hospital trauma care in the areas of professional regulation, the law and ethical theory. Whilst these issues are considered individually, there is overlap between the different areas of regulation, law and ethics, and occasionally contradiction between them.

PROFESSIONAL ACCOUNTABILITY AND REGULATION

Most of those working in the field of pre-hospital trauma care will be subject to professional regulation: doctors by the General Medical Council, paramedics by the Health and Care Professions Council, and nurses by the Nursing and Midwifery Council. Whilst each of these professional groups has a different regulator, the standards the regulators set out as required of their registrants are broadly similar with the protection of the public as a central tenet. In the case of the General Medical Council, this is articulated in the document 'Good Medical Practice' (2); in 'Standards of Conduct, Performance and Ethics' (3) for the Health and Care Professions Council; and 'The Code: Standards of Conduct, Performance and Ethics for Nurses and Midwives' (4) for the Nursing and Midwifery Council.

The published standards of conduct set out the requirements of healthcare professionals in generic terms but must be applied to the specialist field in which the professional is working, in this case pre-hospital trauma care. Professional regulators require

- That registrants are skilled and knowledgeable in their area of practice
- That their skills and knowledge are up to date
- That they act within the limits of their own knowledge and skills

It is incumbent upon registrants to define their scope of practice, in that they must only undertake skills they are competent to perform or make decisions they are competent to make. This is particularly important in specialist areas, such as pre-hospital trauma care where there is a risk of informal and ad hoc development of skills without the appropriate governance arrangements being in place.

Regulators require registrants to work safely and effectively, to engage in effective communication with those they encounter in their professional practice and to provide appropriate supervision of those to whom they have delegated tasks. In highly pressured and time-critical situations, such as are frequently encountered in pre-hospital trauma care, registrants must take care to avoid inappropriate delegation for the sake of expedience. Asking a colleague to undertake a task they are not qualified to, or lawfully permitted to undertake, can expose the patient to increased risk. Allowing a student or trainee to undertake a task they have been taught to do, that will be part of their role and is performed under close supervision is permissible. This is not delegation but supervised practice. The two are not the same and should not be confused.

Professional regulators exercise their duty to protect the public in a number of ways: ensuring those entering the profession have qualified in their discipline and specialism via an approved programme of study, maintaining a register of those eligible to practise in that discipline, and monitoring standards of performance and conduct. In effect the regulator seeks to ensure registrants meet and maintain standards and that they are fit for practice.

CRIMINAL AND CIVIL LAW

LEGAL ACCOUNTABILITY

There is no single legal system operating in the United Kingdom. There are in fact three systems: law applying to England and Wales, Scotland and Northern Ireland. There are some broad principles shared across the different legal systems, but there are also some significant differences.

It is beyond the scope of this chapter to provide an analysis of the differences. The broad principles will be considered in the context of the legal system operating in England and Wales.

In very broad terms, the law can be divided into *criminal law* and *civil law*. Both branches have relevance to those working in pre-hospital trauma care.

Criminal law relates to behaviour that is forbidden by the state and which the state seeks to control by means of punishment. It is designed to maintain order and protect society (5). Criminal offences include assault, homicide, possession and supply of drugs, and driving under the influence of drugs or alcohol.

Civil law relates to matters of concern to individuals rather than the state, for example a contract between two or more individuals. Civil law includes law as it applies to the family, the law relating to property and the area this chapter will concentrate on, the law of tort. The law of tort relates to a wrong affecting an individual or individuals and which has not arisen from a prior agreement. It is there to preserve the rights of the individual (5). Negligence falls within the remit of the law of tort.

Law is derived from two main sources: that created by parliament in the form of Acts of Parliament (statute law) and that created by precedent, following the decisions made by the courts in previous cases, often described as common law or case law.

STATUTE

Those working in the pre-hospital trauma care are subject to the requirements of an extensive and diverse range of statutory legislation. The possession, prescribing and administration of medicines falling within, for example, the Medicines Act 1968 and the Misuse of Drugs Act 1971 which are implemented in orders such as the Prescription Only Medicines (Human Use) Order 1997. Other important legislation relating to clinical care includes the Mental Capacity Act 2005, the Mental Health Act 1983, the Human Rights Act 1998, the Equality Act 2010 and the Children Act 1989.

Other legislation, whilst not directly concerned with clinical care, has clear implications for those working in the field of pre-hospital trauma care, for example the Health and Safety at Work Act 1974, the Health and Social Care Act 2012, the Data Protection Act 1998, Access to Health Records Act 1990 and the Freedom of Information Act 2000. In addition there is a legislation relating to operating and driving an emergency vehicle as well as general road traffic legislation.

COMMON LAW

Civil law is largely underpinned by the law of precedent and is created by the interpretation, by the courts, of legal principles and decisions made by the courts in previous cases. For this reason, the law continues to evolve. However, there are a number of landmark cases which form the basis of legal principles and reasoning. For example, in establishing the minimum standard of care a clinician should provide the courts often follow the principle set out in the case of *Bolam v Friern Hospital Management Committee* (1957). In that case, Mr Justice McNair, when directing the jury, stated that *a doctor is not guilty of negligence if he has acted in accordance with the practice accepted as proper by a responsible body of medical men skilled in that particular art.* Although specific reference is made to doctors, the principle has been applied in respect of many other healthcare professionals. Almost inevitably, the Bolam test has been successfully challenged in the courts in the case of Bolitho (*Bolitho v. City and Hackney Health Authority* [1997]) which established that a judge would be entitled to choose between two bodies of expert opinion and to reject an opinion which is 'logically indefensible' even if it were followed by a body of the profession. Thus *Bolam* can no longer be relied on as a defence, although a judge is likely to override the opinion of a body of professional experts in only the most exceptional circumstances.

CONSENT AND CAPACITY

There is a common law principle that individuals have the right to have their bodily integrity protected against invasion (6), underlining the individual's right to autonomy and self-determination. In accepting this principle, the pre-hospital trauma clinician requires permission or consent in order to lawfully treat the individual. There are of course a small number of circumstances where the clinician can intervene without consent, for example in an emergency and where the patient is unconscious.

It is generally accepted that for consent to be valid there are three basic requirements: consent must be given freely and voluntarily, the individual must have sufficient information on which to base their consent, and they must have sufficient mental capacity to be able to give consent (7).

If, therefore, an individual has the mental capacity to do so, they are free to decide whether they agree to a proposed treatment or not, even if the healthcare professional believes that decision to be unwise. Attempting to persuade an individual to accept a course of action, to the point of coercion, is likely to invalidate consent. The argument that this was done on the basis of acting in the patient's best interest will provide no defence. Patients must be given the freedom to make their own choices. However, in order to make a decision, individuals need information on which to base their decision. The information provided by the clinician must be balanced, allowing the patient to understand the benefits and risks. It is not appropriate to provide the patient with only the benefits of an intervention in order to sway their decision and secure consent to proceed. In accepting that the clinician is bound to provide the patient with sufficient information to make a decision, it is less clear how much information the clinician should provide. The principle is addressed in the case of *Sidaway v Bethlem RHG* (1985) which established that it was not necessary to warn the patient of every risk, but that the patient should be provided with sufficient information for them to reach a balanced decision and the disclosure of risk must be in line with that of a respectable body of medical opinion.

The issue of whether the individual has the mental capacity to give consent is set out in the Mental Capacity Act 2005. The overarching principle in this legislation is that everyone has mental capacity regardless of age or appearance. The act sets out the principles in Box 26.1.

BOX 26.1: Requirements under the Mental Capacity Act 2005

- A person must be assumed to have capacity unless it is established that he lacks capacity.
- A person is not to be treated as unable to make a decision unless all practicable steps to help him to do so have been taken without success.
- A person is not to be treated as unable to make a decision merely because he makes an unwise decision.
- An act done, or decision made, under this act for or on behalf of a person who lacks capacity must be done, or made, in his best interests.
- Before the act is done, or the decision is made, regard must be had to whether the purpose for which it is needed can be as effectively achieved in a way that is less restrictive of the person's rights and freedom of action.

Pre-hospital trauma clinicians are often in the difficult position of having to determine if an individual lacks capacity to allow them to act without consent, in their best interest. In order to establish if an individual has mental capacity, the act deems an individual to lack mental capacity if they cannot

- Understand the information relevant to the decision
- Retain that information
- Use or weigh up that information as part of the process of making the decision
- Communicate their decision, by any means

CONSENT AND CAPACITY: CHILDREN

In law, an adult is a person aged 18 or over, but this does not mean that younger people cannot make autonomous decisions. The principles of the Mental Capacity Act 2005 stand regardless of age.

Children 16 or 17 years old are presumed to have capacity and are able to give consent for treatment, unless they lack capacity for reasons other than age. Whilst the 16 or 17 year old can consent to treatment; their decision to refuse treatment can be overridden by a person with parental responsibility.

The issue of who has parental responsibility is not as clear-cut as it first appears. For example, the father of the child may not have parental responsibility if he was not married to the mother at the time of the birth or is not named on the birth certificate. Parental responsibility under the Children Act 1989 is described in Box 26.2.

BOX 26.2: Responsibility for Children (Children Act 1989)

- A mother always has parental responsibility for her child. Unless this has passed to another agency following statutory intervention.
- A father only has this responsibility if he is married to the mother when the child is born or has acquired legal responsibility for his child by:
  - Jointly registering the birth of the child with the mother (since December 2003)
  - A parental responsibility agreement with the mother
  - A parental responsibility order, made by a court
  - A child arrangements or residence order made by a court.
- A local authority may have responsibility designated to them in a care order in respect of the child (but not where the child is being looked after under section 20 of the Children Act, also known as being 'accommodated' or in 'voluntary care').
- A local authority or other authorised person may hold an emergency protection order in respect of the child.

In respect of same sex civil partners, the biological mother will automatically have parental responsibility. Her partner can acquire parental responsibility if

- She and the mother were in a civil partnership or, deemed to have been in a civil partnership, at the time of the child's birth.
- Her name is registered on the birth certificate.
- She has entered into a parental responsibility agreement with the mother.
- She has obtained a court order for parental responsibility.
- She has a residence order.

In the landmark case of *Gillick v West Norfolk Area Health Authority [1986] AC 112*, Lord Scarman indicated that a child under 16 years may be legally competent to give consent to treatment providing they have 'sufficient understanding and intelligence to enable [them] to understand fully what is proposed'. In interpreting this, the clinician ought to take into account whether the child

- Understands the medical issues including benefit and risk
- Has views of their own and is not just repeating the views of others
- Understands the moral issues of the decision
- Is evidently competent

This, of course, is a complex issue when there is time to make a decision. However, it is significantly more challenging in a time-critical situation requiring important decisions to be made quickly.

The Mental Capacity Act 2005 makes provision for those emergency situations affecting adults and children and where consent cannot be obtained. In such circumstances the clinician can provide necessary clinical care limited to saving a life or preventing significant deterioration. In practice, it is extremely unlikely that a legal challenge would follow treatment given in good faith and in what was believed to be the patient's best interest.

NEGLIGENCE

The matter of clinical malpractice can be dealt with by a number of means, including criminal prosecution, regulatory fitness to practise procedures and civil law, normally within the scope of the law of tort (7).

In order for an individual to succeed in a civil claim of negligence they must demonstrate that they were owed a duty of care by the defendant, that there was a breach in that duty of care and this resulted in them being harmed (7). Some argue that there is a further theoretical construct, that of fault (6).

Simply put, a duty of care is owed to anyone you may foreseeably injure (7). The issue of whether injury was foreseeable was raised in the case of *Donoghue (or McAlister) v Stevenson [1932] AC 562*, where the judge indicated that *'you must take reasonable care to avoid acts or omissions which you can reasonably foresee would be likely to injure your neighbour. Who, then, in law is my neighbour? The answer seems to be persons who are so closely and directly affected by my act that I ought reasonably to have them in contemplation as being so affected when I am directing my mind to the acts or omissions which are called in question'.* In respect of the pre-hospital clinician treating an injured patient, it is apparent that the clinician would owe the patient a duty of care.

Reference has already been made to the Bolam Case (p. 373) which offers the clinician a defence against a claim of clinical negligence if they can demonstrate there is a responsible body of medical (professional) opinion that the clinician's actions were acceptable (7). This issue was evolved in the case of *Bolitho v City and Hackney HA [1997] 4 All ER 771* which introduced a test of logic in that a judge is entitled to take a view that a clinician may not have acted reasonably even if fellow professionals regarded it reasonable if it is not logical to do so.

The matter of harm is tied into the concept of causation, which might be best explained by way of the 'but for' test. The principle being 'but for the actions of the clinician the patient would not have been harmed'. In simple terms had the clinician not done what they did, or omitted to do what they ought to have done, the patient would not have been harmed.

ETHICAL RESPONSIBILITY

It is suggested that in making ethical decisions the clinician should contemplate 'what ought I do?' rather than the 'what will I do?' (8). In order to decide what one ought to do, clinicians need a framework to support ethical decision-making. Ethicists have proposed four key principles worthy of consideration (9), namely autonomy, beneficence, non-maleficence and justice.

AUTONOMY

Autonomy is a principle at the centre of the Mental Capacity Act 2005 but has a broader reach. It is the principle that individuals have the right of self-determination in making decisions for themselves. This includes the notion that an individual is entitled to make decisions the clinician or others might regard as being unwise. In such circumstances clinicians can be tempted into taking an alternative course of action against the patients stated wishes, claiming to be acting in the patient's best interest as a means of justification. Clearly this disregards the individual's right of autonomy and such a course of action may not actually be acting in the patient's best interest.

BENEFICENCE

The principle of beneficence is one of aiming to do good. This must be balanced against the patient's right of autonomy. To that end, the decision to do good or act in the patient's best interests should be patient centred and not clinician centred (10).

NON-MALEFICENCE

Non-maleficence is almost the opposite to the principle of beneficence in that it is the principle of doing no harm. However, it is a principle of balance that accepts harm may not be entirely avoidable, for example the insertion of an intraosseous cannula may necessary to save a life, but may not avoid doing harm such as pain or the introduction of the risk of infection. The balance of beneficence with non-maleficence is about striving to eliminate avoidable harm.

JUSTICE

When regarded from a theoretical perspective, patients would receive all the necessary care to the highest standards available with few if any negative effects. In reality such a situation does not exist, for many reasons, not least because of an environment of finite resources. The principle of justice deals with these issues, incorporating fairness, equality and reasonableness (7).

CONCLUSION

Those involved with pre-hospital trauma care are subject to a degree of scrutiny, guidance and direction, in common with all other healthcare providers. Safe practice (for both patient and doctor) requires a knowledge of legal principles and an awareness of potential ethical challenges. Much of this, however, is common sense: if in doubt, the practitioner should always do what they consider to be best for the patient.

REFERENCES

1. *Oxford Dictionaries.* Accountable (adj.). Accessed December 22, 2014. http://www.oxforddictionaries.com/definition/english/accountable.
2. General Medical Council. Good medical practice. September 2014.
3. Health and Care Professions Council. Standards of conduct, performance and ethics. July 2012.
4. Nursing and Midwifery Council. The Code: Standards of conduct, performance and ethics for nurses and midwives. July 2014.
5. Hope RA, Savulescu J, Hendrick J. *Medical Ethics and Law.* Elsevier Health Sciences, 2008.
6. Mason K, Laurie G. *Mason and McCall Smith's Law and Medical Ethics.* 9th ed. Oxford: Oxford University Press, 2013.
7. Herring J. *Medical Law.* Oxford: Oxford University Press, 2011.
8. Thomson A. *Critical Reasoning in Ethics.* London: Routledge, 2002.
9. Beauchamp TL, Childress JF. *Principles of Biomedical Ethics.* 7th ed. Oxford: Oxford University Press, 2013.
10. Campbell AV, Gillett G, Jones DG. *Medical Ethics.* New York: Oxford University Press, 2005.

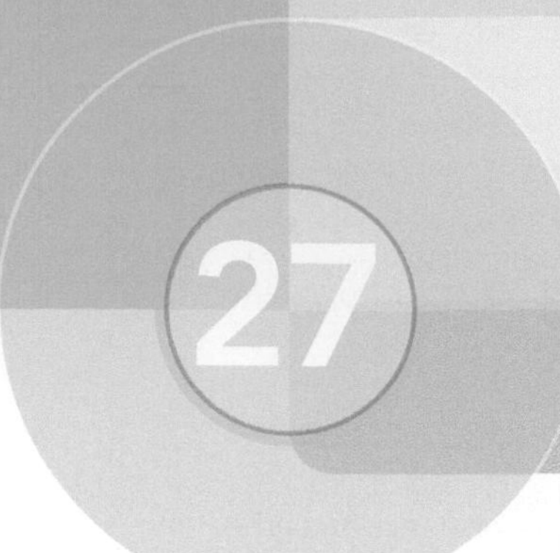

27 Research and audit in pre-hospital care

OBJECTIVES

After completing this chapter the reader will

- Understand what the processes of research and audit entail
- Understand the importance of collecting high-quality clinical data
- Understand how research and audit improve clinical care

INTRODUCTION

Clinicians, educators and researchers in all clinical specialties seek the best outcomes for patients. Those involved in pre-hospital trauma care should be no different. Key to achieving this aim is the use of high-quality, outcome-focused evidence to inform and underpin practice. This important principle is, however, more difficult to adhere to in pre-hospital care than in many other areas of medical practice.

Standard, generally accepted practice in the pre-hospital management of the trauma patient often lacks an evidence base. Where evidence does exist, it is often weak, based on consensus opinion and lacking empirical rigor. The assumption is often made that interventions which have been shown to be effective in hospital will be equally appropriate in immediate care. There are, however, some notable examples of areas of practice supported by high-quality evidence, for example we know that early pre-hospital administration of tranexamic acid to trauma patients with, or at risk of, significant bleeding reduces the risk of death from haemorrhage (1). The challenge here is knowing the extent to which this knowledge has been disseminated and is implemented in practice. We do not know if, internationally, nationally or locally, all eligible patients who would benefit from the treatment are receiving it in line with published guidance.

Research and audit help address some of the challenges, with clinicians using existing research evidence to inform their practice as well as identifying clinical problems which are worthy of investigation. Researchers should be responding to the ideas emerging from practice and developing the evidence which will allow educators to help disseminate their findings. Audit then helps in the implementation of new evidence-based guidelines and the understanding of the extent to which existing evidence-based guidance is implemented in practice.

At least in part because pre-hospital emergency medicine has only recently been accepted as a medical sub-speciality, there is not, as yet, a peer-reviewed journal devoted to this area of practice.

RESEARCH

The word *research* can convey a sense of dry academic work somewhat remote from the real world of clinical practice, yet, when we consider research in the context of evidence-based practice, the benefits for clinicians and for patients become obvious.

Research provides clinicians with the evidence to change practice, to know how effective their intervention or interventions are likely to be, and to understand the likely benefits and risks for patients. In the words of Archie Cochrane, evidence-based health care is *'the conscientious use of current best evidence in making decisions about the care of individual patients or the delivery of health services. Current best evidence is up-to-date information from relevant, valid research about the effects of different forms of health care, the potential for harm from exposure to particular agents, the accuracy of diagnostic tests, and the predictive power of prognostic factors'* (2).

There are thus two groups: the researchers, who produce the evidence through scientific study, and those who consume the evidence, including both clinicians and policy makers. The two are mutually dependent: clinicians identifying aspects of practice where they lack evidence to inform decisions, the researchers undertaking scientific study to answer the questions and the clinicians implementing the findings of the researcher. Whilst the roles are different, it is not uncommon for the clinician and the researcher to be one and the same person.

CLINICAL QUESTIONS

Clinicians can and do encounter situations where they are unsure of the right course of action or which course of action would deliver the greatest benefit or least risk to the patient. In the face of uncertainty, it has been argued that the first step is to translate that uncertainty into answerable clinical questions (3).

For questions to be useful they should be answerable, specific and clearly articulated. With this in mind, questions should be constructed in a structured and reproducible manner. It is not essential that a standard question template is used, but the *three-part question* and the *PICO* question (population [participants], intervention [or exposure for observational studies], comparator and outcomes) are often used.

The three-part question includes the patient characteristic (e.g. adults with penetrating chest injury), an intervention or defining question (e.g. respiratory rate) and an outcome (e.g. survival). This might be constructed into a question such as *'In adults with penetrating trauma to the chest (P) is respiratory rate (I) a good predictor of survival (O)?'*

An alternative that allows for a comparator to be introduced but follows a similar format is the PICO question. The P, I and O are as described in the three-part question, but PICO introduces a comparator. A PICO question might be *'In adult patients with penetrating chest trauma (P) does the administration of intravenous fluids (I) when compared with not administering intravenous fluid (C) improve survival (O)?'*

The question can be made more specific by the addition of the context of care, such as the pre-hospital phase. For example *'In adult patients with penetrating chest trauma (P) does the administration of intravenous fluids in the pre-hospital environment (I) improve survival (O) when compared to withholding intravenous fluid in the pre-hospital environment (C)?'*

Patient or population characteristics, interventions and their comparators are often relatively straightforward to define. Outcome measures can be a little more complex. When formulating the outcome component, it is advantageous that they are patient orientated rather than disease orientated. A disease-orientated outcome might focus on the effect of intervention *X* compared with intervention *Y* in arresting catastrophic external haemorrhage. This outcome measures the control of haemorrhage but does not provide any information on the impact this has on survival. There would be little benefit if haemorrhage were controlled more quickly using a given intervention, but that survival rates using either method were the same. A patient-focused outcome is more concerned with outcomes such as mortality or morbidity. In this case the question may focus on whether intervention *X* resulted in an increased rate of survival to discharge compared with intervention *Y*.

DISCOVERING WHAT IS ALREADY KNOWN

Once properly structured, the question can form the basis of a search of the medical literature to discover if the answer to the question is already known. A well-structured and executed search strategy will help to identify published work that may answer or contribute to answering the question. It is important when searching and reviewing the literature that a distinction is made between opinion and research evidence. Given that the clinician is seeking evidence to support their decision-making, it is the research evidence to which they should be giving weight. They may also wish to restrict their search for evidence to particular types of research which are more robust and scientifically rigorous. This is discussed further in the hierarchy of evidence.

Caution must be exercised when the search reveals a single research report on a particular issue. Some large studies may be sufficiently robust to allow their findings to be used to support clinical decision-making. However, in many cases this evidence does not exist, but there is a body of smaller studies which, when combined, may provide the clinician with the confidence to implement findings.

Many research studies have negative findings, that is they do not prove what it was initially thought they would or they disprove the initial theory. This information can be as important as studies proving the theory. It is as useful to know if an intervention does not improve outcome so we can stop doing it, as it is to know something improves outcome. Unfortunately, negative findings are often not published or may even be suppressed.

COMBINING EXISTING KNOWLEDGE TO PRODUCE ROBUST EVIDENCE

Perhaps the most valuable source of evidence is where the findings of several studies are combined to produce new knowledge and findings that are more robust than any single report. Such studies are termed *systematic reviews*. As the name suggests, a rigorous and systematic search is made of the literature to identify as much published and unpublished evidence on the given issue as possible. This is subjected to detailed analysis and, where appropriate, further statistical testing, in order to generate new knowledge.

Systematic reviews are particularly helpful to the consumers of research in that the reviewers have undertaken the time-consuming processes of developing a search strategy, searching the literature, filtering out weak or irrelevant studies, analysing all of the data and then drawing conclusions. This allows the consumer of the research to access the best available evidence, but in a time-efficient manner.

Systematic reviews take a lot of time and can be expensive to conduct. Furthermore, not all aspects of practice have been investigated in this way. As a result, whilst being potentially very useful, systematic reviews are relatively few in number and will not cover all areas of pre-hospital clinical practice.

GENERATING NEW EVIDENCE

For much of health care practice, there is relatively little research evidence to underpin clinical decisions. Where evidence does not exist, clinical questions may form the basis for scientific research studies.

Although there are many aspects of pre-hospital trauma care that might benefit from the attention of scientific research, there are some issues that cannot be investigated for reasons of cost, practicality or ethics. For example, it might be of value to explore outcome following oxygen therapy in severe trauma by giving some patients 100% oxygen, some 28% oxygen and others no oxygen at all. In reality, it is unlikely that such an investigation could be carried out due to ethical objections. Many would see it as inappropriate to withhold treatment thought to be but not proven to be effective.

It may not be possible for many pre-hospital clinicians to be directly involved in conducting primary research. However, clinicians can be enormously helpful in the identification of practice where they are uncertain of the optimal intervention. Thus they have a vital role in developing clinical questions even if they are unable to find evidence-based answers.

THE HIERARCHY OF EVIDENCE

Pre-hospital clinicians must be alert to the relative value or potency of the evidence they use to inform practice. This is often influenced by the methodological approach or design of the research study. Not all published evidence carries the same weight. Unfortunately much of the evidence underpinning pre-hospital practice is relatively weak.

A number of frameworks are used to rank research evidence in order of its reliability in answering research questions. The Oxford 2011 levels of evidence table is widely used for this purpose (Table 27.1).

SUMMARISING EVIDENCE

It is clearly not practical for clinicians to read all the research evidence relevant to their area of practice, particularly if this involves reading hundreds of individual papers on any given issue. The best solution is summarised evidence, where the work of sourcing and reviewing of the literature is carried out by a review team and the findings published in a digestible form.

Table 27.1 The Oxford Levels of Evidence

Oxford Centre Evidence-Based Medicine 2011 Levels of Evidence					
Question	**Step 1 (Level 1*)**	**Step 2 (Level 2*)**	**Step3 (Level 3*)**	**Step 4 (Level 4*)**	**Step 5 (Level 5*)**
How common is the problem?	Local and current random sample surveys (or censuses)	Systematic review of surveys that allow matching to local circumstances**	Local non-random sample**	Case-series**	n/a
Is this diagnostic or monitoring test accurate? (Diagnosis)	Systematic review of cross-sectional studies with consistently applied reference standard and blinding	Individual cross-sectional studies with consistently applied reference standard and blinding	Non-consecutive studies, or studies without consistently applied reference standards**	Case-control studies, or 'poor or non-independent reference standard'	Mechanism-based reasoning
What will happen if we do not add a therapy? (Prognosis)	Systematic review of inception cohort studies	Inception cohort studies	Cohort study or control arm of randomised trial*	Case-series or case-control studies, or poor quality prognostic cohort study**	n/a
Does this intervention help? (Treatment Benefits)	Systematic review of randomised trials or *n*-of-1 trials	Randomised trial or observational study with dramatic effect	Non-randomised controlled cohort/ follow-up study**	Case-series or case-control, or historically controlled studies**	Mechanism-based reasoning

(*Continued*)

Table 27.1 (Continued) The Oxford Levels of Evidence

Oxford Centre Evidence-Based Medicine 2011 Levels of Evidence					
Question	**Step 1 (Level 1*)**	**Step 2 (Level 2*)**	**Step3 (Level 3*)**	**Step 4 (Level 4*)**	**Step 5 (Level 5*)**
What are the COMMON harms? (Treatment Harms)	Systematic review of randomised trials, systematic review of nested case-control studies, *n*-of-1 trial with the patient you are raising the question about, or observational study with dramatic effect	Individual randomised trial or (exceptionally) observational study with dramatic effect	Non-randomised controlled cohort/ follow-up study (post-marketing surveillance) provided there are sufficient numbers to rule out a common harm. (For long-term harms the duration of follow-up must be sufficient.)**	Case-series, case-control studies, or historically controlled studies**	Mechanism-based reasoning
What are the RARE harms? (Treatment Harms)	Systematic review of randomised trials or *n*-of-1 trial	Randomised trial or (exceptionally) observational study with dramatic effect			
Is this (early detection) test worthwhile? (Screening)	Systematic review of randomised trials	Randomised trial	Non-randomised controlled cohort/ follow-up study**	Case-series, case-control, or historically controlled studies**	Mechanism-based reasoning

Abbreviation: n/a, not applicable.

* Level may be graded down on the basis of study quality, imprecision, indirectness (study PICO does not match questions PICO), because of inconsistency between studies, or because the absolute effect size is very small; level may be graded up if there is a large or very large effect size.

** As always, a systematic review is generally better than an individual study.

The Cochrane Collaborative lead the way in this field, but the Oxford Centre for Evidence-based Medicine also recommends *BMJ Clinical Evidence, NHS Clinical Knowledge Summaries, Dynamed, Physicians Information and Education Resource* and *UpToDate*.

CLINICAL AUDIT

The NHS Clinical Governance Support Team describes clinical audit as *'a quality improvement process that seeks to improve the patient care and outcomes through systematic review of care against explicit criteria and the implementation of change'* (4). To that end clinical audit must be viewed as a part of the clinical governance and quality arrangements of the provider organisation and be considered essential in driving up the standards of pre-hospital trauma care.

A key element of clinical audit is that measurement of performance or compliance is set against agreed standards and criteria. It therefore follows that the routine review of log books or patient report forms, which may be illuminating, does not amount to clinical audit if it is merely a counting exercise. For example, counting the number of times an individual successfully places a peripheral venous cannula may give an indication of levels of activity, but it does not reflect the quality of care or explain whether these interventions were appropriate. If a criteria measure were introduced, such as *'secure venous access was established in all patients with clinical evidence of hypovolaemia within 10 minutes of arrival of the pre-hospital clinician'*, this would provide much more useful information about the quality of service being provided and has a clear link with patient benefit. Log books and patient care forms do provide a useful source of data to inform clinical audit but should not be reduced solely to a simple inventory of the number of times a given procedure has been undertaken.

Provider organisations can, and should, where appropriate, contribute to national clinical audits, providing a local perspective on the national picture of pre-hospital trauma services. However, it is also important for service providers to have a detailed understanding of the quality of care they are providing locally. It is therefore essential that service providers establish an audit programme with local priorities responsive to the needs of local patients and services.

THE AUDIT CYCLE

Clinical audit is typically described as a cyclical process of preparation (standard setting), measurement of current performance, analysis, implementation of change, and re-audit to ensure change of practice. This leads back into the first stage of the next cycle (Figure 27.1).

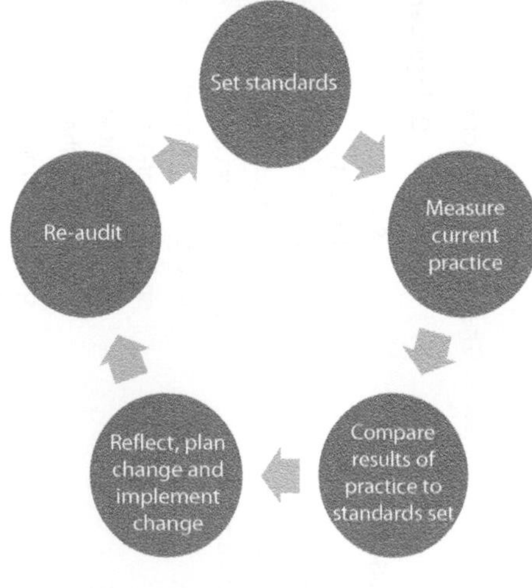

Figure 27.1 The audit cycle.

PREPARATION AND PLANNING

The starting point for anyone engaging in a clinical audit ought to be asking the question *'What needs to be improved and why?'* (5). The answer to the question may reveal a surprising number of issues worthy of investigation, often too many to be answered all at once. It is often useful to start with a blank sheet of paper and invite suggestions for clinical audit from a wide group of stakeholders. This allows a broad perspective rather than the potentially narrow or single perspective of the audit lead. Whilst wide consultation is potentially beneficial in exposing most or all of the areas of concern, in its raw form it is likely to lead to an unmanageable programme of clinical audit. Key themes will emerge and the clinical audit team will be able to establish a programme of clinical audit, prioritised or ranked on the basis of relative importance.

PRIORITIES IN THE CLINICAL AUDIT PROGRAMME

The aspects of practice where compliance with evidence and evidence-based guidelines is sub-optimal might be perfectly clear to an informed observer. This might be the starting point for developing a programme of clinical audit; however, this introduces the risk that less obvious but equally important compliance issues are not identified. It is important that a programme of clinical audit has logic in its prioritisation. The key to informing the prioritisation is the potential impact of non-compliance on patient outcome. It might be appealing to undertake a clinical audit of an area of practice where compliance with guidance is thought to be low compared with an aspect of practice where compliance is moderate to high. However, improving compliance from low to high in a practice of limited consequence for patient outcome has less value than improving compliance from an area of high compliance to 100% compliance where the practice is critical to patient outcome. For example, it might be believed that the age of adult patients was infrequently recorded on the patient care form. Quantifying the extent to which the age was not recorded, providing education to encourage compliance and then demonstrating improvement in compliance might be good practice but is unlikely to make a big impact on patient outcome. Alternatively, it might be noted that most, but not all, seriously injured patients eligible for admission to a trauma centre were considered for transfer to a trauma centre. The consequences of not considering admission to a trauma centre and transporting the patient to a general facility, albeit for a small number of patients, are likely to have a significant impact on patient outcome. In this example it might be expected that all eligible patients are considered for admission to a trauma centre and that anything short of 100% compliance is unacceptable.

Clinical audit programmes should be meaningful and not merely a process of measuring something just because it is measurable; they must focus on measuring something that could lead to patient benefit.

PRACTICE POINT

The key to informing the prioritisation is the potential impact of non-compliance on patient outcome.

PROSPECTIVE OR RETROSPECTIVE CLINICAL AUDIT

Copeland suggests that an audit conducted retrospectively, utilising existing data from clinical records or log books, may be useful in establishing a benchmark or in response to an adverse or serious untoward incident (4). A prospective audit provides greater flexibility and utility in that the audit can set out the data required to assess compliance against a standard rather than attempting to understand compliance using data gathered for another purpose. Using retrospective data may make it impossible to execute certain clinical audits. As with research, reliance on the data you have is inferior to relying on the data you need.

IDENTIFYING THE STANDARDS AGAINST WHICH PERFORMANCE WILL BE MEASURED

The standards against which compliance is measured must be credible and authoritative, as they articulate the expected standard of care in a given situation or for a particular clinical condition.

Ideally the identified standards should be evidence based and nationally agreed, such as the guidelines published by the National Institute for Health and Care Excellence (NICE) or leading specialist bodies such as the British Thoracic Society which produced the 'Guidelines for Emergency Oxygen Use in Adult Patients' (6). In reality, there are significant areas of practice that lack evidence-based guidelines, but which are informed by expert consensus opinion either at a national or local level. It is entirely permissible to use such guidelines as the basis for a clinical audit, provided that the guidance is regarded as credible.

As an underlying principle, the guidance should be able to demonstrate a positive effect on patient outcome. Although some observers do suggest that management-based outcomes, such as cost effectiveness, are appropriate outcome measures in a clinical audit (7).

CRITERIA AGAINST WHICH COMPLIANCE IS MEASURED

It is not sufficient to ask *'Are clinicians following the British Thoracic Society Guidelines for the emergency use of oxygen in adult patients?'*, although that may be the question of interest. It is necessary to define the individual components of care to be measured and the degree of compliance that will be regarded as acceptable. In some cases only 100% compliance will be acceptable, for example 100% of patients with a clinical fracture of the ankle must be assessed for neurovascular function distal to the ankle. In other situations there may be some tolerance in the accepted standard of compliance, for example at least 75% of injured patients have a pain intensity score recorded on the clinical record prior to the administration of analgesia. The extent to which compliance is regarded as acceptable must be determined at this stage and not when the audit has been started. Criteria can be phrased as a series of questions which articulate the desired standard of performance.

It is suggested (7) that to ensure that criteria are robust and reliable, the clinical auditor should consider whether

- It is possible to understand precisely what information is required
- It is possible to obtain the information required to answer the question
- The question is specific enough to give an answer that is useful and meaningful
- The question is sensitive enough to relate solely to the standard being assessed

DATA COLLECTION AND ANALYSIS

Criteria need to be translated into a data collection tool, taking account of the way in which data are to be collected (retrospectively or prospectively). The clinical auditor needs to consider the source of the data, the professional groups who are to be audited and the number of patients or patient episodes to include.

Clinical audits need to be concluded in a timely manner and this should be taken into account when deciding the size of the sample. For procedures or activities that occur frequently it may be possible to audit relatively large numbers of episodes in a short time. Where an intervention or episode occurs infrequently, it might be necessary to compromise on the sample size in order for the audit to be completed in a timely manner. There are circumstances where it is desirable to continue to monitor performance against standards. In this case there should be identified analysis points with the completion of one audit cycle before immediately rolling into the next. It is, however, important that the sample size is sufficient to allow analysis and for the results to be meaningful.

Analysis should be undertaken using a method capable of allowing a comparison to be made between the expected compliance standard and the actual compliance standard. The degree and sophistication of the analysis will be determined by the sample size and local needs.

REPORTING RESULTS AND DEVELOPING AN IMPROVEMENT PLAN

Given that the rational for undertaking a clinical audit is service improvement, it is imperative that the results of the audit are not only communicated but form the basis of a plan of improvement. The analysis is not just about reporting compliance against standards but is crucially also about trying to understand the obstacles and reasons for sub-optimal compliance.

Education is a key to the implementation of any improvement plan, articulating good practice and ways of achieving it. The clinical audit may identify very specific learning needs which are impacting on compliance and require a programme of training or retraining to correct.

RE-AUDIT

The final logical step is to evaluate the effect of the improvement plan through re-audit. Although this is the final step in one cycle, it is also the first step in the next cycle. Achieving maximum compliance is not a reason for complacency: re-audit is a vital part of achieving and maintaining service improvement.

SUMMARY

Both research and clinical audit play an important part in ensuring that seriously injured patients receive the appropriate care based on the best available evidence.

REFERENCES

1. CRASH-2 collaborators, Roberts I, Shakur H, Afolabi A, Brohi K, Coats T, Dewan Y et al. The importance of early treatment with tranexamic acid in bleeding trauma patients: An exploratory analysis of the CRASH-2 randomised controlled trial. *Lancet* 2011;377(9771):1096–1101.

2. Cochrane AL. *Effectiveness & Efficiency: Random Reflections on Health Services*. London: RSM Press, 1999.
3. Geddes J. Asking structured and focused clinical questions: Essential first step of evidence-based practice. *Evidence-Based Mental Health* 1999;2(2):35–36.
4. Copeland G. *A Practical Handbook for Clinical Audit*. London: Clinical Governance Support Team, NHS, 2005.
5. Gillam S, Siriwardena AN. Frameworks for improvement: Clinical audit, the plan-do-study-act cycle and significant event audit. *Quality in Primary Care* 2013;21(2):123–130.
6. O'Driscoll BR, Howard LS, Davison AG, British Thoracic Society. BTS guideline for emergency oxygen use in adult patients. *Thorax* 2008;63(Suppl 6):vi1–vi68.
7. Potter J, Fuller C, Ferris M. *Local Clinical Audit: Handbook For Physicians*. London: Healthcare Quality Improvement Partnership, 2010.

FURTHER READING

Centre for Evidence Based Medicine, http://www.cebm.net
Cochrane Collaborative, http://www.cochrane.org
Healthcare Quality Improvement Partnership, http://www.hqip.org.uk
Institute for Healthcare Improvement, http://www.ihi.org/Pages/default.aspx

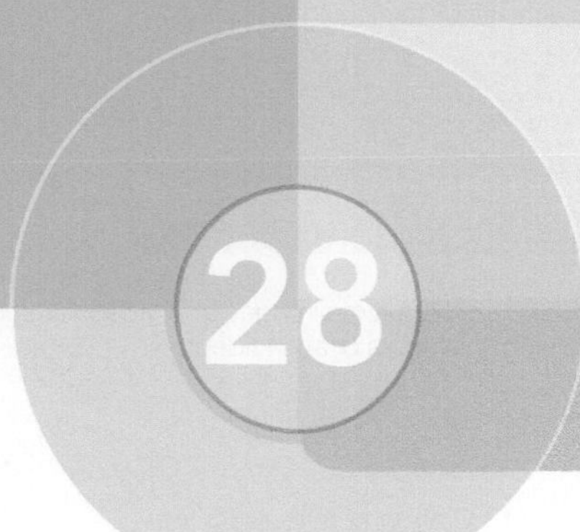

28 Training in pre-hospital emergency medicine (PHEM)

OBJECTIVES

After completing this chapter the reader will be able to

- Understand the origins of the sub-specialty of pre-hospital emergency medicine (PHEM)
- Understand the curriculum framework for PHEM
- Appreciate the role of PHEM within emergency medical systems and trauma networks

INTRODUCTION

Since its inception in 1996, the Faculty of Pre-hospital Care of the Royal College of Surgeons of Edinburgh has been active in articulating the scope of clinical practice underpinning pre-hospital care. Faculty activity has included hosting consensus conferences, developing approval and accreditation systems for training courses, and introducing the concept of a common generic curriculum for all levels of pre-hospital care. The Faculty, in partnership with the British Association for Immediate Care, has also developed the generic short courses (for example the Pre-hospital Emergency Care [PHEC] course) and formal assessments by examination (the Diploma in Immediate Care and Fellowship in Immediate Care) which have become recognised as benchmarks for basic clinical and operational practice. Eligibility to sit the Diploma in Immediate Care has now been extended to nurses and paramedics. In addition to this national educational activity, a number of operational services across the UK developed apprenticeship-style training programmes with the aim of ensuring that doctors and other pre-hospital professionals had the knowledge and skills required to operate safely. In November 2005, the Faculty hosted the first consensus meeting to articulate the competence framework for sub-specialist physician practice in pre-hospital emergency medicine (PHEM). In October 2006, a nationwide questionnaire survey of opinion leaders within UK organisations responsible for pre-hospital care was conducted, and in October 2008 the Faculty established a Curriculum Advisory Group to develop the PHEM curriculum (1,2). The key drivers for PHEM to be developed as a sub-specialist area of medical practice were to (Figure 28.1):

- Meet existing demand for on-scene and in-transit medical support (sometimes referred to as pre-hospital 'enhanced care') (3,4)
- Improve the quality and standards of pre-hospital critical care (5)

- Improve equity of access to on-scene and in-transit medical support (6)
- Improve governance of pre-hospital care and inter-hospital transfer services (7)
- Support the Care Quality Commission essential standards for quality and safety in pre-hospital care
- Improve professional training and development of pre-hospital personnel (8)
- Provide a robust medical incident response (MERIT) capability
- Provide medical leadership for pre-hospital care services and providers

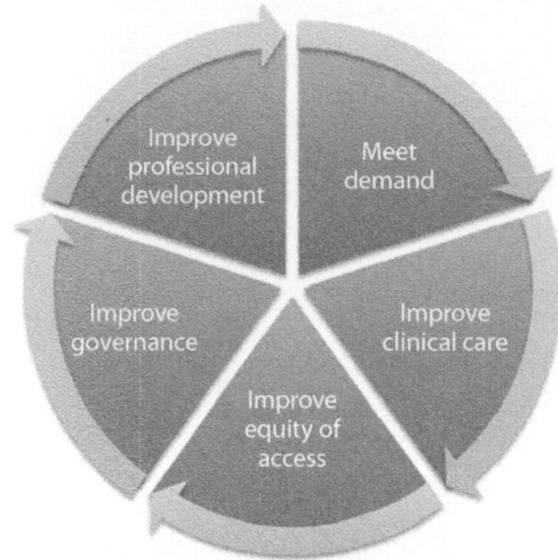

Figure 28.1 Drivers for development of PHEM as a sub-specialist area of medical care.

As a guide, pre-hospital emergency medicine (PHEM) refers to clinical intervention by doctors, and pre-hospital emergency care (PHEC) refers to treatment in the pre-hospital environment more generally. An Intercollegiate Board for Training in PHEM (IBTPHEM) was formed in May 2009. PHEM was subsequently approved by the General Medical Council (GMC) as a medical sub-specialty of emergency medicine and anaesthetics in July 2011 and of acute internal medicine and intensive care medicine in October 2013. There are now PHEM training programmes across the UK with a national recruitment framework and the aim that all UK ambulance services should have consistent immediate access to deployable sub-specialist PHEM services 24 hours a day to support personnel and patients on the ground.

ROLE OF THE PHEM PRACTITIONER

The term *pre-hospital care* covers a wide range of medical conditions, medical interventions, clinical providers and physical locations. Medical conditions range from minor illness and injury to life-threatening emergencies. Pre-hospital interventions therefore also range from simple first aid to advanced emergency care and pre-hospital emergency anaesthesia. Care providers may be lay first responders, ambulance professionals, nurses or physicians of varying backgrounds. All of this activity can take place in urban, rural or remote settings, and is generally mixed with wider out-of-hospital and unscheduled care. The complexity of unscheduled and urgent care provision is illustrated in Figure 28.2.

Another useful way to conceptualise this breadth of clinical providers is to use the levels of practice described in the Skills for Health 'Career Framework for Health' (Figure 28.3). The career framework describes the level of autonomy, responsibility and clinical decision-making expected of a health care professional operating at a particular level.

Sub-specialist PHEM practice relates to the emergency response, primary scene transfer and secondary emergency transfer functions highlighted in Figure 28.2 at the level of the consultant practitioner (level 8) illustrated in Figure 28.3, and thus as described above refers to interventions carried out by doctors. (Pre-hospital emergency care [PHEC] refers to pre-hospital practice more broadly, irrespective of who provides it.) PHEM relates to that area of medical care required for seriously ill or injured patients before they reach hospital (on scene) or during emergency transfer to or between hospitals (in-transit). It represents a unique area of medical

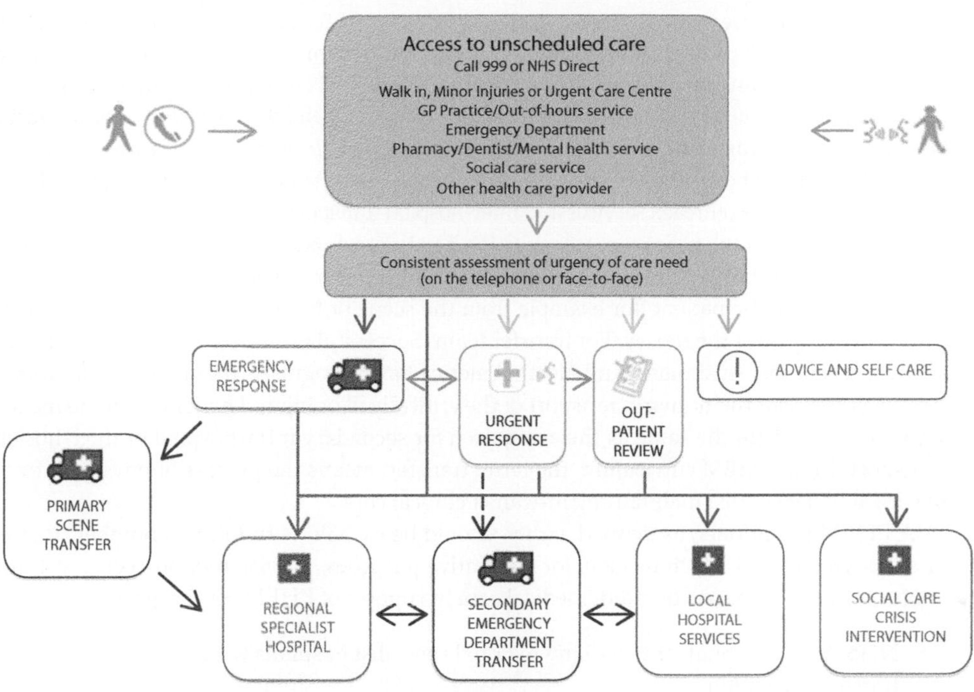

Figure 28.2 Conceptual model of effective urgent care. (Adapted from 'Direction of travel for urgent care: A discussion document', Department of Health, October 2006.)

practice which requires the focused application of a defined range of knowledge and skills to a level not normally available outside hospital.

PHEM encompasses the underpinning knowledge, technical skills and non-technical (behavioural) skills required to provide safe pre-hospital critical care and safe transfer. 'Pre-hospital' refers to all environments outside an emergency department resuscitation room or a place specifically designed for resuscitation and/or critical care in a health care setting. It usually relates to an incident scene but it includes the ambulance environment or a remote medical facility. Implicit in this term is the universal need, for this specific group of patients, for transfer to hospital. Although a component of urgent and unscheduled care (Figure 28.2), PHEM practice relates to a level of illness or injury that is usually not amenable to definitive management in the community setting and is focused on critical care in the out-of-hospital environment.

Critical care refers to the provision of organ and/or system support in the management of severely ill or injured patients. It is a clinical process rather than a physical place, and it requires the application of significant underpinning knowledge and technical skills to a level that is not ordinarily available outside

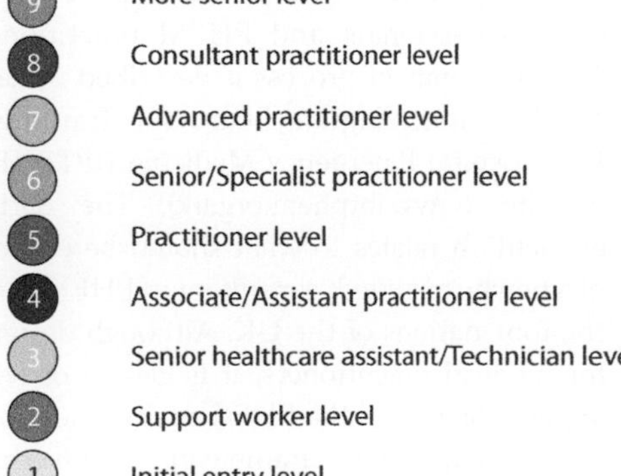
9 More senior level
8 Consultant practitioner level
7 Advanced practitioner level
6 Senior/Specialist practitioner level
5 Practitioner level
4 Associate/Assistant practitioner level
3 Senior healthcare assistant/Technician level
2 Support worker level
1 Initial entry level

Figure 28.3 Skills for Health career framework descriptors.

hospital. Hospital-based critical care is typically divided into three levels: level three (intensive care areas providing multiple organ and system support), level two (high dependency medical or surgical care areas providing single organ or system support) and level one (acute care areas such as coronary care and medical admission units). In the context of PHEM, all three levels of critical care may be required depending on the needs of the patient. In practical terms, the critical care interventions undertaken outside hospital more closely resemble those provided by hospital emergency departments, intensive care outreach services and inter-hospital transport teams.

Transfer refers to the process of transporting a patient whilst maintaining in-transit clinical care. A distinction between retrieval and transport (or transfer) is sometimes made on the basis of the location of the patient (for example from the scene or between hospitals) and the composition or origins of the retrieval or transfer team. Successful pre-hospital emergency medical services in Europe, Australasia and North America have recognised that many of the competences required for the primary transport of the critically ill or injured patient from the incident scene to hospital are the same as those required for secondary intra-hospital or inter-hospital transport. In the PHEM curriculum, the term 'transfer' means the process of physically transporting a patient whilst maintaining in-transit clinical care.

A PHEM practitioner, as defined earlier, should be capable of fulfilling a number of career or employment roles which include, for illustrative purposes, provision of on-scene, in-transit and/or on-line (telephone or radio) medical care in support of PHEM service providers such as

- NHS Acute Hospitals (particularly regional specialist hospitals with an outreach and transfer capability)
- NHS Ambulance Trusts (e.g. as part of regional Medical Emergency Response Incident Teams [MERIT] or their equivalent)
- Defence Medical Services
- Non-NHS independent sector organisations (including immediate care schemes, air ambulance charities, event medicine providers and commercial ambulance and retrieval services)

THE PHEM CURRICULUM

The PHEM curriculum was developed over a considerable time period using consensus development processes with trainees, other healthcare professionals and PHEM practitioners. The development process is described in detail on the Intercollegiate Board for Training in Pre-Hospital Emergency Medicine (IBTPHEM) website (www.ibtphem.org.uk). The derived curriculum relates to what should be expected of a newly 'qualified' consultant in PHEM across the four nations of the UK. Although designed for medical practitioners, it is clearly of wider application within the PHEC environment.

The curriculum framework is illustrated schematically in Figure 28.4. It comprises six sub-specialty-specific, one central and three cross-cutting themes. *Themes* are over-arching

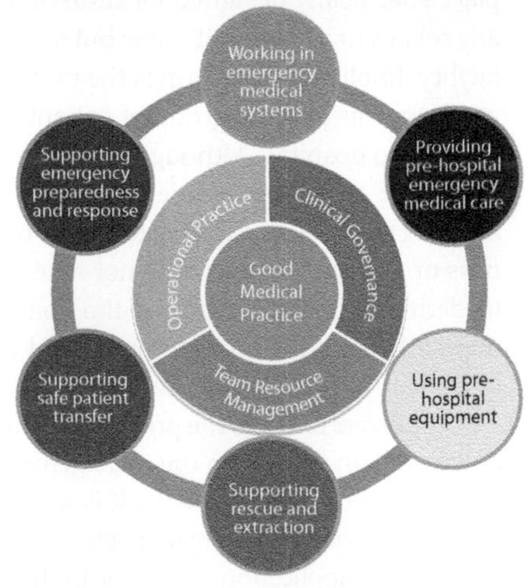

Figure 28.4 Skills for Health career framework descriptors.

areas of PHEM professional practice. The framework diagram illustrates the central importance of *Good Medical Practice* and the relationship between the cross-cutting generic themes of *Operational Practice, Team Resource Management* and *Clinical Governance* to the six specialty-specific themes. The diagram also emphasises the interrelationship of all themes – none stands alone.

Within each theme are a number of discrete work roles or activities which are referred to as 'units'. Each unit contains grouped or related 'elements' of underpinning knowledge, technical skill and behavioural attribute or non-technical skill – otherwise referred to as 'competences'. The full curriculum framework, detailing the elements of underpinning knowledge, technical skill and non-technical skill for each of these themes is available from the IBTPHEM website.

CENTRAL THEME: GOOD MEDICAL PRACTICE (GMP)

Good Medical Practice (GMP) is the term given to the core ethical guidance provided to doctors by the GMC. Other healthcare professional regulators such as the Nursing and Midwifery Council and the Health and Care Professions Council provide similar guidance. GMP sets out the principles and values on which good practice is founded; these principles together describe medical professionalism in action.

CROSS-CUTTING THEME A: OPERATIONAL PRACTICE

Maintaining safe and effective operational practice is a generic or cross-cutting theme of professional practice within PHEM. This theme concerns the knowledge, skills and non-technical skills required to maintain safe and effective operational practice within a pre-hospital emergency medicine service provider.

CROSS-CUTTING THEME B: TEAM RESOURCE MANAGEMENT

Contributing to effective team resource management is a generic or cross-cutting area of professional practice within PHEM. This theme concerns the knowledge, skills and non-technical skills required to work as part of a multi-disciplinary team in the high-hazard, resource-limited, environmentally challenging and time-pressured pre-hospital environment.

CROSS-CUTTING THEME C: CLINICAL GOVERNANCE

Application of clinical governance principles and techniques is a generic or cross-cutting area of professional practice within PHEM. This theme concerns the knowledge, skills and non-technical skills required to ensure that clinical governance principles and mechanisms are applied to clinical practice.

SUB-SPECIALTY THEME 1: WORKING IN EMERGENCY MEDICAL SYSTEMS

Specialist practitioners in PHEM operate within wider emergency medical systems (EMS). These systems have a number of inter-dependent components. Having an understanding of these components, the way in which they interact and the wider regulatory framework surrounding them is essential to effective professional medical practice in this field.

SUB-SPECIALTY THEME 2: PROVIDING PRE-HOSPITAL EMERGENCY MEDICAL CARE

Sub-specialist training in PHEM currently commences after completion of the fourth year of higher specialist training in emergency medicine, anaesthetics, intensive care medicine or acute internal medicine. Trainees therefore have experience of emergency clinical care in the hospital environment. The established principles and techniques used in those settings often need to be modified for effective pre-hospital emergency use. In addition, the provision of emergency medical care in a relatively unsupported environment requires a greater in-depth knowledge of resuscitation in all age groups. The units within this theme reinforce resuscitation concepts learned during higher specialist training and relate them to the pre-hospital operational environment.

SUB-SPECIALTY THEME 3: USING PRE-HOSPITAL EQUIPMENT

Pre-hospital and in-transit emergency care requires use of a wide range of medicines, devices and portable equipment. Practitioners must be competent in both the application and operation of specific equipment items and the principles underlying their function and design.

SUB-SPECIALTY THEME 4: SUPPORTING RESCUE AND EXTRICATION

Pre-hospital emergency medical services are frequently targeted at patients who, because of physical entrapment, physical geography or functional geographic constraints, cannot just be taken to the nearest appropriate hospital. This competence theme focuses on the underpinning knowledge, technical skills and non-technical skills required to manage a trapped patient and effectively interact with professional rescue service personnel at common pre-hospital rescue situations.

SUB-SPECIALTY THEME 5: SUPPORTING SAFE PATIENT TRANSFER

This theme covers the competences required to make destination hospital triage decisions; select the most appropriate transport platform; provide safe, effective and focused in-transit critical care; and ensure that the patients' condition and immediate needs are communicated to receiving hospital clinical staff. As with other competence themes, many of the elements are common across all clinical services.

SUB-SPECIALTY THEME 6: SUPPORTING EMERGENCY PREPAREDNESS AND RESPONSE

This theme encompasses the competences required to ensure that practitioners are appropriately prepared and equipped for larger scale emergency incidents in terms of their understanding of emergency planning and the principles of major incident management.

MEDICAL TRAINING IN PHEM

Doctors in the final years of their training in one of the specialties of acute medicine, anaesthesia, emergency medicine or intensive care medicine can apply to undertake 12 months of

PHEM sub-specialty training in an approved organisation. The IBTPHEM has designed a preferred and unique blended training programme combining training in PHEM and the parent specialty reflecting likely future consultant working patterns.

Training covers the entire PHEM curriculum and is divided into three distinct phases: 1a (initial training, 1 month), 1b (development training, 5 months) and 2 (consolidation training, 6 months). An IBTPHEM residential National Induction Course brings together trainees in phase 1a to familiarise them with the challenges of the pre-hospital environment. The phases allow supervised progression towards competent and more autonomous practice. The gaining of knowledge and skills are assessed continuously by consultant supervisors and formally in the two National Summative Assessments at the end of phases 1 and 2 undertaken by the Royal College of Surgeons of Edinburgh. Success in all these assessments against the curriculum will lead to recognition of sub-specialist status with the GMC. Whilst a fully immersive one-year training programme is provided, alternatives include an 80/20 and 50/50 split between pre-hospital care and base specialty.

It has to be recognised that although this approved training is within National Health Service (NHS) training programmes, it is largely delivered through charitable organisations that provide enhanced care teams by land and air. It is this partnership that has allowed the investment and innovation in PHEM training and the focus on training rather than service provision that is characterised in many other areas of postgraduate training.

The development of sub-specialty training has also required an increase in the number of consultants involved, allowing adequate trainee supervision and training. With increasing number of doctors now with sub-specialty accreditation, the workforce is becoming more qualified and driving a further increase in consultant-led and delivered pre-hospital critical care. In other areas of medicine, this has equated to improved clinical care and better outcomes for patients, and it is reasonable to expect that this will occur in PHEM.

MULTI-PROFESSIONAL PHEM PRACTITIONERS

A large component of the care outlined in Figure 28.2 is provided by ambulance service paramedics. All PHEM training programmes operate medical teams consisting of a physician and a paramedic working together. These paramedics are usually trained to a much higher skill level, and a framework for formalising and recognising this advanced practice is being developed by the College of Paramedics (8).

In November 2015, with close support from the College of Paramedics and Royal College of Nursing, and guidance from the IBTPHEM, the Faculty endorsed the concept of the development of a multi-professional training programme in PHEM and the development of pilot training schemes to test the concept. The Fellowship in Immediate Medical Care is now open to paramedics and nurses.

SUMMARY

The PHEM sub-specialist role is uniquely challenging. The tempo of decision making, the hazards faced at incident scenes, the relatively unsupported and isolated working conditions, the environmental challenges, the resource limitations and the case mix all make this a very different activity compared to in-hospital practice. An investment in training reaps the reward of a motivated, highly skilled individual that is able to better care for patients. The formalisation of PHEM multi-professional training for physicians, paramedics and nurses has only just commenced in the UK and is expected to bring these benefits.

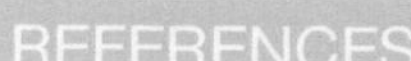

REFERENCES

1. Mackenzie R, Bevan D. For Debate …: A license to practise pre-hospital and retrieval medicine. *Emergency Medicine Journal* 2005;22:286–293.
2. Faculty of Pre-hospital Care. *Pre-hospital and Retrieval Medicine: A New Medical Sub-Specialty?* Edinburgh: Royal College of Surgeons of Edinburgh, 2008.
3. NHS Clinical Advisory Groups Report. Regional networks for major trauma. 2010.
4. Mackenzie R, Steel A, French J, Wharton R, Lewis S, Bates A, Daniels T, Rosenfeld M. Views regarding the provision of prehospital critical care in the UK. *Emergency Medicine Journal* 2009;26:365–370.
5. Hyde P, Mackenzie R, Ng G, Reid C, Pearson G. Availability and utilisation of physician-based pre-hospital critical care support to the NHS ambulance service in England, Wales and Northern Ireland. *Emergency Medicine Journal* 2012;29:177–181.
6. Robertson-Steel I, Edwards S, Gough M. Clinical governance in pre-hospital care. *Journal of the Royal Society of Medicine* 2001;94(Suppl 39):38–42.
7. Clements R, Mackenzie R. Competence in prehospital care: Evolving concepts. *Emergency Medicine Journal* 2005;22:516–519.
8. College of Paramedics. Post-Registration Career Framework. 3rd ed. College of Paramedics, 2015.

FURTHER READING

Information about the Intercollegiate Board for Training in Pre-Hospital Emergency Medicine is available at www.ibtphem.org.uk.

29 Trauma systems

OBJECTIVES

After completing this chapter the reader will

- Understand the organisational context in which UK trauma is managed
- Recognise the importance of systems in offering optimal trauma care
- Recognise and be prepared to promote the features of an effective and safe system

INTRODUCTION

The urgency, multiplicity and complexity of major trauma care demand careful organisation in order to achieve good outcomes. A trauma network is a collaboration between providers commissioned to deliver trauma care services in a geographical area (1). A trauma system is a broader concept that reflects the current view of trauma as a public health disease (2) (Figure 29.1). It is defined as *a public health model for the delivery of optimal trauma care to a specified population* (3). While the emphasis has often been on acute care, its scope must include rehabilitation, re-integration into the community and prevention.

No country has unlimited funds for healthcare. Commissioners rightly demand value for money, but must not undermine safety and quality. Performance and cost-effectiveness are integral aspects of system development. In a national trauma system, it is essential to work to common standards (4) and to achieve a high degree of consistency across individual networks, although there is no single, optimal way of delivering trauma care.

Pre-hospital care is a crucial element of a trauma system. While the details of hospital care are beyond the scope of this book, some aspects are covered generically in this chapter in order to describe trauma systems as a whole.

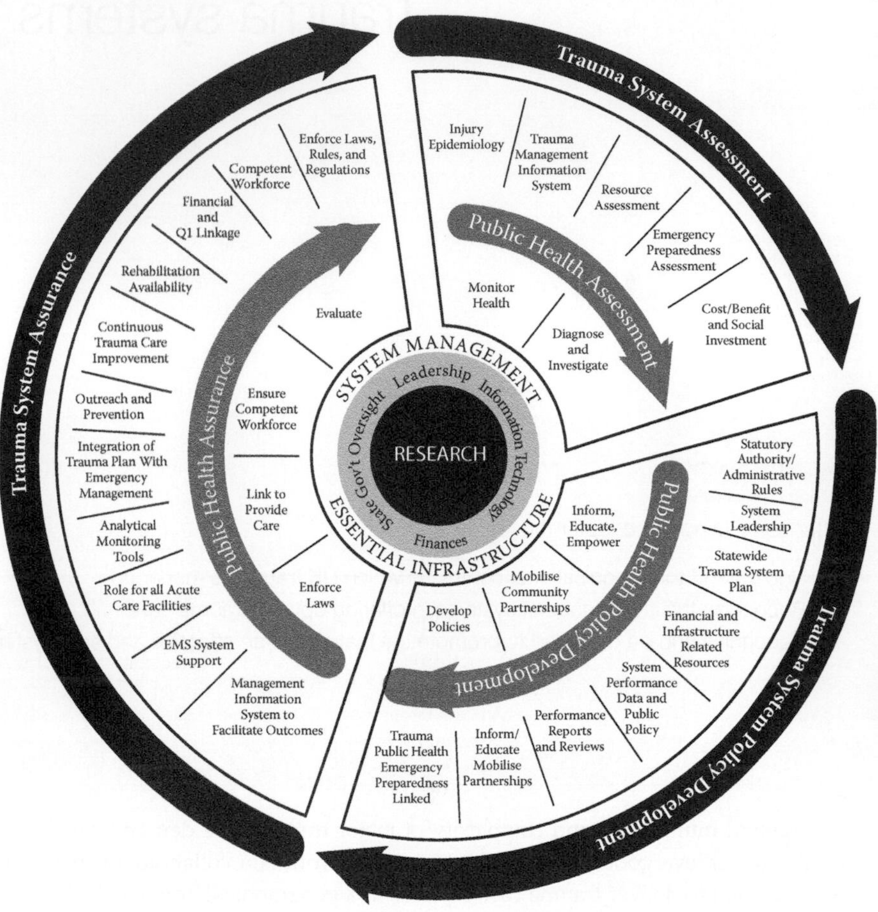

Figure 29.1 Schematic representation of a trauma system. (From Optimal Resources ACSCT. With permission.)

HISTORY

EARLY DEVELOPMENT IN THE UNITED KINGDOM

In 1894, the Manchester Ship Canal was completed, allowing Manchester to become the third largest port in the country, despite being 40 miles inland. Its construction was accompanied by a high incidence of serious injury. The strategic placement of new hospitals with staff trained in injury management and the establishment of temporary treatment centres along the route helped to provide efficient care. Specific transport links were set up to provide rapid access to definitive care. Robert Jones, a pioneer of fracture management, oversaw the system.

The Birmingham Accident Hospital and Rehabilitation Centre was opened as a veterans hospital in the Second World War in 1941 and was used exclusively for trauma patients. It is widely regarded as the forerunner of modern major trauma centres (MTCs). Three surgical teams provided care, each led by two senior trauma surgeons with a senior anaesthetist. The philosophy at the 'Acci' was based on three principles:

- Segregation of the ill from the injured—Only trauma victims were treated at the hospital.
- Continuity of care and unity of control—The same surgical team was responsible for the patient throughout their hospital stay and during rehabilitation.
- Rehabilitation as an integral part of trauma management—Recognising rehabilitation as a pivotal service was visionary.

ADVANCES IN NORTH AMERICA

In 1922, the American College of Surgeons (ACS) established a Committee on Fractures, which diversified to incorporate other types of injury in 1939. In 1950, this evolved into the Committee on Trauma (ACSCOT), which continues to promote high standards in trauma care. Its regularly updated publication *Resources for Optimal Care of the Injured Patient* gives wide-ranging guidance on trauma system components, including those for performance improvement and prevention.

Injury care improved significantly as a result of experience in the Vietnam War (1959–1975). The same principles of care were applied to patients with penetrating injuries in American cities. In 1966, the first civilian trauma centre opened in Cook County, Chicago. In 1969, R. Adams Cowley, who coined the concept of the 'golden hour', established the Shock-Trauma Unit as a standalone trauma hospital in Baltimore, together with a helicopter system serving the whole of Maryland. This was the first region-wide system of care. A funded research programme accompanied these developments.

In 1976, James Styner, an orthopaedic surgeon piloting a light aircraft, crashed his plane into a field in Nebraska. His wife was killed instantly and three of his children sustained critical injuries. The lack of organised care led him to declare, *'When I can provide better care in the field with limited resources than what my children and I received at the primary care facility, there is something wrong with the system and the system has to be changed'.* Within 2 years, he had developed the first *Advanced Trauma Life Support (ATLS)* course (5). By 1980, it had been adopted by the American College of Surgeons. While ATLS focuses on the individual doctor rather than on the team or system, it remains an important training element within trauma systems and has spawned a series of allied courses for nurses, paramedics and battlefield personnel.

In 1979, the mortality in Orange County and San Francisco County in California was reported (6). The improvement in outcome in Orange County after the introduction of an integrated trauma system influenced the development of major trauma systems across the United States and beyond (7,8).

PROGRESS ELSEWHERE

Since the 1960s, a pre-hospital care system has been developed in France. This has matured into the *Service d'Aide Médicale Urgente (SAMU)* (9). While standard operating procedures (SOPs) are now widespread, the SAMU were early implementers of this approach.

In Germany, an efficient system of pre-hospital care has also been developed, based on a dense network of helicopters and fast-response land vehicles (*Notarzteinsatzfahrzeug,* bringing a pre-hospital doctor to the scene, and *Rettungswagen,* serving as a mobile intensive care unit). As in France, doctors are actively engaged in pre-hospital care. In Germany and Austria, specialist trauma surgeons lead the in-hospital trauma service, working closely with anaesthetist-intensivist colleagues. Part of the Austrian system relies on insurance from employers (AUVA: *Allgemeinen Unfallversicherungsanstalt*). This has funded specialist trauma hospitals which resemble updated versions of the Birmingham Accident Hospital. Co-located with the *Ludwig Boltzmann Institute for Experimental and Clinical Traumatology*, the *Lorenz Böhler Trauma Centre* in Vienna has been a centre of excellence in both clinical practice and research for many years.

In the last decade, well-planned trauma systems have emerged in Australia. The best known, the *Victorian State Trauma System* (10) was established in 2000 following a review of trauma and emergency services that found opportunities for improvement at all stages of care and made more than 100 recommendations. The key features of the system include adequate funding, a focus on education and training, improved communications, effective standard operating procedures, an emphasis on research and governance, and designated adult and paediatric trauma centres.

RECENT DEVELOPMENTS IN ENGLAND

Despite early promise, trauma systems were slow to develop further in the United Kingdom. A national pilot project in the North West Midlands in the early 1990s did not reach the mortality reduction target of 30% within three years to support whole-scale national investment in trauma systems, although mortality subsequently halved over a more realistic 7-year period (11,12). Several subsequent reports from professional organisations lobbied for trauma system development, but failed to gain political support.

In 2007, the *National Confidential Enquiry into Patient Outcome and Death (NCEPOD)* published a report titled 'Trauma: Who Cares?' (13), a snapshot that identified serious shortcomings in major trauma care in England. This had a more profound impact. The Parliamentary Public Accounts Committee approved the formal development of a national trauma system in England, overseen by specialised commissioners and underpinned by financial arrangements. A National Clinical Director for major trauma care was appointed and a Clinical Advisory Group (CAG) was established to provide recommendations (1). In 2012, a system of major trauma networks went live in England. Early evidence points to significant improvements within 2 years (14).

In parallel with the governmental support for trauma systems in England, military conflict in Iraq and Afghanistan has been associated with a range of improvements in trauma care that are being transferred to clinical practice in the National Health Service (NHS) (Box 29.1).

BOX 29.1: Civilian Lessons from Military Experience

- Enhanced logistics
- Integrated human factors training
- Regular team practice between busy periods of clinical activity
- Improvements in damage control resuscitation and in the use of blood products
- Near-real-time governance to deal with issues promptly

TRAUMA SYSTEM REQUIREMENTS

GENERAL CHARACTERISTICS OF TRAUMA

Understanding the characteristics and incidence rates of major trauma helps to define trauma system requirements. Six general characteristics of trauma set the scene for system design (Box 29.2).

BOX 29.2: General Characteristics of Trauma

- Severity
- Multiplicity
- Complexity
- Timing
- Urgency
- Chronicity

The overall mortality rate of major trauma is over 10% and it remains the commonest cause of death amongst those under 40 years of age. It frequently occurs out of hours and in a disparate set of urban and rural locations. Its care is often time-critical. This combination has implications for delivering initial care to remote locations and transporting unstable patients to an appropriate hospital in time to treat life- or limb-threatening injuries. Fast vehicles, such as helicopters, have an essential role, especially in rural areas.

Trauma is inherently complex. While some patients sustain single injuries, many have multiple injuries that require multidisciplinary care which must be effectively coordinated and provided in a timely manner. Many injuries fall into the territory of regional specialists, such as neurosurgeons, cardiothoracic surgeons or plastic surgeons, for whom there is too little overall elective and emergency work to justify employing them in every acute hospital. The need to centralise trauma care is a direct consequence.

Most major trauma occurs in the evening and at weekends. The inevitable delay in bringing patients from a remote location or via another hospital in the network skews care in the MTC towards the overnight period. Working 24/7 is a necessity for major trauma, and staffing needs to be adjusted to match workload.

The time course of major trauma care is often prolonged. Anatomical repair and physiological recovery may take weeks, months or longer to achieve. Physical and mental disability may persist for longer still or permanently, constituting a considerable societal burden.

THE FREQUENCY AND TYPES OF MAJOR TRAUMA

In the United Kingdom, major trauma is relatively uncommon. There are about 200 severely injured patients (Injury Severity Score [ISS] >15) per million per year, while appendicitis is about seven times as common (1400 per million per year). For a district hospital serving a population of 250,000, there will be fewer than one major trauma case per week. In the recommended minimum network catchment population of 2 million (see later), there will be about 400 cases/year of severe trauma per annum.

In the United Kingdom, blunt trauma predominates. In most networks, penetrating trauma only accounts for about 3% of major trauma cases, although rates are considerably higher in some inner city areas. In some American cities, in contrast, the percentage may be as high as 30%. In a typical mixed urban and rural area in the United Kingdom, the commonest trauma mechanism is a motor vehicle collision (33%), followed closely by a low-energy fall (<2 metres, 27%), and then by a higher-energy fall (>2 metres, 22%). In moderate trauma (ISS 9–15), more than half the cases result from falls less than 2 metres.

In the United Kingdom, the worst injury in more than 80% of major and moderate trauma cases is to the head, spine or limbs. More than 61% of major trauma involves a serious head injury. Major bleeding from trunk injuries, though less frequent, often requires time-critical surgery (mainly general, vascular or cardiothoracic) or interventional radiology.

In the same typical area, more than 80% of major trauma patients had a serious injury or worse (Abbreviated Injury Scale [AIS] (15) code ≥3) to the head, limbs or spine. This suggests that neurosurgery, orthopaedics and spinal surgery are the three busiest surgical specialties delivering care. Abdominal injuries are less common, with AIS 3+ abdominal injuries occurring in 11% of these patients (just over one per week). In such a population, expertise in damage control surgery must be maintained by continually refreshing training, rather than by ongoing experience.

Major trauma was previously considered to be a disease of young adults. A different age profile is now emerging with a third of patients aged over 65 and a fifth over 80. While the peak incidence still occurs in those aged 15 to 20 years, there is less variation from decade to decade of adult life than previously recognised. Despite the peak in late adolescence and early adulthood, the incidence is much smaller in younger children. Half of the children (0–15 years old) with major trauma are age 13 or over. In patients with major trauma, the mortality in those over 65 is twice that in younger adults. In moderate trauma (for example fractures of the neck or femur), it is 10 times higher than in the younger age group.

THE SIZE OF TRAUMA NETWORKS

It has been recommended (1) that a major trauma network should have a catchment population of at least 2 million in order to have a sufficient caseload to develop a 'trauma culture', as well as to maintain individual experience and expertise. This population also represents the minimum that can support some surgical specialties, such as neurosurgery.

In a typical major trauma network of 2.5 million patients, it is expected that more than 500 patients per year (about 10 per week) will be admitted with an ISS over 15. The Royal College of Surgeons of England recommends that an MTC should admit a minimum of 250 'critically injured' patients per year.

In a frequently quoted study (16), a significantly improved outcome was shown in centres receiving more than 650 cases per year with an ISS >15. However, the improvement was only significant in penetrating torso trauma. The findings cannot be generalised to populations with predominantly blunt trauma.

GENERIC REQUIREMENTS AND GUIDING PRINCIPLES

The overall aims of a major trauma system can be summarised as simple, generic requirements (Box 29.3).

In order to achieve such a system, experience must be concentrated to promote expertise with clear lines of clinical responsibility, there must be continuity of care along the patient's pathway, there must be a focus on rehabilitation, and there must be partnership and cooperation between specialities and NHS trusts. Feedback and governance are essential. For the in-hospital phase, these simple concepts are well illustrated by the 'trauma triangle' (17) (Figure 29.2). While this is described in terms of 'medical' personnel, those in the nursing and allied professions have complementary roles.

BOX 29.3: Aims of a Major Trauma System

- Swift pre-hospital assessment of seriously injured patients
- Immediate life-saving measures when needed and rapid transport to the most appropriate hospital
- Immediate clinical and radiological assessment
- Instant access to damage control resuscitation and surgery or radiological intervention
- Expert, well-coordinated, definitive surgical care with full patient and family engagement
- Intensive care (including specialist intensive therapy unit)
- Reconstructive surgery
- Tailored rehabilitation with full physical and psycho-social support
- Transfer closer to home with continuing rehabilitation support as soon as appropriate

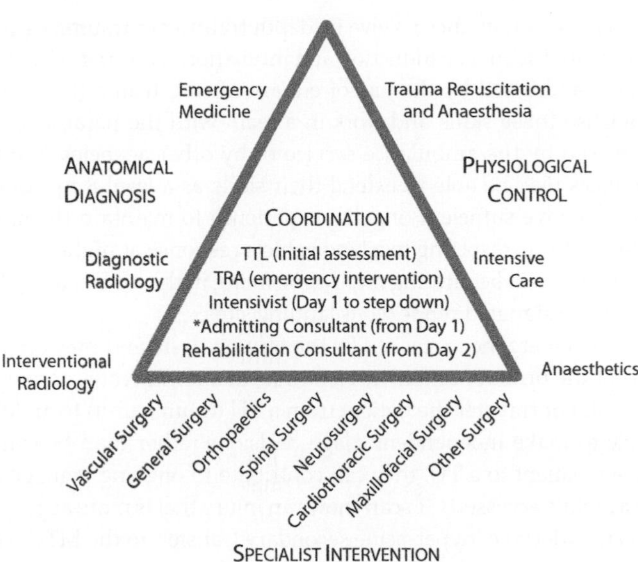

Figure 29.2 The trauma care triangle. The admitting consultant may initially be a dedicated consultant in major trauma care, rather than a specific surgical specialty. Responsibility may be transferred later to a particular specialty depending on current needs and priorities. Children and frail elderly patients may be transferred to the care of paediatricians or geriatricians at an appropriate point on their acute care pathway.

As the bedrock of major trauma care, a full range of surgical specialties sits at the base of the triangle. Interventional radiology is shown at a lower apex of the triangle, providing specialist intervention as well as anatomical diagnosis. Anaesthetists are placed at the other lower apex as they provide physiological control during operative repair and reconstruction.

On reception in hospital, emergency physicians have a particular role in initial anatomical diagnosis, though of course, they will also contribute to or oversee initial physiological control. In more severely injured patients, intensivists have a continuing role in physiological control after the initial interventions. A new subspecialty of trauma resuscitation anaesthetists (TRAs) has been proposed but has yet to become widely accepted (17).

In the pre-hospital phase, an equivalent triangle cannot be drawn. The missing base of the unfinished triangle is a reminder of the frequent need for timely specialist surgical (or radiological) intervention in hospital. The pre-hospital environment with its limited human and physical resources precludes almost all surgical interventions. Pre-hospital coordination may be led by or shared between the leader of the on-scene team (immediate care delivery), the trauma desk paramedic (general guidance, transportation logistics and communication between agencies) and the top cover consultant (senior advice).

FUNDAMENTAL BUILDING BLOCKS

AMBULANCE SERVICES AND ENHANCED CARE TEAMS

Ideally there should be a single service for the entire network. However, some major trauma centres receive patients from across conventional regional boundaries with different ambulance services using different protocols and procedures. Seamless collaboration is required to provide continuity of care.

Ambulance service paramedics receive in-depth training in trauma care, but may lack specific skills such as rapid sequence induction and intubation. This and other related gaps in their skill set are being addressed by the use of enhanced care teams (ECTs) that include senior doctors who practise these skills and work in a team with the paramedics. The doctors may be directly employed by the ambulance service or by other agencies (see following section). Selected paramedics may be able to extend their skills as a level 8 practitioner in the future, but must be able to have sufficient ongoing experience to maintain them. Many ECTs staff a helicopter in the daytime, resorting to a land vehicle response at night or in poor weather conditions. Many services will be offering night-time flying in the future, using lit helipads at acute hospitals and other designated rendezvous landing sites.

ECTs respond to emergencies, tasked by the trauma desk, and may attend the scene of the incident, intercept the primary ambulance en route at a rendezvous, accompany the patient to the primary hospital or transfer the patient from a TU (trauma unit) to an MTC.

ECTs are able to make independent triage decisions rather than be confined to the triage tool. If they take a patient to a TU, they can contribute to ongoing management. If the patient deteriorates or a rapidly accessed CT scan shows an injury that is more appropriately managed in an MTC, they can undertake 'hyper-acute secondary transfer' to the MTC with minimal delay.

ALLIED SERVICES

The police and fire services may reach trauma victims first and need to be trained to initiate care and to work in close cooperation with paramedics and pre-hospital doctors. Other agencies are needed for pre-hospital care in particular terrains, such as search and rescue helicopter services, mountain rescue teams and coastguard services.

Voluntary organisations, such as the *British Association for Immediate Care (BASICS)*, are integrated into the overall plan of care. Following the development of the new specialty of pre-hospital emergency medicine (PHEM), an increasing numbers the doctors engaged in future pre-hospital work may be formally employed by ambulance services or hospitals, rather than working as volunteers.

There are currently 34 charity-funded air ambulances operating across the United Kingdom, some of which benefit from government funding. Their catchment areas are often greater than individual trauma networks. They are able to bring an enhanced care team to the scene, together with resources (such as blood products) that are normally confined to hospitals.

DESIGNATED HOSPITALS FOR MAJOR TRAUMA

One of the key aims of a major trauma service is to centralise the care of the most severely injured patients in hospitals with a full range of surgical and critical care services. Given the pattern of trauma sustained in the United Kingdom, it is essential that the central hospital has neurosurgery and spinal surgery on site. In England, acute hospitals are classified into three different types, depending on their capability for managing major trauma:

- Major trauma centres
- Trauma units
- Local emergency hospitals.

A *major trauma centre (MTC)* (1) is a large, multi-specialty, acute hospital with all of the acute surgical specialties on site, together with resources for delivering critical care and acute rehabilitation. It acts as the central hospital in a major trauma network providing consultant-level care for patients with all types of injury and is optimised for their definitive care.

A *trauma unit (TU)* is an acute hospital in a major trauma network that also provides care for patients with significant injuries, but does not necessarily support certain specialised surgical services, such as neurosurgery, spinal surgery or cardiothoracic surgery. It is optimised for the definitive care of those trauma patients whose injuries lie within the expertise of locally supported specialties, such as orthopaedics and general surgery. It has critical care services on site. The other designated acute facility is the *local emergency hospital (LEH)*. This hospital has not been designated as a TU or MTC and should not receive acute trauma patients, except for those with minor injuries. The LEH still needs to have processes in place to ensure that any seriously injured patients who self-present or who are overlooked in the pre-hospital triage process are transferred promptly and safely to an MTC or TU. The LEH may have a role in the rehabilitation of trauma patients who live locally.

Elsewhere, different hospital classifications are used. In the United States, *Level 1* centres are similar to MTCs, but with specific accreditation criteria and an emphasis on trauma surgeon leadership. *Level 2* centres generally have a full range of surgical specialties, unlike TUs in the UK. They are not required to have an ongoing programme of research or a surgical residency programme. *Level 3* centres are often similar to TUs. Level 4 and level 5 centres are generally found in more remote locations. They are expected to have an ability to carry out advanced trauma life support, but need to transfer out all cases of severe trauma. In this regard, they resemble LEHs.

REHABILITATION UNITS

The chain of trauma care is as strong as its weakest link. Despite the early recognition of their importance, rehabilitation services have been relatively neglected. There are three tiers of rehabilitation service (18):

- Level 3: Local non-specialist rehabilitation
- Level 2: District (250–500,000 population) specialist rehabilitation
- Level 1: Tertiary specialised rehabilitation for complex needs.

Level 2 units have consultants trained and accredited in rehabilitation medicine, who also provide support for the level 3 units. Level 1 units provide high-cost, low-volume services for patients with highly complex rehabilitation needs that are beyond the scope of the local and district specialist services. These are normally provided over a regional population of 1–3 million through specialised commissioning arrangements. The categories of rehabilitation services are further subdivided according to rehabilitation needs. A new national Defence Rehabilitation Centre opened near Loughborough in 2018.

From a major trauma perspective, the focus of attention is on musculoskeletal, brain and spinal rehabilitation. An MTC should be able to provide acute rehabilitation on site in a dedicated clinical area run by consultants in rehabilitation medicine. TUs should be able to provide general rehabilitation within the hospital and should have direct input by rehabilitation consultants. Spinal cord injury rehabilitation is carried out in supra-regional units serving several trauma networks. In addition to defined rehabilitation units, rehabilitation takes place within acute hospitals, in smaller community institutions and at home.

THE TRAUMA PATHWAY

The trauma pathway is summarised in Figure 29.4. Each of these elements is equally important. Historically, the provision of rehabilitation has been the weakest link. The major trauma pathway extends from initial recognition to final rehabilitation. It can be considered in three main phases:

- Recognition and resuscitation
- Repair and reconstruction (definitive care)
- Recovery and rehabilitation

In the field, clinical examination and a high level of suspicion underpin the identification of injuries and physiological derangements, although adjuncts such as ultrasound machines and devices for near-patient testing are becoming increasingly portable and robust enough to allow field use. Recognition of potential major trauma cases in the field is based on the use of a major trauma triage tool.

In hospital, a whole-body, contrast-enhanced, multi-detector CT scan is the default imaging procedure of choice in the severely injured patient (19). Radiation dosage remains an important consideration, especially in younger people. New guidelines (20) indicate how to limit the use of CT in children without unduly missing injuries. Newer scanners use significantly lower doses of radiation than older machines.

A rapidly accessible, dedicated emergency theatre is required to ensure resuscitative surgical interventions can be made whenever they are needed. Surgical expertise must be available 24/7. Similarly, a hybrid interventional radiology (IR) suite and interventional radiologists must be rapidly available to stop bleeding, while maintaining the option of switching to damage control surgery (DCS) in a severely compromised patient without needing to move to a separate location. In DCS, different surgical specialist teams may need to operate sequentially or simultaneously. Definitive surgery can be completed later after a period of physiological stabilisation in the intensive care unit (ICU).

Within an MTC, repair and reconstruction relies on the availability of consultants from a broad range of specialties. Joint operating, simultaneously or sequentially, may be required for optimal care. National standards for managing open limb fractures demand timely collaboration between orthopaedic and plastic surgeons (21). Similarly, craniofacial injuries should be managed jointly between neurosurgeons and maxillofacial surgeons.

There should be 24-hour-a-day dedicated trauma lists in theatres that are separate from the normal emergency theatre. Many repairs and some reconstructions can be undertaken as emergency operations, but complex reconstructions are generally best planned and scheduled.

Recovery from injury takes place in the ICU and on the acute wards and continues after discharge. The clinical environment in this phase should reflect the physiological needs of the patient. Nursing resources should match the indicated level of critical care (22) from level 3 on the ICU with 1:1 nursing, through high-dependency (1:2), to acute ward level 1 (1:4) and level 0 (basic acute ward care). Most MTCs have developed a dedicated admission ward for all significant trauma patients not requiring critical care.

Rehabilitation overlaps with recovery. It is defined as *'the process of assessment, treatment and management by which the individual (and their family/carers) are supported to achieve their maximum potential for physical, cognitive, social and psychological function, participation in society and quality of living'* (23).

Rehabilitation should start as soon as possible and the rehabilitation team should see patients within a day of admission. At the 'R-point' (24), rehabilitation takes over from acute care as the main priority. At this stage, the patient may move to a specific rehabilitation unit or continue to be managed in an acute ward with in-reaching rehabilitation resources. Major trauma in the elderly population was previously under-recognised. As the problems of limited mobility, pain and confusion in frail, elderly trauma patients are similar to those in patients with hip fractures, it is possible and desirable to develop a combined rehabilitation pathway for all these patients.

PRE-HOSPITAL TRIAGE AND TRANSPORT TO THE MOST APPROPRIATE HOSPITAL

Having a high level of suspicion of major trauma and taking the patient to the most appropriate hospital are fundamental to delivering good care. A pre-hospital triage decision tool is used to help direct injured patients to the most appropriate hospital. This guidance will never be perfect, given the limitations of assessment in the challenging pre-hospital environment. A degree of over-triage is inevitable in order to ensure that more than 90% of patients with major trauma are recognised as positive by the triage tool. In order to achieve 90% sensitivity, a low positive predictive value has to be accepted, typically about 30%, that is only 1 in 3 triage-positive patients taken to the MTC turn out to have major injuries after full evaluation in hospital. An example of a trauma triage tool is shown in Figure 29.3. It is derived from the one developed by the American College of Surgeons (25).

Most major trauma systems in England have designated 'trauma desks' within one of the regional ambulance control centres. Experienced paramedics, actively engaged in pre-hospital care in other parts of their job, man the desk 24/7. They deal with all suspected cases of major trauma, acting as initial case managers. Trauma desk staff will offer advice to staff at the scene, select the most appropriate hospital for each patient and may establish conference calls to facilitate decision-making and the sharing of information. This may involve the scene attendants, top-cover consultants and senior clinicians in the receiving hospital (Figure 29.4).

Paramedics or pre-hospital doctors report triage-positive cases to the major trauma desk. The team at the scene or the trauma desk paramedic generally direct these patients to an MTC,

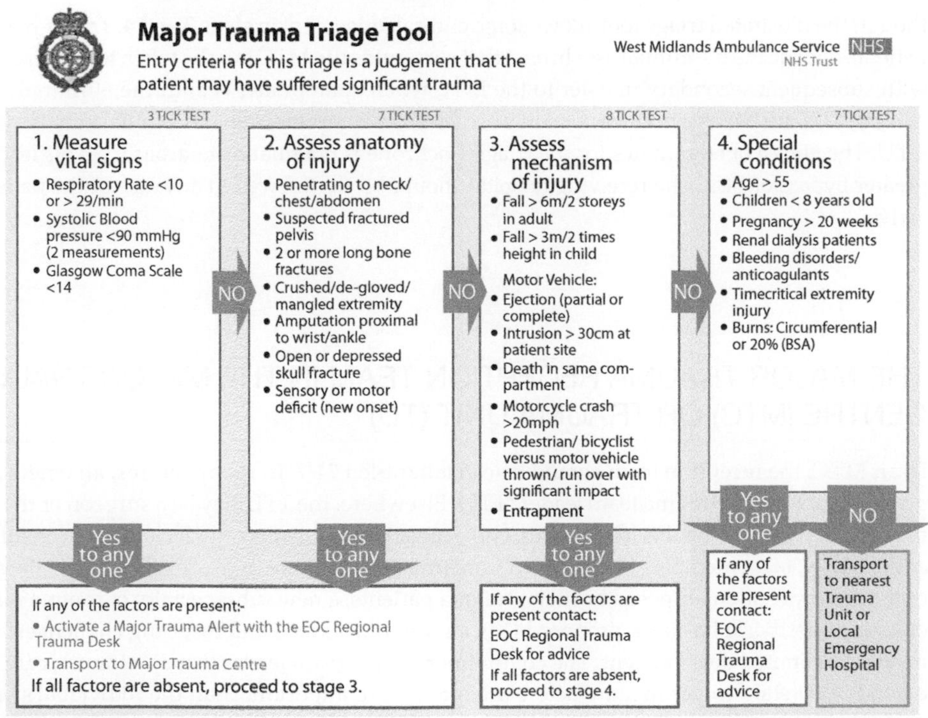

Figure 29.3 Typical major trauma triage tool (derived from the American College of Surgeons).

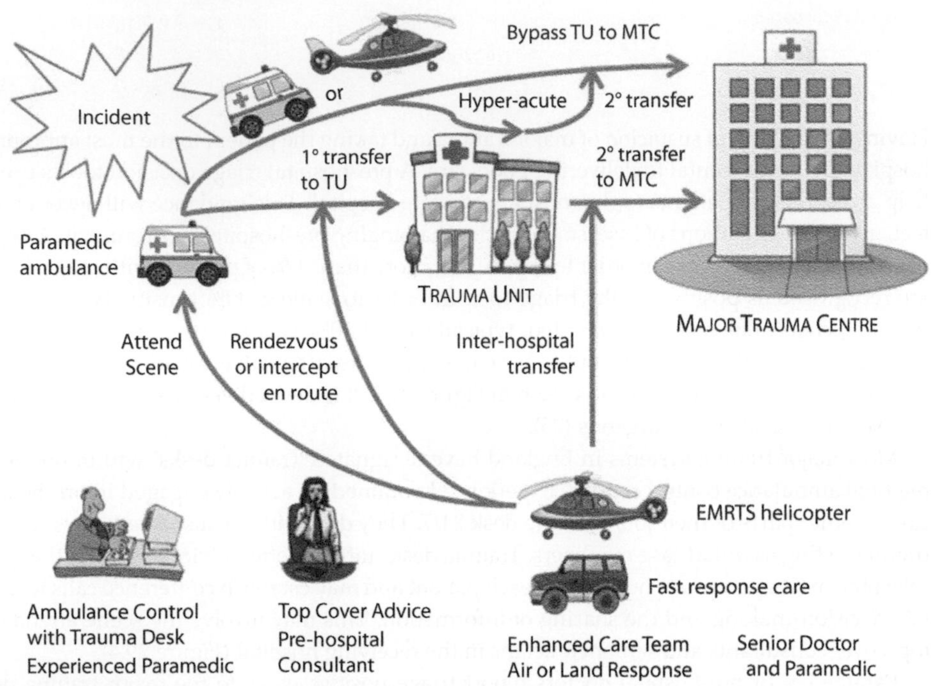

Figure 29.4 Pre-hospital communication, scene attendance and transfer.

though the illustrated triage tool allows some clinical judgement in steps 3 and 4. Triage-positive patients outside the 60-minute 'isochrone' that surrounds the MTC may be taken to a TU instead, with subsequent secondary transfer to the MTC when appropriate. Within the 60-minute isochrone, TUs are bypassed unless patients are severely compromised and significantly closer to a TU. The choice of 60 minutes for the triage isochrone is pragmatic but arbitrary. This leads to greater bypass of TUs. The receiving hospital should be alerted well in advance of the patient's arrival.

MANAGING THE PATIENT

THE MAJOR TRAUMA RECEPTION TEAM IN THE MAJOR TRAUMA CENTRE (MTC) OR TRAUMA UNIT (TU)

In an MTC, the reception team should be consultant-led 24/7. In many centres, an emergency physician acts as the trauma team leader (TTL). Elsewhere, the TTL may be a surgeon or the role may be shared between disciplines. Currently, most trauma teams only include one consultant at the outset, team members being drawn from training grades or non-consultant staff. Because of the airway challenges posed by major trauma patients, a new sub-specialty of trauma resuscitation anaesthesia has been proposed (17), although workload and rostering challenges have resulted in limited development. The commitment of the team leader to major trauma care and a good understanding of human factors are often more important than the individual's background specialty, especially in a largely blunt trauma population, but in most cases the breadth of clinical experience and knowledge of departmental practice makes emergency physicians ideally suited for the role. Specialties not represented in the trauma team should be informed as soon as severe injuries are suspected or identified in their territory. In most MTCs and TUs, the surgical members of the initial reception team are trainees rather than consultants. It is vital to involve the corresponding consultants when any serious injuries are found so that key decision-making and surgical intervention can be undertaken at the consultant level. Similarly, emergency interventional radiology should be carried out at the consultant level. Likewise, the anaesthetist looking after major trauma patients undergoing emergency surgery or radiological intervention should be a consultant. In TUs, the resident TTL is not always a consultant and some specialties (for example neurosurgery and cardiothoracic surgery) are not usually available locally. Prompt referral to the MTC when indicated is therefore essential.

CONSULTATION WITH AND REFERRAL TO THE MTC

For patients who present to TUs, there needs to be a clear, straightforward means of referral and transfer to the MTC. This is illustrated in Figures 29.5 and 29.6.

There are two main approaches to emergency referral from a TU to the MTC. If the patient is considered by the TU team to have injuries that need immediate transfer to the MTC for life-saving intervention, they may be empowered to send the patient to the MTC without prior consultation. This is the full 'open door' or 'send and call' approach, where the referring clinician contacts the receiving TTL as soon as the patient has left (Figure 29.5). The open door arrangement may be modified (as in Figure 29.6) to include immediate contact with the receiving TTL, while simultaneously proceeding with the transfer process. This allows advice to be given that may modify management en route. It may also allow futile situations to be identified before the patient leaves. However, it is essential that no time is lost waiting for the MTC to get back to the TU 'just in case it proves to be futile'.

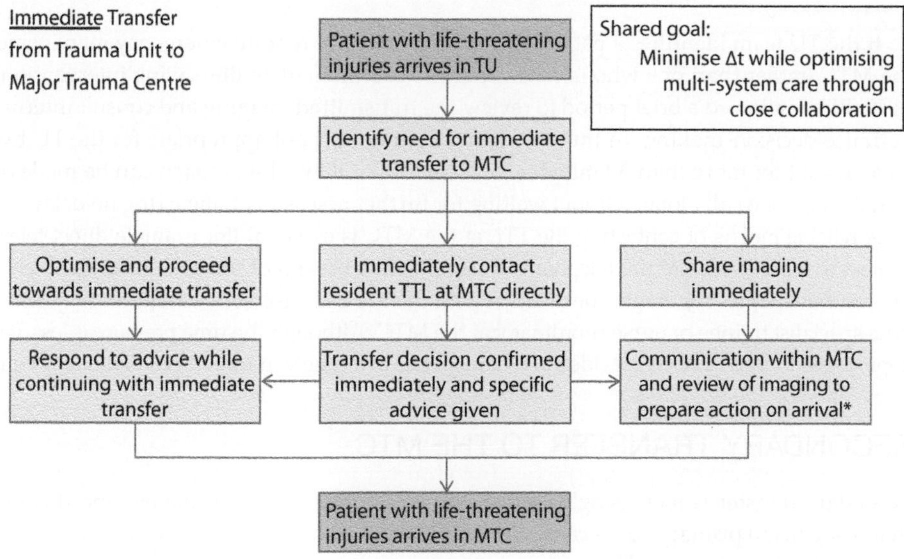

Figure 29.5 Immediate secondary transfer to the MTC. *For critical, time-dependent interventions, it is imperative not to cause unnecessary delay. Occasionally, subsequent MTC review may identify a reason not to transfer, for example futility in an un survivable condition. The transfer can still be aborted if the patient has not yet left the TU.

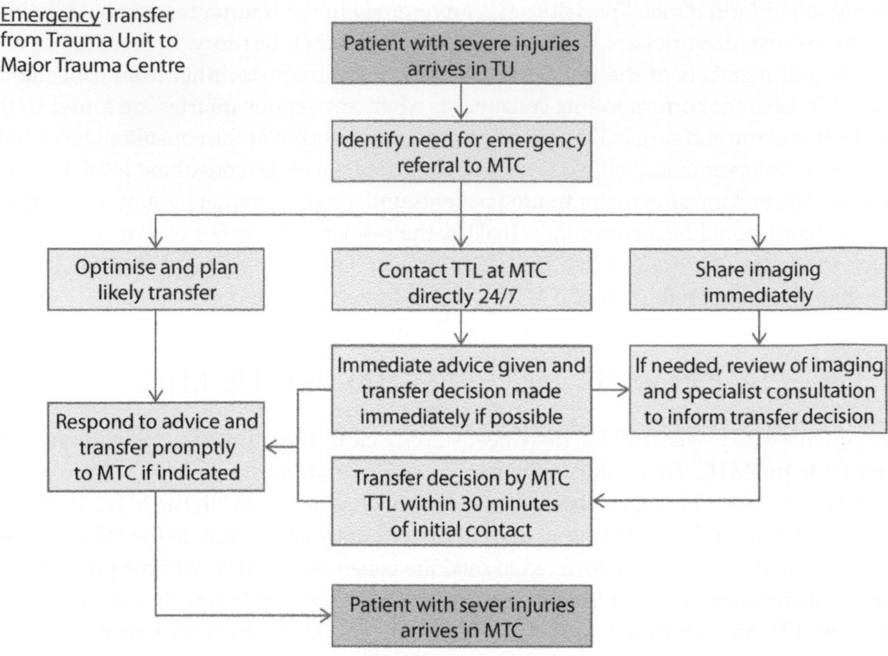

Figure 29.6 Emergency secondary transfer to the MTC. For immediate and emergency referral of severely injured patients, the TTL is contacted directly by the referring clinician in the TU or by the Ambulance Service Trauma Desk. The CT and other images are transmitted to the imaging PACS system in the MTC, so that the TU imaging can be viewed on the MTC's own system by the receiving team. PACS, picture archiving and communication system, is a medical imaging technology that provides economical storage of and convenient access to images from multiple modalities (source machine types).

If the TU team identifies a patient who may or may not require emergency management in the MTC (rather than one who is considered to need immediate life-saving intervention), the MTC TTL is allowed a brief period to review the transmitted imaging and consult internally to optimise decision-making. In this emergency setting, it is not appropriate for the TU team to have to wait for more than 30 minutes for a decision. Often, the decision can be made on the initial telephone call alone, without waiting for further assessment, incurring no delay at all.

A reliable means of contacting the TTL at the MTC is essential (for example direct telephone contact to a personal internal telephone or pager with a backup of the emergency (red) phone in the resuscitation room). Acute consultation with the MTC for less serious injuries may take place via a specialist trainee or nurse coordinator at the MTC. Although the time pressure is less, it is still appropriate for the MTC to provide a senior response in a timely manner to consultation requests.

SECONDARY TRANSFER TO THE MTC

Secondary transfer is increasingly carried out as 'retrieval' by the same enhanced care team that responds to primary scene calls in the network. This spares the TU from losing personnel for transfer; however, the TU must maintain the training and capability to transfer patients in case the retrieval team is already engaged on a separate mission. If an enhanced care team decides to take a patient to a TU, but serious injuries that are more appropriately managed in the MTC are identified on arrival there, 'hyper-acute secondary transfer' is indicated. For this to be effective, the TU reception team must act quickly and efficiently to carry out clinical examination and a CT scan, so that little overall time is lost.

RESPONSIBILITY AND REVIEW AFTER ADMISSION TO THE MTC

Each MTC will ensure that arrangements are in place for effective coordinated patient care. The coordination role is particularly important when multiple specialties are involved.

In some centres, major trauma acute care/rehabilitation coordinators review care and engage with patients, families, and the medical and nursing teams. Clinical coordination may lie with a multidisciplinary team, or a single nominated specialty.

DISCHARGING PATIENTS FROM THE MTC TO A TU

One of the commonest delays in the system of care is discharging patients from the MTC to a TU or from the MTC or TU to a separate rehabilitation unit. Current standards are for a TU or general rehabilitation unit to receive a patient within 2 days of being declared ready to transfer. For a specialised rehabilitation unit, the transfer should take place within 1 day. Lack of capacity often leads to delay.

MAKING THE SYSTEM WORK

A number of important additional elements are critical to trauma system success; these are listed in Box 29.4.

BOX 29.4: Features of an Effective Trauma System

- Funding
- Capacity and flow management
- Peer review
- National trauma registry reporting
- Organisational structure
- Leadership and involvement culture
- Multi-disciplinary team meetings
- Near-real-time reporting and governance
- Policies and procedures
- Education and training

FUNDING

The resources required for major trauma care are expensive. Cost-effective business management must go hand in hand with clinical expertise. Currently, there is a 'best practice tariff' for major trauma that must be captured diligently and accurately to help fund the service.

CAPACITY AND FLOW MANAGEMENT

Trauma is episodic with diurnal, weekly and seasonal patterns. This variation in workload can be challenging to institutions with fixed facilities and staffing. Occupancy planning to provide a degree of slack and escalation policies for effective surge control are essential ingredients of MTC and network management. Similar considerations apply to the provision of paramedic ambulances and enhanced care team helicopters.

PEER REVIEW

Review of MTC, TU and network performance by senior clinicians from equivalent institutions and health service officials is an important external quality control process. Nationally agreed measures (4), developed by a national clinical reference group, are used as the basis of the assessments.

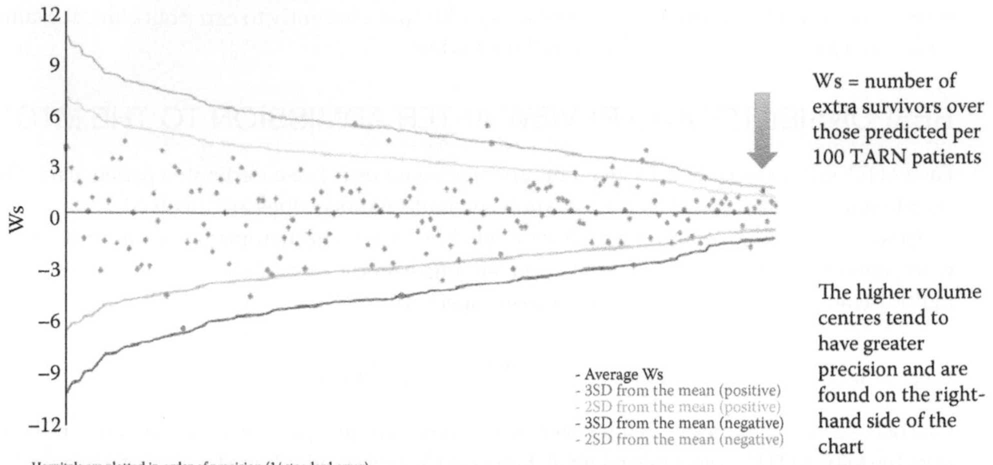

Figure 29.7 TARN funnel plot showing comparative performance of the various MTCs and TUs.

NATIONAL TRAUMA REGISTRY REPORTING

In the United Kingdom, the *Trauma Audit & Research Network (TARN)* (26) has developed and maintains a national trauma registry. It produces regular, comparative outcome reports based on the number of unexpected survivors per 100 patients enrolled onto the database – the W_s statistic. This is weighted to adjust for the different severity profiles of patients seen in different MTCs or TUs. The results are presented as a funnel plot to allow visualisation of relative performance (Figure 29.7).

TARN also produces a quarterly dashboard report to show comparative performance in terms of specific processes (rather than outcome) such as whether a consultant team leader is available within 5 minutes of the patient's arrival in hospital. The outcome reports and dashboards are scrutinised as part of peer review.

ORGANISATIONAL STRUCTURE

Although it is critical that a trauma system is clinically focused, organisational structures play an important role in maintaining stakeholder engagement and optimising overall care. It is essential for the network to have a defined influence, so that it cannot be ignored by individual trusts or other supporting organisations.

Within the MTC, the major trauma service is often aligned managerially with a particular service, such as the emergency department or orthopaedic service. As major trauma impinges on a wide range of specialties, it is wise to set up a separate group to oversee care within the MTC, chaired by a senior clinician from outside the directorate in which major trauma sits. Rather than making the organisation more complicated than it needs to be, these complementary structures promote stakeholder engagement and representation.

LEADERSHIP AND INVOLVEMENT CULTURE

Leadership and involvement culture are key parts of an effective trauma system that must be transmitted to new members of staff, including trainees rotating through the various elements of the system, by the example and enthusiasm of senior permanent staff. They are promoted through network and council meetings, multi-disciplinary team meetings, the governance process and education.

MULTI-DISCIPLINARY TEAM MEETINGS

Trauma care is inherently multi-disciplinary. Face-to-face multi-specialty clinical meetings are essential for coordinating care. There should be a daily multi-specialty meeting to discuss recent admissions and new problems or changing plans in other patients. In addition, the main individual surgical specialties need to hold weekly meetings between consultants, nurses, therapists and coordinators. Similar procedures must be in place for established pre-hospital care schemes.

NEAR-REAL-TIME REPORTING AND GOVERNANCE

Accurate information is central to clinical management and governance. Near-real-time information can be fed back to clinicians and used to report and address any issues raised, while the patient is still in hospital. There must also be a coordinated system of collating issues so that trends can be followed and kept on a risk register until resolved. The World Health Organization has recommended that local governance meetings take place every week in busy institutions and that deaths panels (where fatalities are scrutinised by peers) should meet between monthly and quarterly (27).

Governance meetings involving all groups involved in patient care must take place locally both within the MTCs and TUs. Pre-hospital providers must be invited and encouraged to attend. Governance meetings should also take place at a network level.

In the United Kingdom, TARN provides some of the aggregated data for governance, in the form of W_s charts, dashboards and other material. In the United States, the American College of Surgeons has developed a trauma quality improvement programme (ACS TQIP® (28)) involving more than 200 participating trauma centres.

POLICIES AND PROCEDURES

Major trauma networks should develop a handbook of policies and procedures that are easily accessible physically or on the institutional intranet. While some policies may be tailored to specific hospitals or services, most policies should be shared for consistency across the network.

EDUCATION AND TRAINING

Education is central to performance. It is also a major source of staff motivation and satisfaction. Standardised trauma courses, such as the *Advanced Trauma Life Support (ATLS)* and *the European Trauma Course (ETC)*, need to be combined with regular informal teaching and bespoke specialist courses to provide staff with a wide range of opportunities. Specific courses for paramedics, nurses and allied professions for pre-hospital and in-hospital practice are equally important.

The importance of human factors in the aircraft industry was recognised after an air crash in 1978 when the plane ran out of fuel while the flight crew was trying to solve a landing gear problem. Within a year, the American National Transportation Board (NTSB) recommended *crew (or cockpit) resource management (CRM)* training for all airline crews. The National Aeronautics and Space Administration (NASA) immediately endorsed the CRM approach. Improvements in inter-personal communication, leadership and decision-making were demonstrated, and the principles were recognised to be transferrable to other environments where time-critical decisions are made (29,30).

The importance of non-technical factors in causing errors, omissions and delays in acute trauma care has been increasingly recognised. A working definition of human factors in healthcare is *'enhancing clinical performance through an understanding of the effects of teamwork, tasks, equipment, workspace, culture, organisation on human behaviour and abilities, and application of that knowledge in clinical settings'* (31).

CONTINUING DEVELOPMENT

IMPROVEMENT, INNOVATION AND RESEARCH

Trauma systems are not static. The governance process strives for improvement. Innovation should be encouraged, but without losing the quality afforded by consistency and reliability. Research provides the foundation for future practice. While randomised, controlled trials represent a gold standard; they are often difficult to carry out in emergency situations and especially in the pre-hospital environment. Research projects require adequate case numbers to demonstrate important findings with convincing statistical significance. Multi-centre or multi-network projects facilitate this and are more likely to attract funding.

PREVENTION

No system is complete until it embraces prevention. Adolescents are one of the most vulnerable groups. Their immature judgement of risk, combined with peer pressure, demands an education programme that is carefully pitched in order to influence behaviour. Meeting face-to-face with major trauma victims of their own age brings major trauma to their attention. Such encounters need to be handled carefully, so that they do not trigger denial or fuel a risk-taking culture. Alcohol and drug awareness is a key part of any trauma prevention programme and should not be limited to adolescents and young adults.

The elderly are particularly vulnerable to low-energy falls, particularly if they are receiving anticoagulant medication. Falls prevention programmes in frail, elderly people are well established, but there is a need to address the risk of injury in fitter elderly people who are more active than in previous generations.

Car and road design remain important elements of a prevention strategy. Nanotechnology, new materials and intelligent movement sensors will have an important future role. Here too, human factors must not be ignored. A careful balance must be struck between limiting individual freedom and promoting safety, so that individuals learn about risk and are not driven to rebel with other forms of high-risk or reckless behaviour.

CONCLUSION

The best care for the injured can only be achieved by the implementation and maintenance of an effective trauma system. Pre-hospital care is now recognised to be an essential component of such a system, not only for the provision of care before patients arrive in hospital, but also as a resource for ensuring that patients are matched with the most appropriate receiving facility. Inevitably, such systems are complex, however, and they will only function well if all their potential elements are funded, integrated and appropriately governed. In addition, every individual involved as part of such a system must know their own role, the roles and skills of those they work with, and must ensure that their practice remains up to date.

REFERENCES

1. Regional Networks for Major Trauma. NHS Clinical Advisory Groups Report, Department of Health, September 2010. www.gov.uk/government/publications/regional-trauma-networks-clinical-advisory-group-document.
2. Committee on Trauma, American College of Surgeons. Resources for optimal care of the injured patient. 2014. https://www.facs.org/quality-programs/trauma/vrc/resources. (Original diagram: U.S. Department of Health and Human Services, Health Resources and Services Administration. Model Trauma System Planning and Evaluation. Rockville, MD: U.S. Department of Health and Human Services, 2006. Available at www.facs.org/quality-programs/trauma/tsepc/resource.)
3. The Intercollegiate Group on Trauma Standards. *Regional trauma systems: Interim guidance for commissioners*. London: The Royal College of Surgeons of England, December 2009.
4. Major trauma measures, Trauma Quality Improvement Network System (TQuINS), National Peer Review Programme, NHS England. www.tquins.nhs.uk/?menu=resources.
5. Styner R. *The light of the moon: Life, death and the birth of advanced trauma life support*. Lulu Press, 2007.
6. West JG, Trunkey DD, Lim RC. Systems of trauma care: a study of two counties. *Archives of Surgery* 1979;114:455–460.
7. West JG, Cales RH, Gazzaniga AB. Impact of regionalization: The Orange County experience. *Archives of Surgery* 1983;118:740–744.
8. Cales RH. Trauma mortality in Orange County: The effect of implementation of a regional trauma system. *Annals of Emergency Medicine* 1984;13:1–10.
9. SAMU. www.samu-de france.fr/en/System_of_Emergency_in_France_MG_0607.
10. Victorian State Trauma System. www.health.vic.gov.au/trauma/.
11. Nicholl J, Turner J, Dixon S. The cost-effectiveness of the regional trauma system in the North West Midlands. School of Health and Related Research (SCHARR), University of Sheffield, 1995. www.sheffield.ac.uk/scharr/.
12. Oakley PA, MacKenzie G, Templeton J, Cook AL, Kirby RM. Longitudinal trends in trauma mortality and survival in Stoke-on-Trent 1992–1998. *Injury* 2004;35:379–385.
13. National Confidential Enquiry into Patient Outcome and Death (NCEPOD). Trauma: Who cares? A report of the National Confidential Enquiry into Patient Outcome and Death (NCEPOD), 2007. www.ncepod.org.uk/2007t.htm.
14. Cole E, Lecky F, West A, Smith N, Brohi K, Davenport R. The impact of a pan-regional inclusive trauma system on quality of care. *Annals of Surgery* 2016;264(1):188–194.
15. Abbreviated Injury Scale, Association for the Advancement of Automotive Medicine. www.aaam.org/about-ais.html.
16. Nathens AB, Jurkovich GJ, Maier RV, Grossman DC, MacKenzie EJ, Moore M, Rivara FP. Relationship between trauma center volume and outcomes. *Journal of the American Medical Association (JAMA)* 2001;285:1164–1171.
17. Oakley P, Dawes R, Thomas R. The consultant in trauma resuscitation and anaesthesia. *British Journal of Anaesthesia* 2014;113:207–210.
18. Turner-Stokes L. Specialist neuro-rehabilitation services: Providing for patients with complex rehabilitation needs. British Society for Rehabilitation Medicine. www.bsrm.co.uk/publications/Levels_of_specialisation_in_rehabilitation_services5.pdf.
19. RCR guidelines. www.rcr.ac.uk/docs/radiology/pdf/BFCR(11)3_trauma.pdf.

20. CT in children. www.rcr.ac.uk/docs/radiology/pdf/BFCR(14)8_paeds_trauma.pdf.
21. British Orthopaedic Association Standards for Trauma. www.boa.ac.uk/publications/boa-standards-trauma-boasts/.
22. Levels of Critical Care for Adult Patients. Intensive Care Society Standards, 2009. www.ics.ac.uk/.
23. Definition of rehabilitation by Turner-Stokes. www.england.nhs.uk/commissioning/spec-services/npc-crg/group-d/d02/.
24. Rehabilitation for patients in the acute care pathway following severe disabling illness or injury: BSRM core standards for specialist rehabilitation. Working Party of the British Society of Rehabilitation Medicine, October 2014. www.bsrm.co.uk/publications/.
25. Centers for Disease Control and Prevention (CDC). Guidelines for field triage of injured patients. Recommendations of the National Expert Panel on Field Triage, 2011. *MMWR Morbidity and Mortality Weekly Report* 2012;61:1–21.
26. Trauma Audit and Research Network. www.tarn.ac.uk/.
27. World Health Organization. Guidelines for trauma quality improvement programmes. 2009. www.who.int/violence_injury_prevention/services/traumacare/traumaguidelines/en/
28. The American College of Surgeons Trauma Quality Improvement Program (ACS TQIP®). www.facs.org/quality-programs/trauma/tqip/.
29. Carayon P, Tosha B. Wetternecka TB, Rivera-Rodriguez AJ, Hundt AS, Hoonakker P, Holden R, Gurses AP. Human factors systems approach to healthcare quality and patient safety. *Applied Ergonomics* 2014;45:14–25.
30. Catchpole K. Spreading human factors expertise in healthcare: Untangling the knots in people and systems. *BMJ Quality and Safety* 2013;22:793–797.
31. Catchpole K. Towards a working definition of human factors in healthcare. Clinical Human Factors Group. http://chfg.org/definition/towards-a-working-definition-of-human-factors-in-healthcare.

Appendix A: Practical procedures in thoracic trauma

NEEDLE THORACOCENTESIS

PROCEDURE

1. Identify the 2nd intercostal space in mid-clavicular line, remembering that the 2nd rib joins the sternum at the sternal angle and that the 2nd intercostal space is below this rib and above the 3rd rib (Figure A.1).
2. Clean the skin with an alcohol wipe.
3. Insert a large bore cannula (>4.5 cm in length) perpendicularly into the chest (Figure A.2).
4. Remove the metal needle (trochar) leaving the cannula in place and uncapped. Air should be heard to escape, but this is not invariable. If the procedure has been successful, the patient's condition and vital signs will rapidly begin to improve.
5. If there is a possibility that the cannula is not long enough and tension pneumothorax is still strongly suspected, push the cannula hard into the chest wall, indenting the skin, as this will create a little extra length. It is essential to be aware of the risk of going too medial with the possibility of injury to great vessels (1).
6. If the procedure is unsuccessful using these landmarks, it should be repeated in the finger thoracostomy area (see next section).

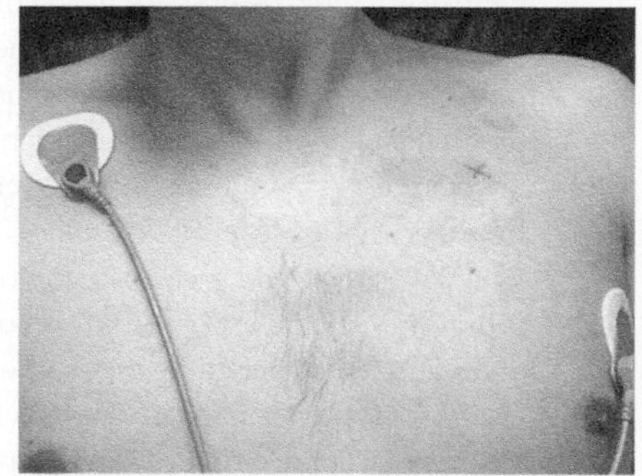

Figure A.1 Correct site for (initial attempt) needle thoracostomy.

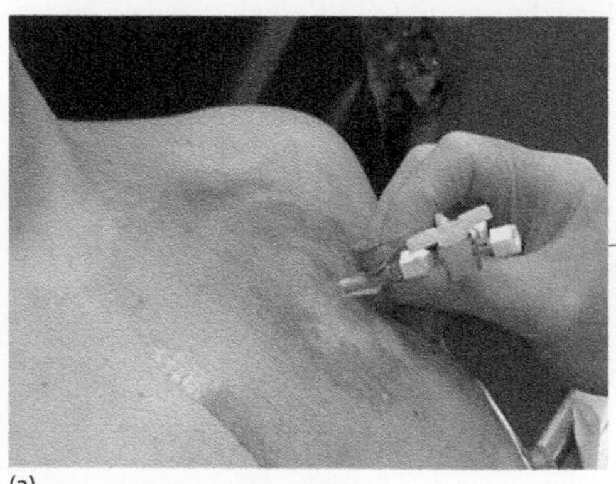

(a)

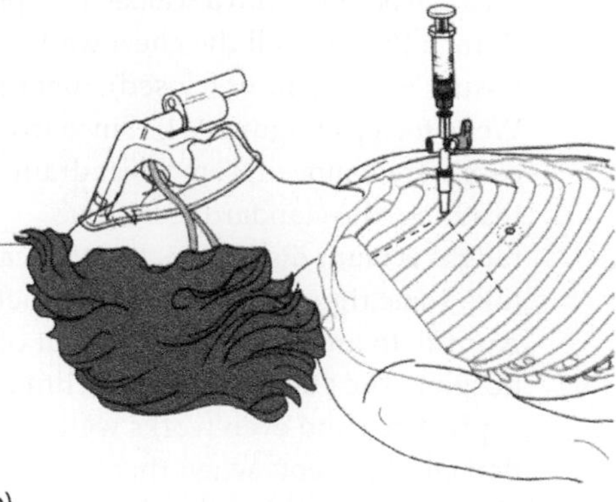

(b)

Figure A.2 (a,b) Correct insertion technique in 2nd intercostal space mid-clavicular line.

FINGER THORACOSTOMY

INTRODUCTION

Finger thoracostomy is the first half of putting in a chest drain, that is it is gaining access to the pleural space. It is an important (and a change in emphasis) to consider this as a procedure in its own right. This is because it is possible to gain access to the pleural space in less than 20 seconds if the practitioner does not worry about the chest drain itself – this can come later. A finger thoracostomy can also be performed using the equipment in a standard suture kit.

This is a painful procedure and unless the patient is anaesthetised, adequate local anaesthetic infiltration around the site of the thoracostomy and down to the pleura is required in addition to parenteral analgesia. When traumatic cardiac arrest has occurred, injection of local anaesthetic must be omitted and the procedure performed with the minimum delay.

PROCEDURE

1. Identify 4th intercostal space mid-axillary line, which is in the 'safe triangle' (Figure A.3). If the nipple is used as a marker of the 5th intercostal space in the male, the space must be traced along the rib edge as it rises moving laterally; simply extending a line laterally from the nipple will indicate a space which is too low. For this reason, the spaces are best counted down from the manubriosternal junction and then followed along the rib edge above when the collect space is identified.
2. As far as possible create clean conditions – sterility is not practically achievable pre-hospital. In practice, this means a minimum of Betadine® spray, and gloves; sterile towels. It should be remembered that empyema is the most serious of complications post-thoracostomy with rates (after tube insertion) varying from 1% to 25% (2,3). The use of prophylactic antibiotics does not reduce the risk of empyema (4).
3. If the patient is not anaesthetised, as stated above, adequate local anaesthesia and analgesia are essential. The use of ketamine should be considered.
4. Use a scalpel to make a 1 inch (2½ cm) cut in the skin along the line of the intercostal space. This can be done with a scalpel or by pinching the skin and cutting with scissors.
5. 'Punch through' all the chest wall tissues with a pair of (closed) Spencer Wells forceps (Figure A.4). Since trocars were removed from chest drain teaching, the standard technique taught is blunt dissection, but this can take some time and is often extremely painful. In an unstable patient out of hospital, the punch through technique is preferred and even works well in flail chest patients when there is little structural support to the chest wall. This is called a 'punch' as the force is applied very quickly and deliberately.

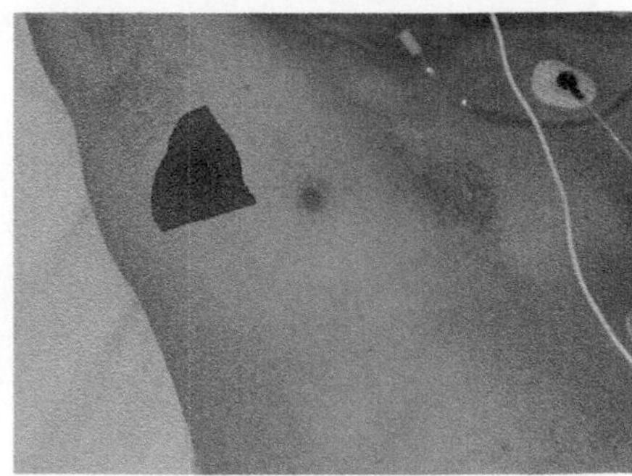

Figure A.3 The safe triangle for finger thoracostomy.

Because the forceps are held 4 to 5 cm down the shaft, there is no risk of damage to the mediastinal structures.

6. By rotation and gently opening and closing the forceps, enlarge the hole through the chest wall and pleura.
7. Insert finger into pleural cavity, then perform a 360° finger sweep to free the lung from any chest wall adhesions. Exclude bowel in the chest and feel for lung touching the tip of finger. Feeling the lung touch the finger excludes an advanced tension pneumothorax. Care must be taken to avoid lacerating the inserted finger on fractured rib ends.
8. Dress the thoracostomy hole with sterile/dry gauze (or see later).
9. If the patient is not being ventilated, a suitable one-way valve must be applied.

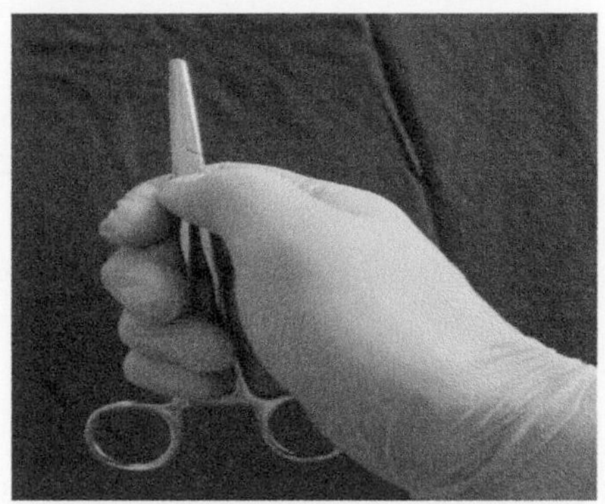

Figure A.4 The correct way to hold the Spencer Wells forceps in order to perform a safe punch through. The closed pair of forceps is held in the dominant hand grasping the arms of the forceps. The hand hold should be about 4–5 cm away from the points of the forceps, but judged according to the estimated thickness of the patient's chest. They may need to be farther in an obese patient or if there is considerable surgical emphysema. The points of the forceps are placed against the intercostal muscles or overlying fat in the correct place for the thoracostomy, and the soft tissues punched through into the pleural cavity in one swift movement.

PRACTICE POINT

There is no place for underwater drainage systems in pre-hospital care.

CLAMSHELL THORACOTOMY

PROCEDURE

1. Identify the patient who fits the inclusion criteria:
   - Penetrating trauma to the chest within the 'cardiac box' (Figure A.5)
   - Signs of life within previous 5 minutes

   Having identified the need for thoracotomy, make the decision to proceed. Don't delay and don't start CPR.
2. Attempt a sterile field, but under no circumstances delay the procedure.
3. Put on double gloves; there is a high risk of injury to the hands from sharp rib ends.
4. Delegate someone else to look after
   - Endotracheal intubation
   - Intravenous access
   - Sedation/analgesia (which will be required if the procedure is successful and the patient starts re-perfusing their brain)
5. Perform bilateral finger thoracostomies in the posterior axillary line, 4th intercostal space using the technique described earlier.
6. Pause for 15 seconds to see if patient has improved from relief of a tension pneumothorax. If not, carry on.

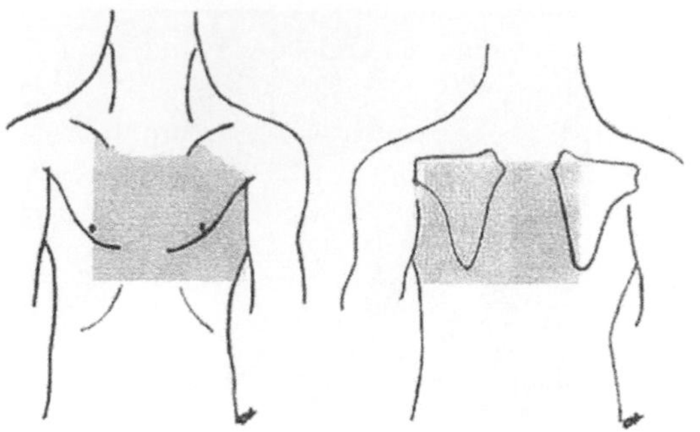

Figure A.5 The 'cardiac box'.

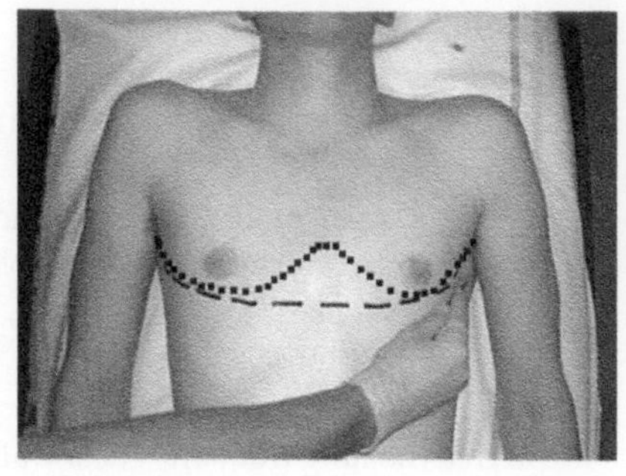

Figure A.6 Thoracotomy line. The correct line is the dotted one, the dashed line is incorrect.

7. Cut along the 4th intercostal space from the lateral end of one of the thoracostomies towards the sternum. It is important to remember that the plane of this is not an axial/cross section of the patient's chest and that the intercostal space drops downwards as it extends forwards out of the axillary area. Failure to do this will lead to the need to cut through ribs (Figure A.6). Cut through the skin and intercostal muscles together using Tuff Cut® scissors, joining the thoracostomies. Take care not to damage structures deep to chest wall.
8. Cut through sternum with the scissors and along the intercostals space to the other thoracostomy, joining the thoracostomies and taking care not to damage structures deep to chest wall. The use of a Gigli saw to cut the sternum is not recommended as it takes considerably longer and is likely to result in the spraying of tissue and blood.
9. Pull clamshell open leading to extension of thoracic spine. Be careful to avoid injury on cut ends of sternum/ribs.
10. Use an assistant or a retractor to open the clamshell (Figure A.7).
11. Look for cardiac amponade (a tense blue blood-filled sack).
12. If tamponade is found, relieve it by picking up the most anterior part of the pericardium (this will avoid the phrenic nerve) with a pair of tissue forceps, snipping the pericardium, extending the cut superiorly staying as anterior as possible and scooping out any clot, being careful not to 'deliver the heart' anteriorly which will kink the great vessels.
13. Observe to see if heart beats. If the heart it is fibrillating, flick it.
14. Gently obstruct the cardiac hole either by placing a finger over it, suturing or stapling the hole or inserting a Foley catheter into the hole followed by balloon inflation and very gentle traction. The Foley catheter technique risks enlarging the hole if too much traction is used.
15. In the pre-hospital environment, do not attempt to suture a hole unless experienced in this technique
16. Give blood if available.
17. Expedite transfer to a major trauma centre.

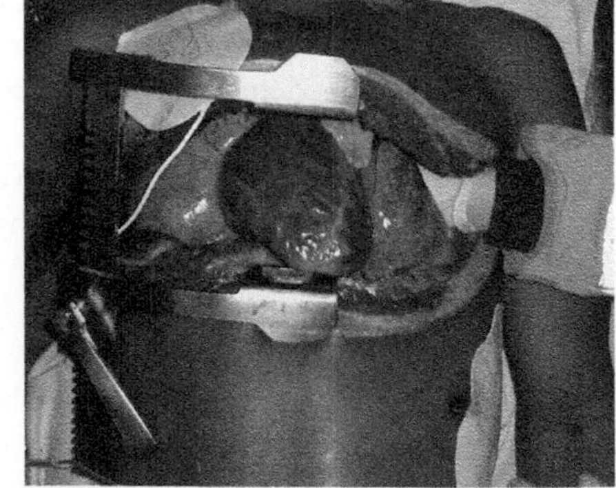

Figure A.7 Clamshell thoracotomy with no intra-pericardial injury. Note the hand compressing the descending aorta against the vertebral column.

NOTES

Cardiac massage may be required as may adrenaline, but the greatest chance of survival is with patients who spontaneously regain output (and consciousness) after relief of their tamponade. Digital compression of the aorta is possible if major abdominal or pelvic bleeding is suspected, but if this is required in pre-hospital care, the outcome is likely to be very poor.

REFERENCES

1. ED Docs get it wrong a lot. *Emergency Medicine Journal* 2005;22:788.
2. Bailey RC. Complications of tube thoracostomy in trauma. *Journal of Accident and Emergency Medicine* 2000;17:111–114.
3. Eddy AC, Lunag K, Copass M. Empyema thoracis in patients undergoing emergent closed tube thoracostomy for thoracic trauma. *American Journal of Surgery* 1989;157(7):494–497.
4. Maxwell RA, Campbell DJ, Fabian TC, Croce MA, Luchette FA, Kerwin AJ, Davis KA, Nagy K, Tisherman S. Use of presumptive antibiotics following tube thoracostomy for traumatic hemopneumothorax in the prevention of empyema and pneumonia – A multi-center trial. *Journal of Trauma* 2004;57(4);742–748.

Appendix B: Traumatic cardiac arrest

TRAUMATIC CARDIAC ARREST: 2 Hs and 2 Ts

For most pre-hospital clinicians, traumatic cardiac arrest is a situation that is very rarely encountered. However, when it is, rapid decisions are required if a successful outcome is to be achieved. In the pre-hospital environment access to skilled assistance may be limited, although this will depend on the circumstances. As a consequence the necessary procedures may need to be carried out in sequence, rather than parallel, and according to a protocol with which the clinician must be completely familiar, even if the skills themselves are rarely practised. If there are multiple rescuers, effective clear leadership is essential. Attendance at a suitable cadaver-based training course is recommended.

In essence in *traumatic* rather than *medical* cardiac arrest, there are 2 Hs and 2 Ts.

2 Hs and 2 Ts

The causes of traumatic cardiac arrest mean that such situations must be managed very differently to cardiac arrest from medical causes. Traumatic cardiac arrest arises from one (or more) of the following mechanisms:

2 Ts

- Tension pneumothorax
- Tamponade (pericardial; usually due to penetrating cardiac trauma)

2 Hs

- Hypoxia (usually airway obstruction, but may be reflex after head injury)
- Haemorrhage (massive haemorrhage from external or internal sources)

Immediate effective identification and management of these conditions is essential. If this is not possible, the only hope lies in immediate evacuation to hospital.

INITIAL ASSESSMENT

A rapid initial assessment looking for an obvious cause is mandatory. This will confirm (or eliminate) the presence of cardiac arrest (in practice often a very low cardiac output state): or an airway obstruction or massive external haemorrhage may be obvious, or a penetrating injury such as a knife wound in the precordium may be found.

STEP 1: IDENTIFY AND CONTROL LIFE-THREATENING EXTERNAL BLEEDING

Direct pressure and elevation (where appropriate) or a tourniquet must be immediately applied. Haemostatic dressings may be applied in traumatic cardiac arrest, but initial control of haemorrhage will be by pressure through the dressings. Whilst external bleeding is being managed, intravenous access can be gained and fluids, ideally blood products, administered. External jugular or femoral access may be easier in the shutdown patient and early resort to intraosseous access may buy time. Early vascular access is the priority in traumatic cardiac arrest, especially due to haemorrhage. Even in cases of tamponade or pneumothorax, access will be needed for induction of anaesthesia or analgesia. In traumatic cardiac arrest in children, *intraosseous access is first line*, venous access can follow. In adults, a large bore line should be inserted in the external jugular or femoral vein. Intraosseous access is unlikely on its own to allow administration of sufficient volumes of fluid but may buy time and allow some refilling, thus making cannulation easier.

In most cases, there will be no life-threatening external haemorrhage, in which case, having ensured that access is being obtained and fluids commenced, move to step 2.

STEP 2: ENSURE THE AIRWAY IS PATENT AND PROTECTED, THEN ADMINISTER HIGH FLOW OXYGEN WITH VENTILATORY SUPPORT IF NEEDED

The normal stepped airway care sequence must be followed, beginning with simple airway manoeuvres. If there is no return of spontaneous circulation once the airway is clear, prehospital emergency anaesthesia (PHEA) will be necessary. Once the airway is clear and protected, move on to step 3.

STEP 3: IDENTIFY LIFE-THREATENING CHEST TRAUMA

The next intervention will depend on whether advanced surgical trauma skills are available. If they are, bilateral finger thoracostomies should be performed with scalpel and blunt finger dissection in the 5th intercostal space just anterior to the mid-axilla line producing a 2.5 cm incision on each side. If thoracostomy/thoracotomy are not possible, bilateral needle thoracocentesis should be performed. If there is no rapid improvement in the patient's condition, rapid infusion of blood products (or less ideally fluids) to achieve a palpable pulse and transfer to hospital is essential. Evacuation should not be delayed whilst gaining vascular access.

If the patient recovers spontaneous cardiac output and respiratory effort, and especially if signs suggest that a tension pneumothorax has been effectively treated, go to step 4.

If this is not the case, and if there is major bleeding from the thoracostomies or evidence of a penetrating chest wound, and cardiac arrest continues, a clamshell thoracotomy should be performed. This will allow management of life-threatening pulmonary haemorrhage (which will be seen from the thoracostomy incisions) or tamponade from penetrating trauma. If neither are present, go to step 4.

The clamshell thoracotomy is achieved by extending each thoracostomy incision with Tuff Cut™ shears, which should be used to cut the sternum. The cut must follow the curve of the intercostal space and must avoid the neurovascular bundle. Once the chest is open (an assistant will need to hold the thoracotomy open to allow effective access), pericardial tamponade, if present, can be relieved and the cardiac wound may then be closed with a suture (or staple) or by using a Foley catheter inserted through the wound and then inflated and with gentle traction applied. Very gentle traction is applied to the catheter in order to ensure closure of the wound without pulling the balloon through the defect and enlarging it. Blood products or other fluids may be infused via the cardiac wound using the end of the giving set without a cannula.

There is no role for needle pericardiocentesis in traumatic cardiac arrest.

There may also be a posterior cardiac wound as a result of transfixion of the heart which will also require closure. Whilst these injuries are being managed, the heart should be handled as little as possible.

Formal surgical equipment is not usually available in the pre-hospital environment but if a clamp is available, it can be used to control haemorrhage from a lobe of the lung or a non-crushing clamp can be placed across the hilum. The hilar twist manoeuvre can be performed by dividing the inferior pulmonary ligament and rotating the lower lobe of the lung anteriorly over the upper lobe and will effectively control major pulmonary haemorrhage on that side. Once inside the chest, if no evidence of massive intrathoracic bleeding or penetrating chest trauma is found or such bleeding has been controlled, go to step 4.

STEP 4: IDENTIFY AND MANAGE HAEMORRHAGE INTO THE ABDOMEN OR PELVIS

The presence of internal haemorrhage other than in the chest is often presumptive and must be deduced based on the physical signs and mechanism of injury, or the failure of the patient to improve with appropriate interventions. There may be pattern bruising, abrasions and lacerations over the abdomen and pelvis, abdominal pain (pre-arrest), abdominal distension, or in the case of pelvic injury, pelvic disruption, blood at the urethral meatus, evidence of perineal trauma or scrotal injury in males.

Where pelvic or abdominal haemorrhage is suspected to be the cause of cardiac arrest, the management is urgent and vigorous fluid replacement, ideally with blood. The pelvis must not be 'sprung'. Pelvic instability is an unreliable sign and springing may exacerbate any bleeding. *In all suspected cases, a pelvic binder must be correctly applied.*

If a thoracostomy has been performed, some control of lower torso haemorrhage can be achieved by applying manual pressure on the descending aorta within the thorax. Laparotomy has no role in the pre-hospital management of cardiac arrest. Go to step 5.

STEP 5: IDENTIFY AND MANAGE (OR EXCLUDE) LONG BONE FRACTURES

Long bone fractures causing sufficient haemorrhage to result in cardiac arrest are very rare and usually obvious. If compound and causing massive bleeding, they will have been managed as part of step 1. Commercial splints should be applied, using traction splintage for femoral fractures. If pelvic fracture is possible, this will influence the choice of splint, suggesting use of a splint that does not provide traction against the symphysis. Go to step 6.

STEP 6: RAPID TRANSPORT TO THE NEAREST MAJOR TRAUMA CENTRE

If no treatable cause has been found, or all possible treatment has been carried out, or if spontaneous circulation has returned, the patient must be transported immediately to a major trauma centre. In some circumstances, there may be a role for a temporary stop at a trauma unit prior to transfer to a more distant major trauma centre. Some traumatic arrests will be due to devastating head injury, but only rarely is this diagnosis possible in the pre-hospital environment. Otherwise the only appropriate course is to treat other salvageable causes first.

CPR

The role of cardiopulmonary resuscitation in traumatic cardiac arrest is controversial. What is absolutely clear, however, is that chest compressions alone will be entirely futile if the cause of the cardiac arrest is not addressed. There is also a role for supported ventilation once an obstructed airway has been cleared and whilst tension pneumothorax or untreated tamponade are managed or active bleeding from a site which can be controlled is stopped. Remember that positive pressure ventilation may exacerbate pneumothorax if there is an ongoing bronchial or pulmonary leak, or may result in systemic air embolus if there is a vascular communication. If there are insufficient assistants, however, attention must focus primarily on identifying and managing the cause of the arrest.

CPR does have a role after all these have been corrected, or non-compressible haemorrhage has been identified and blood products or fluids are being infused. Before this, CPR can impede clinical assessment and make procedures such as vascular access more difficult. If the clinical skill set available does not allow the performance of a clamshell thoracotomy and tamponade is suspected (other causes can be temporarily managed by clearing the airway, finger thoracotomy and administration of blood or fluid), then CPR should be promptly commenced and continued until arrival in hospital. IV fluids will increase preload in low cardiac output states and may increase cardiac output although consideration should be given to dilution of haemoglobin and clotting factors, potential exacerbating oxygen delivery and traumatic coagulopathy.

RETURN OF SPONTANEOUS CIRCULATION (ROSC)

Effective resuscitation may result in rapid return of consciousness and spontaneous cardiac output. Pre-hospital emergency anaesthesia must therefore be available. Judicious ketamine and appropriate maintenance of paralysis is most appropriate. If a thoracotomy has been performed, return of spontaneous circulation (ROSC) is likely to result in bleeding from the internal mammary and other smaller vessels at the incision/blunt dissection margins. Significant bleeding can be controlled by the use of artery forceps.

Index

Page numbers followed by f and t indicate figures and tables, respectively.

F

G

H

J

K

L

T

X

Y

Z